T0358922

Controversies in ACL Reconstruction

Editor

DARREN L. JOHNSON

CLINICS IN
SPORTS MEDICINE

www.sportsmed.theclinics.com

Consulting Editor
MARK D. MILLER

January 2017 • Volume 36 • Number 1

ELSEVIER

1600 John F. Kennedy Boulevard • Suite 1800 • Philadelphia, Pennsylvania, 19103-2899

http://www.theclinics.com

CLINICS IN SPORTS MEDICINE Volume 36, Number 1
January 2017 ISSN 0278-5919, ISBN-13: 978-0-323-48271-4

Editor: Lauren Boyle
Developmental Editor: Donald Mumford

Clinics in Sports Medicine (ISSN 0278-5919) is published quarterly by Elsevier Inc., 360 Park Avenue South, New York, NY 10010-1710. Months of issue are January, April, July, and October. Business and Editorial Offices: 1600 John F. Kennedy Blvd., Ste. 1800, Philadelphia, PA 19103-2899. Customer Service Office: 3251 Riverport Lane, Maryland Heights, MO 63043. Periodicals postage paid at New York, NY and additional mailing offices. Subscription prices are $343.00 per year (US individuals), $627.00 per year (US institutions), $100.00 per year (US students), $389.00 per year (Canadian individuals), $774.00 per year (Canadian institutions), $235.00 (Canadian students), $475.00 per year (foreign individuals), $774.00 per year (foreign institutions), and $235.00 per year (foreign students). Foreign air speed delivery is included in all *Clinics* subscription prices. All prices are subject to change without notice. **POSTMASTER:** Send address changes to *Clinics in Sports Medicine*, Elsevier Health Sciences Division, Subscription Customer Service, 3251 Riverport Lane, Maryland Heights, MO 63043. Customer Service (orders, claims, online, change of address): Elsevier Health Sciences Division, Subscription Customer Service, 3251 Riverport Lane, Maryland Heights, MO 63043. **Tel: 1-800-654-2452 (U.S. and Canada); 314-447-8871 (outside U.S. and Canada). Fax: 314-447-8029. E-mail: journalscustomerservice-usa@elsevier.com (for print support); journalsonlinesupport-usa@ elsevier.com (for online support)**.

Reprints. For copies of 100 or more of articles in this publication, please contact the Commercial Reprints Department, Elsevier Inc., 360 Park Avenue South, New York, NY 10010-1710. Tel.: 212-633-3874; Fax: 212-633-3820; E-mail: reprints@elsevier.com.

Clinics in Sports Medicine is covered in *MEDLINE/PubMed (Index Medicus) Current Contents/Clinical Medicine, Excerpta Medica,* and *ISI/Biomed.*

Contributors

CONSULTING EDITOR

MARK D. MILLER, MD
S. Ward Casscells Professor; Head, Division of Sports Medicine, Department of
Orthopaedic Surgery, University of Virginia, Charlottesville, Virginia; Team Physician,
James Madison University, Harrisonburg, Virginia

EDITOR

DARREN L. JOHNSON, MD
Medical Director of Sports Medicine; Professor and Chairman, Division of Sports
Medicine, Department of Orthopaedic Surgery, University of Kentucky School of
Medicine, Lexington, Kentucky

AUTHORS

MARCIO ALBERS, MD
Research Fellow, Department of Orthopaedic Surgery, University of Pittsburgh,
Pittsburgh, Pennsylvania

ANNUNZIATO AMENDOLA, MD
Chief, Division of Sports Medicine; Professor, Department of Orthopaedic Surgery,
DUMC, Duke University, Durham, North Carolina

ALLEN F. ANDERSON, MD
Orthopaedic Surgeon, Tennessee Orthopaedic Alliance, Nashville, Tennessee

CHRISTIAN N. ANDERSON, MD
Orthopaedic Surgeon, Tennessee Orthopaedic Alliance, Nashville, Tennessee

CHRISTOPHER A. ARRIGO, MS, PT, ATC
Owner and Clinical Director, Advanced Rehabilitation, Tampa, Florida

JAMES R. BAILEY, MD
Fellow, Orthopaedics, Duke University Medical Center, Durham, North Carolina

BARTON R. BRANAM, MD
Assistant Professor, Division of Sports Medicine, Department of Orthoapedic Surgery,
College of Medicine, University of Cincinnati, Cincinnati, Ohio

ROBERT T. BURKS, MD
Professor, Department of Orthopedic Surgery, University of Utah, Salt Lake City, Utah

TOM CHAO, MD
Kern Medical Center, Bakersfield, California

MATTHEW D. CRAWFORD, MD
Department of Orthopaedic Surgery, DUMC, Duke University, Durham, North Carolina

KEVIN M. DALE, MD
Fellow, Orthopaedics, Duke University Medical Center, Durham, North Carolina

LEE H. DIEHL, MD
Assistant Professor, Department of Orthopaedic Surgery, DUMC, Duke University, Durham, North Carolina

KYLE R. DUCHMAN, MD
Department of Orthopaedics & Rehabilitation, University of Iowa Hospitals and Clinics, Iowa City, Iowa

FREDDIE H. FU, MD, DSc (Hon), DPs (Hon)
Department of Orthopaedic Surgery, University of Pittsburgh, Pittsburgh, Pennsylvania

ALAN GETGOOD, MPhil, MD, FRCS (Tr&Orth), DipSEM
Consultant Orthopaedic Surgeon, Department of Surgery, Fowler Kennedy Sport Medicine Clinic, Western University, London, Ontario, Canada

BENJAMIN HERMAN, MD, FRCSC
Orthopaedic Sport Medicine Fellow, Department of Surgery, Fowler Kennedy Sport Medicine Clinic, Western University, London, Ontario, Canada

SEBASTIÁN IRARRÁZAVAL, MD
Assistant Professor, Department of Orthopedic Surgery, Pontificia Universidad Católica de Chile, Santiago, Chile

DARREN L. JOHNSON, MD
Medical Director of Sports Medicine; Professor and Chairman, Division of Sports Medicine, Department of Orthopaedic Surgery, University of Kentucky School of Medicine, Lexington, Kentucky

CHRISTOPHER C. KAEDING, MD
Judson Wilson Professor, Department of Orthopaedic Surgery; Director, Sports Medicine Center; Head Team Physician, Department of Athletics, The Ohio State University, Columbus, Ohio

NICHOLAS I. KENNEDY, BA
Oregon Health and Science University, Portland, Oregon; Research Assistant, Steadman Philippon Research Institute, Vail, Colorado

CHRISTOPHER M. LAPRADE, BS
Medical College of Wisconsin, Milwaukee, Wisconsin

ROBERT F. LAPRADE, MD, PhD
Steadman Clinic; Chief Medical Officer, Steadman Philippon Research Institute, Vail, Colorado

BENJAMIN LÉGER-ST-JEAN, MD
Fellow, Sports Medicine Center, The Ohio State University, Columbus, Ohio

ROBERT LITCHFIELD, MD, FRCSC
Consultant Orthopaedic Surgeon & Medical Director, Department of Surgery, Fowler Kennedy Sport Medicine Clinic, Western University, London, Ontario, Canada

T. SEAN LYNCH, MD
Center for Shoulder, Elbow, and Sports Medicine, Columbia University Medical Center, New York, New York

ROBERT A. MAGNUSSEN, MPH, MD
Assistant Professor, Department of Orthopaedics, The Ohio State University, Columbus, Ohio

CHAITU S. MALEMPATI, DO
Assistant Professor of Orthopaedic Surgery and Sports Medicine, Division of Sports Medicine, Department of Orthopaedic Surgery, University of Kentucky School of Medicine, Lexington, Kentucky

LUCAS S. MARCHAND, MD
Resident, Department of Orthopedic Surgery, University of Utah, Salt Lake City, Utah

ADAM V. METZLER, MD
Division of Sports Medicine, Commonwealth Orthopaedic Centers, Edgewood, Kentucky

MARK D. MILLER, MD
S. Ward Casscells Professor; Head, Division of Sports Medicine, Department of Orthopaedic Surgery, University of Virginia, Charlottesville, Virginia; Team Physician, James Madison University, Harrisonburg, Virginia

CLAUDE T. MOORMAN III, MD
Professor, Orthopaedics, Duke University Medical Center, Durham, North Carolina

DUSTIN L. RICHTER, MD
Sports Medicine Fellow, Department of Orthopaedic Surgery, University of Virginia, Charlottesville, Virginia

KURT P. SPINDLER, MD
Cleveland Clinic Sports Health Center, Garfield Heights, Ohio

CHRISTOPHER J. UTZ, MD
Assistant Professor, Division of Sports Medicine, Department of Orthoapedic Surgery, College of Medicine, University of Cincinnati, Cincinnati, Ohio

BART VUNDELINCKX, MD
Orthopaedic Sport Medicine Fellow, Department of Surgery, Fowler Kennedy Sport Medicine Clinic, Western University, London, Ontario, Canada

BRIAN C. WERNER, MD
Assistant Professor, Department of Orthopaedic Surgery, University of Virginia, Charlottesville, Virginia

KEVIN E. WILK, PT, DPT, FAPTA
Associate Clinical Director; Physiotherapy Associates, Champion Sports Medicine; Director of Rehabilitative Research, American Sports Medicine Institute, Birmingham, Alabama

JAMES D. WYLIE, MD, MHS
Fellow, Department of Orthopedic Surgery, University of Connecticut, Farmington, Connecticut

Contents

Anterior cruciate ligament (ACL) injuries are increasingly common in the United States. This may be related to the increase in high school sports participation, particularly in female athletes. A significant proportion of these injuries are caused by noncontact mechanisms. The incidence of these noncontact injuries may be significantly reduced by enrolling young athletes in jump-training programs. The diagnosis of ACL injuries involves a focused history and physical examination, which can provide a high index of suspicion. Although radiographs are important to rule out associated injuries, the gold standard for diagnosis of ACL injuries is MRI, which has shown excellent accuracy.

The anterior cruciate ligament (ACL) is one of the more studied structures in the knee joint. It is not a tubular structure, but is much narrower in its midsubstance and broader at its ends, producing an hourglass shape. The ACL is composed of 2 functional bundles, the anteromedial and posterolateral bundles, that are named for their location of insertion on the anterior surface of the tibial plateau. Although the relative contribution in terms of total cross-sectional area of the ACL has been noted to be equal in regards to each bundle, dynamically these bundles demonstrate different properties for knee function.

Anterior cruciate ligament (ACL) injuries are common and affect a young, active patient population. Despite much research, ACL reconstruction graft choice remains a topic of debate. Based on the best available evidence, autograft seems to be superior to allograft for ACL reconstruction in young, active patients. Future high-level studies are required in order to better define the role of allograft in ACL reconstruction. As graft choice is often influenced by surgeon preference, it is important that surgeons understand the current literature as well as the goals of their patients.

Intrasubstance tears of the anterior cruciate ligament (ACL) are being diagnosed with increasing frequency in the skeletally immature. Management options include nonoperative/early surgical, or delayed surgical reconstruction. Nonoperative/delayed reconstruction results in worse functional outcomes than early reconstruction. Physicians are faced with a treatment dilemma; clinical and basic science studies have demonstrated risk of limb-length discrepancy and angular deformity with ACL reconstruction. Vertical drill tunnels decrease physeal damage and minimize growth deformity; however, this technique results in nonanatomic ACL graft placement. All-epiphyseal reconstruction avoids damage to the growth plate. These techniques are biomechanically superior to extraarticular and modified physeal-sparing procedures.

Anterior cruciate ligament (ACL) ruptures are some of the most common sports-related injuries. Treatment of these injuries with ACL reconstruction has evolved over the last several decades. Anatomic single-bundle ACL reconstruction offers an accurate and reproducible method to reproduce native knee anatomy, restore knee kinematics, and ultimately restore function and decrease long-term degenerative effects. The importance of adequate arthroscopic visualization and a thorough understanding of the native anatomic ACL landmarks are discussed in this article. Furthermore, surgical technique, pearls, pitfalls, potential complications, rehabilitation, and outcomes are reviewed.

Anterior cruciate ligament (ACL) reconstruction is a commonly performed procedure. Drilling the femoral tunnel independent of the tibial tunnel has become popular as surgeons strive to create tunnels in the anatomic locations of the femoral and tibial attachments of the native ligament. The 2-incision technique effectively and reproducibly accomplishes this goal. The 2-incision technique for ACL reconstruction is a valuable tool in the skillset of the reconstructive knee surgeon. Indications for the 2-incision surgery are reviewed in detail. Furthermore, technical tips, complications, and outcomes are discussed.

▶ Video content accompanies this article at http://www.sportsmed. theclinics.com.

The medial collateral ligament (MCL) is the most commonly injured ligament of the knee. The anterior cruciate ligament (ACL) is the most commonly injured ligament in conjunction with the MCL. Most MCL injuries can be treated nonoperatively, whereas the ACL often requires reconstruction. A good physical examination is essential for diagnosis, whereas radiographs and MRI of the knee confirm diagnosis and help guide treatment planning. Preoperative physical therapy should be completed before surgical management to allow for return of knee range of motion and an attempt at MCL healing.

Posterolateral knee injuries occur more commonly than in the past. These injuries most commonly occur concurrent with cruciate ligament tears. The main stabilizers of the posterolateral knee are the fibular collateral ligament, the popliteus tendon, and the popliteofibular ligament. These static stabilizers function to prevent increased varus, external rotation, and coupled posterolateral rotation of the knee. The most important clinical tests to diagnose posterolateral knee injuries are the varus stress test, posterolateral drawer, and dial tests. Varus stress radiographs are key objective means to diagnose these injuries. Anatomic-based reconstructions have been validated to restore stability and improve outcomes.

Varus malalignment and an increased tibial slope can result in instability in an anterior cruciate ligament (ACL)–deficient knee. Malalignment can also be a cause of recurrent instability following ACL reconstruction. Varus malalignment can contribute to loosening or failure of primary ACL reconstruction and contribute to progressive medial compartment arthritis. High tibial osteotomies performed in conjunction with ACL reconstruction can improve alignment, restore anterior knee stability, and help reduce the advancement of arthritis.

After anterior cruciate ligament (ACL) rupture, anteroposterior and rotational laxity in the knee causes instability, functional symptoms, and damage to other intra-articular structures. Surgical reconstruction aims to restore the stability in the knee, and to improve function and ability to participate in sports. It also protects cartilage and menisci from secondary injuries. Because of persistent rotational instability after ACL reconstruction, combined intra-articular and extra-articular procedures are more commonly performed. In this article, an overview of anatomy,

CLINICS IN SPORTS MEDICINE

THE CLINICS ARE AVAILABLE ONLINE!
Access your subscription at:
www.theclinics.com

CLINICS IN SPORTS MEDICINE

FORTHCOMING ISSUES

April 2017
Facial Injuries in Sports
Michael J. Stuart, Editor

July 2017
Articular Cartilage
Eric McCarty, Editor

October 2017
The Female Athlete
Siobhan M. Statuta, Editor

RECENT ISSUES

October 2016
Return to Play following
Musculoskeletal Injury
Darren L. Johnson, Editor

July 2016
Hip Arthroscopy

April 2016
Ethics in Sports Medicine
Stephen R. Thompson, Editor

January 2016
Prakash Singh

RELATED INTEREST

Foot and Ankle Clinics, June 2016 (Vol. 21, Issue 2)
New Ideas and Techniques in Foot and Ankle Surgery
John G. Anderson and Donald R. Bohay, Editors
Available at: http://www.foot.theclinics.com/

THE CLINICS ARE AVAILABLE ONLINE!
Access your subscription at:
www.theclinics.com

Foreword

Anterior Cruciate Ligament

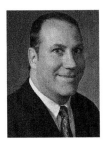

Mark D. Miller, MD
Consulting Editor

Dr Johnson put together a great treatise on managing anterior cruciate ligament (ACL) injuries. Interestingly, he and I were fellows together almost a quarter of a century ago, when we both thought that this topic was "solved." In fact, our mentor, Dr Freddie Fu, would encourage us to move quickly through these cases, noting "if you go fast you cannot make a mistake." Imagine my surprise many years later when Dr Fu, speaking as a visiting professor, advised my fellows to slow down and carefully look at the ACL anatomy before proceeding with reconstruction. As is so often the case with Dr Freddie Fu, he was onto something, and he literally schooled an international audience of ACL surgeons on the importance of restoring ACL anatomy.

This issue outlines our current understanding on managing ACL injuries in the twenty-first century. Darren has assembled a literal "Who's Who" of ACL surgeons to completely update the readers on this evolving topic. The issue begins with making the diagnosis, proceeds with a review of ACL anatomy (fittingly, by Dr Fu), reviews options for graft selection, discusses pediatric ACL injuries, reviews ACL treatment options (single bundle, two incision, and so forth), provides guidance on complex cases (malalignment, combined posterolateral corner injuries, and revision surgery), introduces controversies regarding extra-articular augmentation, and concludes with recommendations for rehabilitation and return to play.

Many questions remain, and we still haven't "solved" the ACL paradigm. I applaud Dr Johnson for brilliantly documenting the state-of-the-art regarding our current knowledge on the management of ACL injuries. I join him in recognizing and applauding our mentor, Dr Freddie Fu, for his passion in encouraging ACL surgeons worldwide to slow

Clin Sports Med 36 (2017) xiii–xiv
http://dx.doi.org/10.1016/j.csm.2016.10.002
0278-5919/17/© 2016 Published by Elsevier Inc.

down, appreciate anatomy, and continue our quest to become better ACL surgeons and get the athletes we treat back to their preinjury status.

Mark D. Miller, MD
S. Ward Casscells Professor
Head, Division of Sports Medicine
Department of Orthopaedic Surgery
University of Virginia
Team Physician, James Madison University
400 Ray C. Hunt Drive, Suite 330
Charlottesville, VA 22908-0159, USA

E-mail address:
mdm3p@virginia.edu

Preface

Management of the Anterior Cruciate Ligament Deficient Knee

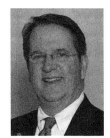

Darren L. Johnson, MD
Editor

I am very honored to be able to serve as the editor for this outstanding issue of *Clinics in Sports Medicine* on the management of the anterior cruciate ligament–deficient knee. I am confident that if you were to pool the editors-in-chief of our major orthopedic peer-reviewed journals, anterior cruciate ligament as a submission for publication would probably be the number one topic of submissions. Clearly, there is great interest in this topic given the number of anterior cruciate ligament disruptions that happen annually in this country. It seems that number is increasing each and every year. Over the last 30 years of orthopedic management of this complex problem, much has changed; much is currently being investigated, and we have much to learn moving forward. Over the last 10 years, there has been a renowned focus with respect to detailed anterior cruciate ligament anatomy as it pertains to our surgical reconstruction techniques. I think clearly that Dr Freddie Fu from the University of Pittsburgh was instrumental in getting all of us surgeons in North America to refocus on the detailed anatomy of the anterior cruciate ligament attachment sites. I clearly think and believe that this renowned focus on what Dr Freddie Fu has taught us has enabled us to become better anterior cruciate ligament surgeons. We should all be thankful to him for starting this discussion in this country over 10 years ago. However, there is much to be learned moving forward in improving our results of anterior cruciate ligament surgery. Having been an anterior cruciate ligament surgeon myself over the last 23 years, I am still humbled and perplexed by this unique problem that I see in the office on a weekly basis. Clearly all of my patients do not do well and not all of them return to anterior cruciate ligament–dependent sports at their previous level. For me personally, I have learned a great deal by the contributions of this distinguished group of authors. I am confident that I am a better physician in managing anterior cruciate ligament–deficient knee problems having read in great detail this outstanding issue.

Clin Sports Med 36 (2017) xv–xvi
http://dx.doi.org/10.1016/j.csm.2016.10.001
0278-5919/17/© 2016 Published by Elsevier Inc.

sportsmed.theclinics.com

I have asked a special group of authors to contribute their knowledge and expertise to this issue of *Clinics in Sports Medicine*. As I am sure you'll testify, they have done a simply remarkable job. These authors have contributed much of their academic careers to what we know about anterior cruciate ligament injury and its management. They are on the cutting edge of making advancements in the treatment of this unique challenge, which we have not solved yet. I want to personally thank each and every contributor for donating their valuable time and energy to this educational effort. It is a true honor of mine to have worked with this special unique group in making this a tremendous success. I hope you enjoy this issue as much as I have enjoyed putting it together. I sincerely hope that it enables you to provide better care to the patients we are so lucky to have served. We as well as our patients will benefit tremendously.

Darren L. Johnson, MD
Director of Sports Medicine
Department of Orthopaedic Surgery
University of Kentucky School of Medicine
Lexington, KY 40536-0284, USA

E-mail address:
dljohns@uky.edu

Epidemiology and Diagnosis of Anterior Cruciate Ligament Injuries

 CrossMark

Christopher C. Kaeding, MD[a,b,*], Benjamin Léger-St-Jean, MD[c],
Robert A. Magnussen, MPH, MD[d]

KEYWORDS

- ACL • Epidemiology • History • Physical examination • Mechanism of injury
- Diagnostic imaging

KEY POINTS

- The incidence of anterior cruciate ligament injuries is 120,000 annually in the United States, and slowly increasing, especially among female athletes. Forty-one percent of these injuries are from noncontact mechanisms.
- The incidence of ACL noncontact injuries may be significantly reduced by enrolling young athletes in jump-training programs.
- Key questions to include on history taking are presence of continuous effusion, popping sensation during trauma, and sensation of giving way.
- The most accurate physical examination test is the Lachman test.
- Although radiographs are important to rule out associated injuries, the gold standard for diagnosis of ACL injuries is MRI, which has shown excellent accuracy.

INTRODUCTION

More than 120,000 anterior cruciate ligament (ACL) injuries occur every year in the United States, mostly during the high school and college years.[1] The incidence of these injuries is slowly increasing, especially in females. This is likely caused by their increasing participation in high school and other organized sports. In addition, several studies have shown that female athletes are at an increased risk of ACL injury in sex-comparable sports.[1] The reason for this increased risk is likely multifactorial including

Disclosure Statement: The authors have nothing to disclose.
[a] Department of Orthopaedic Surgery, Sports Medicine Center, The Ohio State University, 2050 Kenny Road, Columbus, OH 43221, USA; [b] Department of Athletics, The Ohio State University, 2050 Kenny Road, Columbus, OH 43221, USA; [c] Sports Medicine Center, The Ohio State University, 2050 Kenny Road, Columbus, OH 43221, USA; [d] Department of Orthopaedics, The Ohio State University, 2050 Kenny Road, Columbus, OH 43221, USA
* Corresponding author. 2050 Kenny Road, Columbus, OH 43221.
E-mail address: Christopher.kaeding@osumc.edu

Clin Sports Med 36 (2017) 1–8
http://dx.doi.org/10.1016/j.csm.2016.08.001
0278-5919/17/© 2016 Elsevier Inc. All rights reserved.

such factors as genetic predisposition, hormone levels, narrower notch width, and differences in cutting and landing biomechanics. Diagnosis of these injuries in the acute setting is challenging as the physical examination is less reliable because of joint swelling and muscle guarding. Nonetheless, a focused history and physical examination are essential tools in diagnosing an ACL injury. Radiographs are useful to rule out associated injuries, but the gold standard to diagnose an ACL injury is MRI, which has been shown to have excellent sensitivity and specificity. A better understanding of the risk factors for injury and more accurate diagnoses could facilitate prevention of ACL injuries in active individuals and thus minimize subsequent meniscal and cartilage damage in patients that are ACL deficient.

EPIDEMIOLOGY

Knee injuries in high school athletes account for 60% of sport-related surgeries.[2,3] According to some studies, ACL injuries may account for 50% of all of these knee injuries.[4] According to the Centers for Disease Control and Prevention, in 2006 ACL reconstruction surgery costs were estimated to be nearly $1 billion.[5] More recently, epidemiologic studies have shown that female high school athletes have a 2.1- to 3.4-fold increased risk of ACL injury for sex-comparable sports.[5,6]

To provide an evidence-based incidence and yearly risk of ACL tears in high school athletes, Gornitzky and colleagues[1] performed a systematic review and meta-analysis. In their study, they found an overall incidence in females of 0.081 ACL injuries per 1000 exposures for all sports combined. The riskiest sports for women were soccer and basketball with a risk of having an ACL injury of 1.1% and 0.9% per season, respectively. In male athletes, the overall incidence of ACL injuries was 0.05 per 1000 exposures. The riskiest sports were football and lacrosse with 0.8% and 0.4% risk of having an ACL injury per season, respectively. Female athletes had an overall higher rate of injury per exposure (relative risk, 1.57; 95% confidence interval [CI], 1.35–1.82) than male athletes and in comparable sports, such as soccer and basketball, the rates were much higher (3.7 and 3.8, respectively). When one considers these sport-specific seasonal risks in the context of a multisport athlete over a 4-year span, overall risk of suffering an ACL tear during a high school career can reach 5% to 10%.

Many studies have reported that most ACL injuries are by noncontact mechanisms.[7–9] These findings were challenged in a recent study performed in 100 US high schools by Joseph and colleagues[5] from 2007 to 2012 where they reported that 58.8% of ACL injuries occurred as a result of a contact mechanism. Regardless of the true percentage of noncontact ACLs, a significant proportion of ACL injuries are caused by noncontact mechanisms, making these injuries a major focus for prevention efforts. In a retrospective study focused only on noncontact primary ACL injuries, Beynnon and colleagues[6] showed that college athletes had significantly higher injury risk than high school athletes after adjustment for sport and sex (relative risk, 2.38; 95% CI, 1.55–3.64).

When considering patients that have had a previous ACL reconstructions, studies have provided two important findings. The first is that in the first 2 years of surgery, patients have a similar risk of injuring their contralateral ACL or tearing their graft.[10] The second finding is that patients who have had a previous ACL injury have a significantly increased risk of having a second ACL injury with rates ranging from 4- to 25-fold.[11] It has been shown that returning to a high level of activity after an ACL reconstruction is a strong risk factor for retearing the graft.[12,13] These epidemiologic studies are incredibly important in identifying risk factors involved in ACL injury and providing information to patients and families regarding their individual risk profiles and possible modification of these factors to decrease the risk of subsequent ACL injury. Small graft size has also been shown to be a risk factor for ACL graft retear.[14]

MECHANISM OF INJURY

Landing or plant-and-cut maneuvers are frequently regarded as the main sporting tasks responsible for ACL injuries.[8,15,16] Epidemiologic studies and video analysis of ACL injuries have led researchers to compare differences between males in females in terms of landing mechanics and overall lower limb alignment profiles.[17,18] In a prospective study focusing on female athletes, Hewett and colleagues[18] prescreened 205 female athletes looking at three-dimensional kinematics and joint loads during a jump landing task. They found that the nine athletes who eventually had an ACL injury had greater knee abduction angles (8°), 2.5 times greater knee abduction moments, and 20% greater ground reaction forces at landing compared with their teammates who did not have injuries.[11] These factors have been identified as independent predictors of ACL injury.[18]

Studies focused on cutting tasks have shown that coronal plane hip motions, specifically adduction, are primarily responsible for increased knee abduction.[19,20] Reduced hip and knee flexion during landing are also considered risk factors for ACL injury because this limb position puts greater loads on static joints restraints (ligaments, capsule) rather dynamic restraints (muscles, tendons).[21–24] Just as sagittal and coronal mechanics are important, transverse plane mechanics are also involved in ACL injury mechanisms. Internal rotation at the hip may contribute to knee valgus[19,25] and internal rotation of the tibia causes significant increases in ACL strain.[26–29] Therefore, when combining these three movement planes, the typical noncontact ACL injury would occur in the context of a female athlete landing from a jump with her hip relatively extended and internally rotated, her knee in near full extension and valgus with her tibia internally rotated, and her foot planted.

In addition to considering limb position, several researchers have focused their efforts on neuromuscular control of the lower limb.[11,30] Some of the neuromuscular risk factors associated with ACL injury are elevated quadriceps to hamstring muscle activation,[31,32] early activation of the hamstrings when the foot contacts the ground,[33] and greater quadriceps and gluteus maximus activation with reduced hamstring and gastrocnemius activation.[34] Although most of the risk factors of ACL injury have to do with lower limb mechanics and kinematics, some authors have suggested that upper limb kinematics may also have a role to play in knee valgus loading.[35]

A better understanding of knee kinematics has allowed researchers to develop successful prevention programs, reducing the risk of noncontact ACL injuries by roughly 50%.[11] In a 2012 meta-analysis of ACL injury prevention programs,[36] the authors found that the younger the athletes, the more effective the program was at preventing injuries. This finding is not surprising considering that most of the postural and dynamic risk factors for ACL injury seem to develop as a normal maturation process in women. Preventive programs should therefore be instituted in the preadolescent or early adolescent phase before athletes develop "pathologic" neuromuscular activation patterns and kinematics.

HISTORY AND PHYSICAL EXAMINATION

The typical history of a patient with an ACL injury involves either a noncontact deceleration, jumping, cutting action, or a direct impact on the knee.[37] Obviously, many other mechanisms may also result in ACL injury, and in many cases patients are not able to recall exactly what happened. Common patient descriptions include feeling that the knee hyperextended or temporarily "popped out of its socket."

Studies have focused on the accuracy of specific elements of a patient's history and physical examination that could predict ACL injury.[38–40] These studies must be interpreted carefully because most of these studies are subject to bias, in particular verification bias. An example of this is a retrospective study on patients who have already undergone MRI and arthroscopy for a knee injury. These patients were probably more likely to have ACL injuries than the patients that did not have advanced imaging.

A 2010 cross-sectional analysis by Wagemakers and colleagues[40] found 10 determinants in the history and physical examination that showed a statistically significant association with ACL injury. After multivariate analysis, four determinants explained 41% of the variance in the model: (1) presence of continuous effusion (odds ratio [OR], 4.4; 95% CI, 1.4–14.5), (2) popping sensation during trauma (OR, 6.1; 95% CI, 1.9–19.5), (3) giving way (OR, 3.5; 95% CI, 1.1–10.9), and (4) a positive anterior drawer test (OR, 6.4; 95% CI, 1.8–23.0). When considered in association, the presence or absence of all three elements mentioned in the history results in a positive predictive value of 83% and negative predictive value of 81%. In this scenario, adding a positive anterior drawer test did not result in higher predictive values. However, in many cases, these three elements are not all positive or negative, necessitating a heavier reliance on physical examination findings.

In a 2006 meta-analysis including 28 studies, Benjaminse and colleagues[38] compared the accuracy of the anterior drawer test, Lachman test, and pivot shift tests. In their study, the Lachman test was the most accurate test with a positive likelihood ratio of 10.2 (95% CI, 4.6–22.7) and a negative likelihood ratio of 0.2 (95% CI, 0.1–0.3). The specificity of the pivot shift was high at 98% (95% CI, 96–99) but the sensitivity was low at 24% (95% CI, 21–27). This finding is not surprising considering that the pivot shift is a hard test to perform in the acute setting because of patient guarding. As for the anterior drawer test, the sensitivity and specificity of this test was shown to be dependent on the timing of the injury. In acute injuries, the sensitivity was only 49% (95% CI, 43–55) and specificity was 58% (95% CI, 39–76), whereas in chronic injuries the results were 92% (95% CI, 88–95) and 91% (95% CI, 87–94), respectively.

When extrapolating these results to a specific patient population, one can calculate pretest and posttest probabilities of ACL rupture. As an example, according to a study by Noyes and colleagues,[41] 44% of patients who suffered an acute knee injury with significant swelling had an ACL injury. In this patient population, a patient with a positive Lachman test would now have an 88% chance of having an ACL injury. However, if the Lachman test were negative, the chance of having an ACL rupture would be only 7%.

In some unique cases, such as with patients with large legs, it may be difficult to perform these tests. To find a better diagnostic test for ACL injuries, Lelli and colleagues[42] introduced a new test, the lever sign. To perform this test, the patient lays supine and a fist is placed underneath the proximal aspect of the calf muscle to act as a fulcrum. A downward force is then applied to the thigh with the other hand and the examiner observes if the heel of the foot rises off the table. If the heel rises, it is believed that the ACL is intact and transmits the downward force from the femur to the tibia and through the fulcrum at the calf. If the heel does not rise against gravity, it is believed that the ACL is not functional, either stretched or torn. In their pilot study, the sensitivity and specificity of this test were 100%. These results have not been replicated in other studies to date and one should be careful before concluding that this test is perfect. However, this test might be an interesting alternative in patients where the more traditional tests are hard to perform or inconclusive.

DIAGNOSTIC IMAGING AND ANCILLARY TESTS

In any acute knee injury, orthogonal anteroposterior and lateral knee radiographs are always indicated as a first step to rule out fractures and associated injuries.[43] Tibial eminence fractures visible on radiograph are considered bony equivalents to an ACL injury and the Segond fracture, which is an avulsion fracture of the lateral capsule from the tibial plateau, is pathognomic of an ACL injury.[37] In most cases, plain radiographs are normal aside from the presence of effusion and therefore the most helpful diagnostic imaging modality is MRI.[37] Studies have reported variability in accuracy (82%–100%),[44–46] sensitivity, and specificity of MRI in the diagnosis of ACL injury.[47–49] Interestingly, in more recent studies, the level of diagnostic accuracy has not significantly improved with higher-field MRI machines, evolving from 93% accuracy with 0.2 T to 95% with 3.0 T MRIs.[48,49] To improve accuracy, more radiologists ask for oblique coronal and sagittal views that allow full-length views of the ACL in one frame. In a 2014 study,[47] three experienced orthopedic surgeons retrospectively reviewed the records of 54 patients who had undergone both MRI and knee arthroscopy. They compared the diagnostic accuracy of MRI with and without oblique images. The accuracy improved from 80% to 91%, suggesting that these sequences may helpful in diagnosing more subtle tears. Stress radiographs and knee ligament arthrometers, such as the KT-1000 and KT-2000 (MEDmetric Corporation, San Diego, CA), are additional tools that can assist in diagnosis of ACL tears but are currently mainly used for research purposes.[37]

SUMMARY

ACL injuries are a major burden on the US health care system with annual costs averaging $1 billion. A significant proportion of these injuries are caused by noncontact mechanisms and jump-training-type prevention programs are effective at reducing the incidence of these injuries, especially when instituted early in the development of the athlete. A focused history and physical examination may strongly suggest an ACL injury, but the preoperative diagnostic gold-standard for diagnosis remains MRI.

REFERENCES

1. Gornitzky AL, Lott A, Yellin JL, et al. Sport-specific yearly risk and incidence of anterior cruciate ligament tears in high school athletes: a systematic review and meta-analysis. Am J Sports Med 2015. [Epub ahead of print].

2. Ingram JG, Fields SK, Yard EE, et al. Epidemiology of knee injuries among boys and girls in US high school athletics. Am J Sports Med 2008;36:1116–22.

3. Powell JW, Barber-Foss KD. Injury patterns in selected high school sports: a review of the 1995-1997 seasons. J Athl Train 1999;34:277.

4. Risberg MA, Lewek M, Snyder-Mackler L. A systematic review of evidence for anterior cruciate ligament rehabilitation: how much and what type? Phys Ther Sport 2004;5:125–45.

5. Joseph AM, Collins CL, Henke NM, et al. A multisport epidemiologic comparison of anterior cruciate ligament injuries in high school athletics. J Athl Train 2013;48: 810–7.

6. Beynnon BD, Vacek PM, Newell MK, et al. The effects of level of competition, sport, and sex on the incidence of first-time noncontact anterior cruciate ligament injury. Am J Sports Med 2014;42:1806–12.

7. Arendt E, Dick R. Knee injury patterns among men and women in collegiate basketball and soccer NCAA data and review of literature. Am J Sports Med 1995;23:694–701.

8. Boden BP, Dean GS, Feagin JA, et al. Mechanisms of anterior cruciate ligament injury. Orthopedics 2000;23:573–8.

9. Mountcastle SB, Posner M, Kragh JF, et al. Gender differences in anterior cruciate ligament injury vary with activity epidemiology of anterior cruciate ligament injuries in a young, athletic population. Am J Sports Med 2007;35:1635–42.

10. Wright RW, Dunn WR, Amendola A, et al. Risk of tearing the intact anterior cruciate ligament in the contralateral knee and rupturing the anterior cruciate ligament graft during the first 2 years after anterior cruciate ligament reconstruction: a prospective MOON cohort study. Am J Sports Med 2007;35:1131–4.

11. Hewett TE, Myer GD, Ford KR, et al. The 2012 ABJS Nicolas Andry Award: the sequence of prevention: a systematic approach to prevent anterior cruciate ligament injury. Clin Orthop Relat Res 2012;170:2930–10.

12. Borchers JR, Pedroza A, Kaeding C. Activity level and graft type as risk factors for anterior cruciate ligament graft failure: a case-control study. Am J Sports Med 2009;37:2362–7.

13. Kaeding CC, Pedroza AD, Reinke EK, et al. Risk factors and predictors of subsequent ACL injury in either knee after ACL reconstruction: prospective analysis of 2488 primary ACL reconstructions from the MOON Cohort. Am J Sports Med 2015;43:1583–90.

14. Mariscalco MW, Flanigan DC, Mitchell J, et al. The influence of hamstring autograft size on patient-reported outcomes and risk of revision after anterior cruciate ligament reconstruction: a Multicenter Orthopaedic Outcomes Network (MOON) Cohort Study. Arthroscopy 2013;29:1948–53.

15. Krosshaug T, Nakamae A, Boden BP, et al. Mechanisms of anterior cruciate ligament injury in basketball video analysis of 39 cases. Am J Sports Med 2007;35:359–67.

16. Olsen O-E, Myklebust G, Engebretsen L, et al. Injury mechanisms for anterior cruciate ligament injuries in team handball a systematic video analysis. Am J Sports Med 2004;32:1002–12.

17. Paterno MV, Schmitt LC, Ford KR, et al. Biomechanical measures during landing and postural stability predict second anterior cruciate ligament injury after anterior cruciate ligament reconstruction and return to sport. Am J Sports Med 2010;38:1968–78.

18. Hewett TE, Myer GD, Ford KR, et al. Biomechanical measures of neuromuscular control and valgus loading of the knee predict anterior cruciate ligament injury risk in female athletes a prospective study. Am J Sports Med 2005;33:492–501.

19. Powers CM. The influence of abnormal hip mechanics on knee injury: a biomechanical perspective. J Orthop Sports Phys Ther 2010;40:42–51.

20. Imwalle LE, Myer GD, Ford KR, et al. Relationship between hip and knee kinematics in athletic women during cutting maneuvers: a possible link to noncontact anterior cruciate ligament injury and prevention. J Strength Cond Res 2009;23:2223.

21. Hewett TE, Myer GD, Ford KR. Anterior cruciate ligament injuries in female athletes. Part 1: mechanisms and risk factors. Am J Sports Med 2006;34:299–311.

22. Decker MJ, Torry MR, Wyland DJ, et al. Gender differences in lower extremity kinematics, kinetics and energy absorption during landing. Clin Biomech 2003;18: 662–9.

23. Schmitz R, Thompson T, Riemann B, et al. Gender differences in hip and knee kinematics and muscle preactivation strategies during single leg landings. J Athl Train 2002;37:S-20.

24. Yu B, Garrett WE. Mechanisms of non-contact ACL injuries. Br J Sports Med 2007;41:i47–51.

25. McLean SG, Huang X, van den Bogert AJ. Association between lower extremity posture at contact and peak knee valgus moment during sidestepping: implications for ACL injury. Clin Biomech 2005;20:863–70.

26. Withrow TJ, Huston LJ, Wojtys EM, et al. The effect of an impulsive knee valgus moment on in vitro relative ACL strain during a simulated jump landing. Clin Biomech 2006;21:977–83.

27. Markolf KL, Burchfield DM, Shapiro MM, et al. Combined knee loading states that generate high anterior cruciate ligament forces. J Orthop Res 1995;13:930–5.

28. Oh YK, Lipps DB, Ashton-Miller JA, et al. What strains the anterior cruciate ligament during a pivot landing? Am J Sports Med 2012;40:574–83.

29. Shin CS, Chaudhari AM, Andriacchi TP. Valgus plus internal rotation moments increase anterior cruciate ligament strain more than either alone. Med Sci Sports Exerc 2011;43:1484–91.

30. Griffin LY, Agel J, Albohm MJ, et al. Noncontact anterior cruciate ligament injuries: risk factors and prevention strategies. J Am Acad Orthop Surg 2000;8:141–50.

31. Brown T, McLean SG, Palmieri-Smith RM. Associations between lower limb muscle activation strategies and resultant multi-planar knee kinetics during single leg landings. J Sci Med Sport 2014;17:408–13.

32. Zebis MK, Andersen LL, Bencke J, et al. Identification of athletes at future risk of anterior cruciate ligament ruptures by neuromuscular screening. Am J Sports Med 2009;37:1967–73.

33. Cowling EJ, Steele JR. Is lower limb muscle synchrony during landing affected by gender? Implications for variations in ACL injury rates. J Electromyogr Kinesiol 2001;11:263–8.

34. Walsh M, Boling MC, McGrath M, et al. Lower extremity muscle activation and knee flexion during a jump-landing task. J Athl Train 2012;47:406–13.

35. Donnelly CJ, Lloyd DG, Elliott BC, et al. Minimizing valgus knee loading during sidestepping: implications for ACL injury risk. J Biomech 2012;45:1491–7.

36. Myer GD, Sugimoto D, Thomas S, et al. The influence of age on the effectiveness of neuromuscular training to reduce anterior cruciate ligament injury in female athletes a meta-analysis. Am J Sports Med 2013;41:203–15.

37. Terry M. Campbell's operative orthopedics. JAMA 2009;301:329–30.

38. Benjaminse A, Gokeler A, van der Schans CP. Clinical diagnosis of an anterior cruciate ligament rupture: a meta-analysis. J Orthop Sports Phys Ther 2006;36: 267–88.

39. Swain MS, Henschke N, Kamper SJ, et al. Accuracy of clinical tests in the diagnosis of anterior cruciate ligament injury: a systematic review. Chiropr Man Therap 2014;22:25.

40. Wagemakers HP, Luijsterburg PA, Boks SS, et al. Diagnostic accuracy of history taking and physical examination for assessing anterior cruciate ligament lesions of the knee in primary care. Arch Phys Med Rehabil 2010;91:1452–9.

41. Noyes FR, Bassett R, Grood E, et al. Arthroscopy in acute traumatic hemarthrosis of the knee. Incidence of anterior cruciate tears and other injuries. J Bone Joint Surg Am 1980;62:687–95.

42. Lelli A, Di Turi RP, Spenciner DB, et al. The "lever sign": a new clinical test for the diagnosis of anterior cruciate ligament rupture. Knee Surg Sports Traumatol Arthrosc 2016;24:2794–7.

43. Shea KG, Carey JL. Management of anterior cruciate ligament injuries: evidence-based guideline. J Am Acad Orthop Surg 2015;23:e1–5.

44. Quinn S, Brown T, Szumowski J. Menisci of the knee: radial MR imaging correlated with arthroscopy in 259 patients. Radiology 1992;185:577–80.

45. Vahey T, Broome D, Kayes K, et al. Acute and chronic tears of the anterior cruciate ligament: differential features at MR imaging. Radiology 1991;181:251–3.

46. Lee JK, Yao L, Phelps CT, et al. Anterior cruciate ligament tears: MR imaging compared with arthroscopy and clinical tests. Radiology 1988;166:861–4.

47. Kosaka M, Nakase J, Toratani T, et al. Oblique coronal and oblique sagittal MRI for diagnosis of anterior cruciate ligament tears and evaluation of anterior cruciate ligament remnant tissue. Knee 2014;21:54–7.

48. Cotten A, Delfaut E, Demondion X, et al. MR imaging of the knee at 0.2 and 1.5 T: correlation with surgery. AJR Am J Roentgenol 2000;174:1093–7.

49. Van Dyck P, Vanhoenacker FM, Lambrecht V, et al. Prospective comparison of 1.5 and 3.0-T MRI for evaluating the knee menisci and ACL. J Bone Joint Surg Am 2013;95:916–24.

Gross, Arthroscopic, and Radiographic Anatomies of the Anterior Cruciate Ligament

Foundations for Anterior Cruciate Ligament Surgery

Sebastián Irarrázaval, MD[a], Marcio Albers, MD[b], Tom Chao, MD[c],
Freddie H. Fu, MD[b],*

KEYWORDS

- Anterior cruciate ligament • Anatomy • Double bundle • Arthroscopy • Embryology

KEY POINTS

- The understanding of the double bundle anatomy of the anterior cruciate ligament (ACL) is the key to performing an individualized anatomic ACL reconstruction.
- The arthroscopic view during ACL reconstruction grants a 10 times magnification that allows excellent anatomic landmarks identification.
- Respecting the variation of ACL anatomy makes every case technically unique and ensures that optimum treatment is tailored to all patients.

INTRODUCTION

Anterior cruciate ligament reconstruction (ACLR) is one of the most common orthopedic procedures, with more than 130,000 ACLRs performed annually in the United States alone.[1] The objective of ACLR is to reestablish knee function and prevent future meniscal and chondral damage, which can lead to secondary degenerative changes in the knee joint.[2–4] Approaches to ACLR surgery are governed by the principle of restoring native anatomy, which in turn may better replicate normal knee function.

Anatomic ACLR is based on the following 4 fundamental principles: (1) restore the anteromedial (AM) and posterolateral (PL) bundles, the 2 functional anterior cruciate ligament (ACL) bundles; (2) restore native ACL insertion sites by aligning the tunnels in proper anatomic positions; (3) correctly tension each bundle; and (4) adapt ACLR to each patient, thus ensuring that tunnel diameter and graft size are dictated by the characteristics of their native insertion sites.[5] The concept of anatomic ACLR

[a] Department of Orthopedic Surgery, Pontificia Universidad Católica de Chile, Santiago, Chile; [b] Department of Orthopaedic Surgery, University of Pittsburgh, Pittsburgh, PA, USA; [c] Kern Medical Center, Bakersfield, CA, USA
* Corresponding author. Department of Orthopaedic Surgery, University of Pittsburgh, Kaufman Medical Building, Suite 1011, 3941 5th Avenue, Pittsburgh, PA 15203.
E-mail address: ffu@upmc.edu

Clin Sports Med 36 (2017) 9–23
http://dx.doi.org/10.1016/j.csm.2016.08.002
0278-5919/17/© 2016 Elsevier Inc. All rights reserved.

has received considerable attention because the biomechanical and clinical results of this approach have been correlated with better outcomes than nonanatomic ACLR.[6-13] Because of the importance of understanding the detailed anatomy of the ACL in order to perform anatomic ACLR, this article aims to clarify the microscopic and macroscopic anatomy of this ligament.

HISTORY OF ANTERIOR CRUCIATE LIGAMENT ANATOMY

The earliest known description of the human ACL was recorded around 3000 BC on an Egyptian papyrus scroll. During the Roman era, Claudius Galen (199–129 BC) described the knee ligaments, terming the ACL the "ligamenta genu cruciate."[14] In 1543, Andreas Vesalius completed the first known formal anatomic study of the human ACL in his book De Humani Corporis Fabrica Libris Septum.

For about 400 years, the ACL was thought of a single homogenous structure. Two bundles of the ACL were described for the first time in 1836 by Weber and Weber.[15] Despite other subsequent descriptions of the two-bundle anatomy by Palmer,[16] Abbott and colleagues,[17] and Girgis and colleagues,[18] the discovery did not become well known for many decades. These first reports characterized the ACL bundles based on their relative tibial insertion sites, with the resulting AM and PL bundle nomenclature still in use today. Although it is now widely accepted that the ACL is composed of 2 bundles,[19] there is a considerable amount of variation regarding the relative sizes of the AM and PL bundles depending on the type of study (ie, fetal, arthroscopic, or cadaveric).

More recently, Norwood and Cross[20] and Amis and Dawkins[21] described a third ACL bundle termed the intermediate bundle. Because the anatomic and biomechanical properties of the intermediate bundle are most similar to the AM bundle, the intermediate bundle is commonly considered part of the AM bundle.

EMBRYONIC ANTERIOR CRUCIATE LIGAMENT ANATOMY

The ACL begins to appear in the fetus as early as week 8 of the gestation period.[22-26] The ACL likely originates in the embryo as a ventral condensation of the fetal blastoma that then migrates posteriorly with the development of the intercondylar space.[27] Similarly, knee menisci may originate from the same process as the ACL, which would give further support to the idea that these structures function interdependently with one another. Another proposed method for fetal ACL formation is a confluence between ligamentous collagen fibers and periosteum fibers.[28] Following initial ligament formation, no major organizational or compositional changes occur throughout the remainder of fetal development.[22]

The AM and PL bundles of the ACL begin to become apparent by week 16 of gestation.[22,24-26,29] The fetal ACL is similar to the adult ligament, but differs in that the bundles are more parallel in orientation and the femoral origins are broader in size.[30] Histologically, the fetal ACL demonstrates a higher amount of cellularity and vascularity.[29] The 2 bundles in the fetal ACL are separated by a membranous septum, similar to the adult ligament[29] (Fig. 1).

MICROSCOPIC ANATOMY AND HISTOLOGY OF THE ANTERIOR CRUCIATE LIGAMENT

The ACL is an intra-articular, extrasynovial structure enveloped by 2 synovial layers.[14,19,31,32] This ligament is composed of numerous dense connective tissue fascicles predominantly composed of type I collagen and, secondarily, of type III collagen.[14,33,34] As stated earlier, a septum of connective tissue–containing vascular-derived stem cells separates the AM and PL bundles.[35] This membrane contains

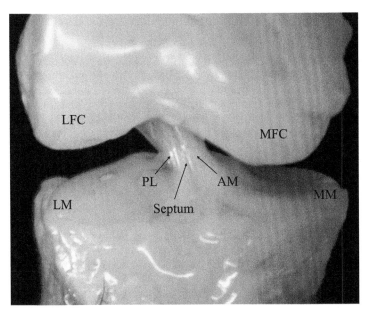

Fig. 1. Sixteen weeks of gestational age fetus knee showing the ACL bundle anatomy. LFC, lateral femoral condyle; LM, lateral meniscus; MFC, medial femoral condyle; MM, medial meniscus.

periligamentous vessels that transversely penetrate the ligament and anastomose with a longitudinal network of endoligamentous vessels that vascularize the ACL[36] (**Fig. 2**).

The ACL insertion site is divided into a 4-layered structure with mixed histology, where chondrocyte-like cells are integrated with typical-appearing tenocytes.[14,19,32,33] These layers include ligamentous, fibrocartilaginous, and mineralized fibrocartilage, in addition to a subchondral bone plate.[37] The gradual transition of the layers acts to dissipate force transmitted through the ACL, thereby preventing excessive stress to act at the insertion sites.[14,31,33,37]

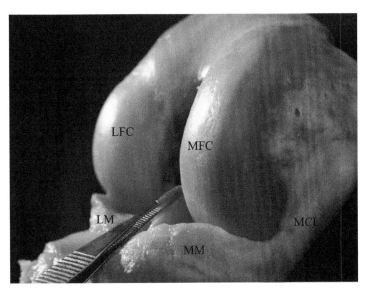

Fig. 2. ACL synovial membrane. MCL, medial collateral ligament.

MACROSCOPIC ANATOMY OF THE ANTERIOR CRUCIATE LIGAMENT

The ACL originates on the medial surface of the lateral femoral condyle and runs an oblique course within the knee joint, going from a lateral and posterior to a medial and anterior position before inserting into a broad area of the central tibial plateau (**Fig. 3**). The average total intra-articular length of the ligament is approximately 32 mm (range 22–41 mm), a length that may vary depending on the position of the knee.[14,21,37] ACL length is shortest at 90° of flexion and can increase by 18.8 ± 10.1% during unloaded extension.[38] Application of an anterior or combined rotational load can increase ACL length during extension by almost 5%.[38]

Cross-sectional areas of the ligament vary over the length of the ACL, with a midsubstance cross-section measuring approximately 44 mm², whereas the origin and insertion sites of the ACL can be more than 3 times this area.[18,39] Considering that the geometry of soft tissue structures, such as the ACL, is largely dictated by loading and orientation, the precise cross-sectional area of the midsubstance is debatable.[39–44] Quantitative in situ analysis of ACL measurements by Fujimaki and colleagues[38] found the ACL cross-section at the isthmus to be the smallest in extension (39.9 ± 13.7 mm²), although this increased with flexion of the knee (40.0 ± 12.1 mm² at 90°).

As the ligament inserts along both the femoral condyle and the tibial plateau, the ends of the ligament fan out in a manner that reproduces an hour-glass shape. Notably, this anatomic phenomenon causes the isthmus to be less than half the area of the insertion sites,[38] a fact that must be recognized during reconstruction because ligamentous cross-sectional area may directly play a role in the absorption of kinematic forces in the knee joint.[14,38,39]

Anatomy of Anterior Cruciate Ligament Bundles

The ACL comprises the AM and PL bundles, so termed based on the relative insertion sites on the tibia (**Fig. 4**). Both bundles can be observed arthroscopically, particularly with the knee held in 90° to 120° of flexion. Anatomic studies have characterized the

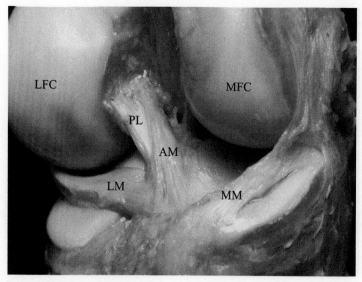

Fig. 3. ACL macroscopic anatomy.

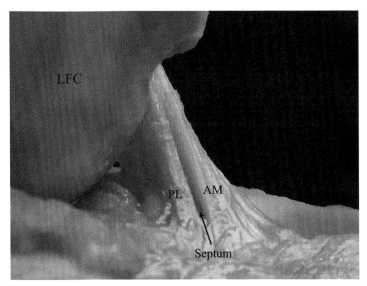

Fig. 4. ACL AM and PL bundles separated by the septum.

individual properties of the AM and PL bundles. In particular, the AM bundle is approximately 38 mm in length,[18,37] whereas the PL bundle is approximately 17.8 mm in length.[45] Despite these differences, the AM and PL bundles have similar cross-sectional diameters.[18,37,39,45,46]

Anatomy of Anterior Cruciate Ligament Insertions

The femoral origin of the ACL is an ovoid area averaging 18 mm in length and 11 mm in width.[47] Within this area, the AM bundle is located on the proximal portion of the medial wall of the lateral femoral condyle, whereas the PL bundle occupies a more distal position near the anterior articular cartilage surface of the lateral femoral condyle (**Fig. 5**). Two bony ridges define the femoral attachment site: the lateral intercondylar ridge and the lateral bifurcate ridge. The lateral intercondylar ridge, also called the resident's ridge, is an important landmark to recognize during ACLR as the native ACL always inserts inferior to this ridge.[48,49] The equally important lateral bifurcate ridge runs perpendicular to the lateral intercondylar ridge and separates the AM and PL bundles.[48]

Harner and colleagues[39] studied the origin and insertion of the AM and PL bundles using a laser micrometer system and concluded that each bundle occupies approximately 50% of the total femoral origin, with cross-sectional footprints measuring 47 ± 13 mm^2 and 49 ± 13 mm^2 for the AM and PL bundles, respectively. Mochizuki and colleagues[50] contradicted these results, observing that the AM bundle origin was 1.5 times larger than the origin of the PL bundle, although a less sensitive methodology was used to make these measurements.

On the tibia, the AM and PL bundle insertions are localized over a broad area between the medial and lateral tibial spines. Within this area, the AM bundle insertion occupies an anterior and medial position, whereas the PL bundle insertion is located more posteriorly and laterally (**Fig. 6**). The ACL tibial insertion has an average anteroposterior length of 11 mm (range 9–13 mm) and an average medial-lateral width of 17 mm (range 14–20 mm). The overall size of the tibial insertion is approximately 120% of the femoral origin. However, as is the case with the femoral origin, the

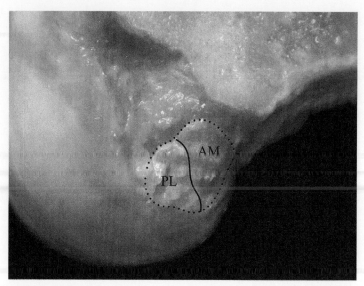

Fig. 5. Femoral insertion site.

2 bundles share approximately equal tibial insertion site areas, where the AM bundle occupies 56 ± 21 mm^2, and the PL bundle occupies 53 ± 21 mm^2.[39] However, not only does size vary among individuals but also the footprint shape differs as well, which may alter the average cross-sectional area calculated over the tibia.[18,32,33,47,51–53]

Both bundles have a close anatomic relation with the lateral meniscus. Posteriorly, fibers of the PL bundle are in close proximity to the posterior root of the lateral meniscus. In some individuals, the bundle may attach to the meniscus itself (**Fig. 7**).

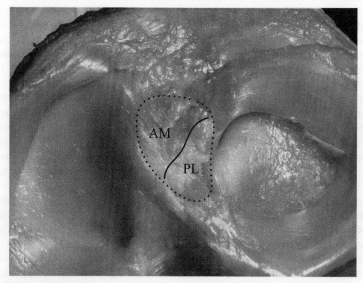

Fig. 6. Tibial insertion site.

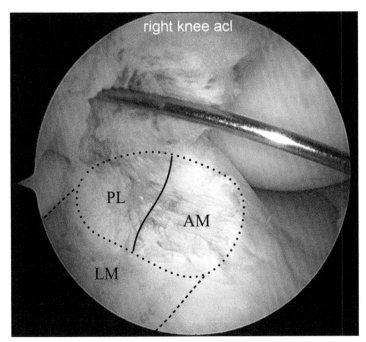

Fig. 7. Arthoscopic view of the anterior horn of the lateral meniscus relation with the ACL tibial insertion site.

Similarly, the AM bundle may have attachments to the anterior horn of the lateral meniscus. Quantitative analysis of the ACL insertion site shows that ACL intrusion onto the anterolateral meniscal root can reach 63.2% of the root attachment.[54]

Many different anatomic landmarks can be used to arthroscopically identify the tibial insertion site. The most commonly described landmarks are the anterior horn of the lateral meniscus and anterior edge of the posterior cruciate ligament. However, these are soft tissue structures that may have a varying anatomic relation with the ACL.[55] Other landmarks to take into account are the medial and lateral tibial eminences.[12,50,56] The ACL center is positioned 5.7 ± 1.1 mm anterior to a projected line from the apex of the medial tibial eminence.[55] Therefore, the tibial insertion site of the ACL may be reliably identified based on the location of the medial tibial eminence.[55]

The shape of the tibial insertion site is a topic of debate. Indeed, a recent study showed that the shape of the tibial insertion site varies when inspected after transection arthroscopically. More specifically, in 51% of cases, the shape is elliptical; in 33%, it is triangular, and in 16%, it is C-shaped.[57]

Anterior Cruciate Ligament Neurovascular Anatomy

Proximally, the ACL receives its blood supply from the middle genicular artery, which feeds a synovial plexus around the ligament.[33] Distally, the medial and lateral inferior genicular arteries supply the plexus, although to a lesser degree.[31,33,58] Furthermore, watershed areas exist around the insertion sites and along the anterior aspect of the distal third of the ligament, as supported by immunohistochemical analysis.[33,58]

Approximately 1% of the area of the ACL consists of neural tissue supplied by branches of the tibial nerve.[31] This neural tissue serves many functions within the

ACL. For example, perivascular neural elements surround the vascular plexus and assist in vasomotor control, whereas other nerve fibers transmit slow pain impulses.[59] Surrounding the synovium are slow- and rapid-adapting mechanoreceptors. The slow-adapting mechanoreceptors relay information about motion, position, and joint rotation, and the rapid-adapting mechanoreceptors detect tension changes within the ligament.[60,61] After ACL rupture, residual mechanoreceptors within the torn stumps may still function in proprioception.[62,63] However, the extent of residual function if this stump is preserved requires further research to determine its significance.

Anterior Cruciate Ligament Functional Anatomy

The AM and PL bundles change their alignment in respect to each other as the knee moves from extension to flexion. The femoral insertion sites are vertically oriented when the knee is fully extended, and, consequently, the 2 ACL bundles are oriented in parallel. As the knee moves to 90° of flexion, the AM bundle insertion site on the femur rotates posteriorly and inferiorly, in contrast to the femoral insertion of the PL bundle, which rotates anteriorly and superiorly. These modifications orient the femoral footprints more horizontally, causing the 2 bundles to twist around each other and become crossed. When the knee is flexed, the femoral insertion of the PL bundle is anterior to the AM bundle. This crossing pattern and the different lengths of each bundle have implications for the tensioning pattern of the overall ligament and each individual bundle.

In a study by Gabriel and colleagues,[64] forces were measured in each bundle while exerting an anterior tibial load of 134 N over several flexion angles. Force was also measured under a combined rotatory load over 10 Nm of valgus and 5 Nm of internal tibial torque. These assessments showed that the PL bundle is tightest in extension (in situ force of 67 ± 30 N) and becomes relaxed as the knee is flexed. When flexed and not stretched, the PL bundle shortens by 1.5 to 7.1 mm.[65,66] The PL bundle also tightens during internal and external rotation by ≈ 2.7 mm.[67] Conversely, the AM bundle is more relaxed in extension and reaches maximum tension as the knee approaches 60° of flexion (in situ force of 90 ± 17 N).[21,64] Compared with extension, at 90° of flexion, the AM bundle stretches by about 3.3 mm.[65,66,68,69]

Knee Bony Anatomy Related to the Anterior Cruciate Ligament

Just as ACL size varies among individuals, so does the bony anatomy, although the relationship of ACL size and intercondylar width may not hold a direct relationship. As such, patients can have a relatively large ACL within a very small intercondylar space. A small notch-width index, or the ratio of the notch width to epicondylar width, is linked to an increased likelihood of ACL rupture.[70,71]

Anterior Cruciate Ligament Radiographic Anatomy

To evaluate ACL anatomy, MRI is the most reliable imaging technique. MRIs can visualize the 2 bundles in the sagittal plane and in parallel orientation with the knee extended, in addition to showing the PL bundle in the coronal plane. The double-bundle structure can be more easily appreciated with higher resolution images, such as those obtained at a magnet strength of 1.5 T (**Fig. 8**).

Traditionally, ACL tunnel locations in preparation for reconstruction have been determined from plain radiographs, with several methods existing for the intraoperative radiographic evaluation of the tunnels.[72–77] Nevertheless, this technique provides a 2-dimensional projection of 3-dimensional bone geometry. Therefore, this method is not fully reliable because femoral rotation can influence the measured size of the

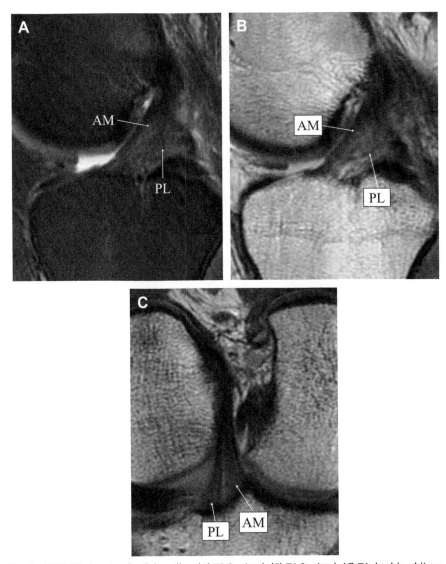

Fig. 8. ACL MRI showing both bundles. (*A*) T2 Sagittal. (*B*) T1 Sagittal. (*C*) T1 double oblique.

condyles, leading to inaccurate results.[78,79] Consequently, bony and soft tissue anatomic landmarks should be used to determine tunnel positions during ACLR.

Currently, 3-dimensional computed tomography (CT) reconstruction is the standard for postoperative tunnel position evaluation. There are 2 main methods to measure the femoral tunnel positions (ie, sagittal cut) and one method for measuring tibial tunnel positions (ie, axial cut). On the femoral side, the quadrant method references the Blumensaat line, which is understood as the most anterior (ie, superior) aspect of the notch (**Fig. 9**). The anatomic coordinate axes method is based on a report by Watanabe and colleagues,[80] who described tunnel position relative to the border between the medial wall and articular surface of the lateral condyle.

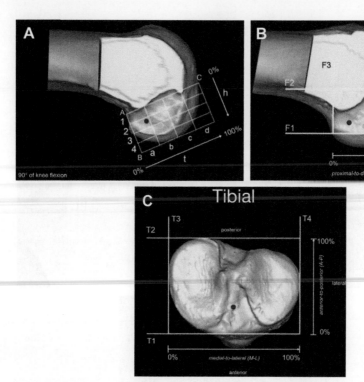

Fig. 9. Three-dimensional CT evaluation of the femoral and tibial tunnel location. Anatomic AM tunnel position: (*blue*); anatomic PL tunnel position: (*green*). (*A*) Quadrant method (for femoral side): the locations of the femoral tunnels are established within a 4 × 4 grid, which is oriented along the most anterior edge of the notch roof, parallel (t) and perpendicular (h) to the Blumensaat line. (*B, C*) Anatomic coordinate axes method (for the femoral and tibial sides): the locations of the tunnels are determined in the axial and sagittal planes, aligned with the respective bone anatomic axes. Lines: F1—posterior border of the medial wall of the lateral condyle; F2—most anterior point of the notch; F3—proximal border of the notch; F4—distal point of the notch roof; T1—anterior border of the tibial plateau; T2—most posterior border of the tibial plateau; T3—medial border of the tibial plateau; T4—lateral border of the tibial plateau. Axes: Femoral side—posterior-to-anterior (P-A) = F1 to F2; proximal-to-distal (Pr-D) = F3 to F4. Tibial side: anterior-to-posterior (AP) = T1 to T2; medial-to-lateral (ML) = T3 to T4. (*Adapted from* Forsythe B, Kopf S, Wong AK, et al. The location of femoral and tibial tunnels in anatomic double-bundle anterior cruciate ligament reconstruction analyzed by three-dimensional computed tomography models. J Bone Joint Surg Am 2010;92:1418–26; and Kopf S, Forsythe B, Wong AK, et al. Nonanatomic tunnel position in traditional transtibial single-bundle anterior cruciate ligament reconstruction evaluated by three-dimensional computed tomography. J Bone Joint Surg Am 2010;92:1427–31.)

SUMMARY

Detailed knowledge of ACL anatomy is essential for achieving anatomic surgical reconstruction, which is based on the native anatomy of this ligamentous structure. The anatomy of the ACL is complex because this ligament does not have a cylindrical, but rather hourglass shape, with different dimensions in regards to femoral insertion, tibial insertion, and the isthmus. Furthermore, the dimensions and shape of the mid-substance depend on the degree of knee flexion.

Soft and bony anatomic references of the knee are critical for proper positioning of the femoral and tibial tunnels during ACLR. Among the radiological tools available for assessing the ACL, preoperative MRI and postoperative CT are reliable tests for evaluating the anatomy and tunnel positioning of this ligament, respectively.

The goal of understanding ACL anatomy during ACLR is to restore the patient's knee kinematics, thereby improving function, conferring stability to the knee, and decreasing long-term degenerative changes. Although the current body of knowledge regarding the ACL is extensive, it remains incomplete. Further research will provide a better understanding of rotational stability and knee kinematics in those with an intact and reconstructed ACL.

REFERENCES

1. Mall NA, Chalmers PN, Moric M, et al. Incidence and trends of anterior cruciate ligament reconstruction in the United States. Am J Sports Med 2014;42(10): 2363–70.
2. Beynnon BD, Johnson RJ, Abate JA, et al. Treatment of anterior cruciate ligament injuries, part 2. Am J Sports Med 2005;33(11):1751–67.
3. Beynnon BD, Johnson RJ, Abate JA, et al. Treatment of anterior cruciate ligament injuries, part I. Am J Sports Med 2005;33(10):1579–602.
4. Jacobsen K. Osteoarthrosis following insufficiency of the cruciate ligaments in man. A clinical study. Acta Orthop Scand 1977;48(5):520–6.
5. Fu FH, van Eck CF, Tashman S, et al. Anatomic anterior cruciate ligament reconstruction: a changing paradigm. Knee Surg Sports Traumatol Arthrosc 2015; 23(3):640–8.
6. Allen CR, Giffin JR, Harner CD. Revision anterior cruciate ligament reconstruction. Orthop Clin North Am 2003;34(1):79–98.
7. Harner CD, Giffin JR, Dunteman RC, et al. Evaluation and treatment of recurrent instability after anterior cruciate ligament reconstruction. Instr Course Lect 2001; 50:463–74.
8. Heming JF, Rand J, Steiner ME. Anatomical limitations of transtibial drilling in anterior cruciate ligament reconstruction. Am J Sports Med 2007;35(10): 1708–15.
9. Kopf S, Forsythe B, Wong AK, et al. Nonanatomic tunnel position in traditional transtibial single-bundle anterior cruciate ligament reconstruction evaluated by three-dimensional computed tomography. J Bone Joint Surg Am 2010;92(6):1427–31.
10. Shen W, Forsythe B, Ingham SM. Application of the anatomic double-bundle reconstruction concept to revision and augmentation anterior cruciate ligament surgeries. J Bone Joint Surg Am 2008;90(Suppl 4):20–34.
11. Steiner ME, Battaglia TC, Heming JF, et al. Independent drilling outperforms conventional transtibial drilling in anterior cruciate ligament reconstruction. Am J Sports Med 2009;37(10):1912–9.
12. van Eck CF, Lesniak BP, Schreiber VM, et al. Anatomic single- and double-bundle anterior cruciate ligament reconstruction flowchart. Arthroscopy 2010;26(2): 258–68.
13. Zantop T, Diermann N, Schumacher T, et al. Anatomical and nonanatomical double-bundle anterior cruciate ligament reconstruction: importance of femoral tunnel location on knee kinematics. Am J Sports Med 2008;36(4):678–85.
14. Zantop T, Petersen W, Sekiya JK, et al. Anterior cruciate ligament anatomy and function relating to anatomical reconstruction. Knee Surg Sports Traumatol Arthrosc 2006;14(10):982–92.

15. Weber W, Weber E. Mechanik der menschlichen Gehwerkzeuge. Dieterichsche Buchhandlung, Göttingen [Weber W, Weber E. Mechanics of the human walking apparatus, 1992 (trans: Maquet P, Furlong R). Springer, Berlin]. 1836.

16. Palmer I. On the injuries to the ligaments of the knee joint: a clinical study. Acta Chir Scand 1938;81(Suppl 53):1–282.

17. Abbott LC, Saunders JB, Bost FC, et al. Injuries to the ligaments of the knee joint. J Bone Jt Surg 1944;26:503–21.

18. Girgis FG, Marshall JL, Monajem A. The cruciate ligaments of the knee joint. Anatomical, functional and experimental analysis. Clin Orthop Relat Res 1975;(106):216–31.

19. Bicer EK, Lustig S, Servien E, et al. Current knowledge in the anatomy of the human anterior cruciate ligament. Knee Surg Sports Traumatol Arthrosc 2010;18(8): 1075–84.

20. Norwood LA, Cross MJ. Anterior cruciate ligament: functional anatomy of its bundles in rotatory instabilities. Am J Sports Med 1979;7(1):23–6.

21. Amis AA, Dawkins GP. Functional anatomy of the anterior cruciate ligament. Fibre bundle actions related to ligament replacements and injuries. J Bone Joint Surg Br 1991;73(2):260–7.

22. Gardner E, O'Rahilly R. The early development of the knee joint in staged human embryos. J Anat 1968;102(Pt 2):289–99.

23. O'Rahilly R. The early prenatal development of the human knee joint. J Anat 1951; 85(2):166–70.

24. Haines RW. The early development of the femoro-tibial and tibio-fibular joints. J Anat 1953;87(2):192–206.

25. Merida-Velasco JA, Sanchez-Montesinos I, Espin-Ferra J, et al. Development of the human knee joint ligaments. Anat Rec 1997;248(2):259–68.

26. Ratajczak W. Early development of the cruciate ligaments in staged human embryos. Folia Morphol (warsz) 2000;59(4):285–90.

27. Ellison AE, Berg EE. Embryology, anatomy, and function of the anterior cruciate ligament. Orthop Clin North Am 1985;16(1):3–14.

28. Behr CT, Potter HG, Paletta GA Jr. The relationship of the femoral origin of the anterior cruciate ligament and the distal femoral physeal plate in the skeletally immature knee. An anatomic study. Am J Sports Med 2001;29(6):781–7.

29. Ferretti M, Levicoff EA, Macpherson TA, et al. The fetal anterior cruciate ligament: an anatomic and histologic study. Arthroscopy 2007;23(3):278–83.

30. Tena-Arregui J, Barrio-Asensio C, Viejo-Tirado F, et al. Arthroscopic study of the knee joint in fetuses. Arthroscopy 2003;19(8):862–8.

31. Arnoczky SP. Anatomy of the anterior cruciate ligament. Clin Orthop Relat Res 1983;(172):19–25.

32. Petersen W, Tillmann B. Anatomy and function of the anterior cruciate ligament. Der Orthopade 2002;31(8):710–8 [in German].

33. Petersen W, Tillmann B. Structure and vascularization of the cruciate ligaments of the human knee joint. Anat Embryol (Berl) 1999;200(3):325–34.

34. Strocchi R, de Pasquale V, Gubellini P, et al. The human anterior cruciate ligament: histological and ultrastructural observations. J Anat 1992;180(Pt 3):515–9.

35. Matsumoto T, Ingham SM, Mifune Y, et al. Isolation and characterization of human anterior cruciate ligament-derived vascular stem cells. Stem Cell Dev 2012;21(6): 859–72.

36. Dodds JA, Arnoczky SP. Anatomy of the anterior cruciate ligament: a blueprint for repair and reconstruction. Arthroscopy 1994;10(2):132–9.

37. Fu FH, Bennett CH, Lattermann C, et al. Current trends in anterior cruciate ligament reconstruction. Part 1: biology and biomechanics of reconstruction. Am J Sports Med 1999;27(6):821–30.
38. Fujimaki Y, Thorhauer E, Sasaki Y, et al. Quantitative in situ analysis of the anterior cruciate ligament: length, midsubstance cross-sectional area, and insertion site areas. Am J Sports Med 2016;44(1):118–25.
39. Harner CD, Baek GH, Vogrin TM, et al. Quantitative analysis of human cruciate ligament insertions. Arthroscopy 1999;15(7):741–9.
40. Dargel J, Schmidt-Wiethoff R, Feiser J, et al. Relationship between human femorotibial joint configuration and the morphometry of the anterior cruciate ligament. Arch Orthop Trauma Surg 2011;131(8):1095–105.
41. Dienst M, Schneider G, Altmeyer K, et al. Correlation of intercondylar notch cross sections to the ACL size: a high resolution MR tomographic in vivo analysis. Arch Orthop Trauma Surg 2007;127(4):253–60.
42. Iriuchishima T, Yorifuji H, Aizawa S, et al. Evaluation of ACL mid-substance cross-sectional area for reconstructed autograft selection. Knee Surg Sports Traumatol Arthrosc 2014;22(1):207–13.
43. Katouda M, Soejima T, Kanazawa T, et al. Relationship between thickness of the anteromedial bundle and thickness of the posterolateral bundle in the normal ACL. Knee Surg Sports Traumatol Arthrosc 2011;19(8):1293–8.
44. Noguchi M, Kitaura T, Ikoma K, et al. A method of in-vitro measurement of the cross-sectional area of soft tissues, using ultrasonography. J Orthop Sci 2002; 7(2):247–51.
45. Kummer BYM. Funktionelle anatomie der kreuzbaender. Arthroskopie 1988;1:2–10.
46. Andersen HN, Dyhre-Poulsen P. The anterior cruciate ligament does play a role in controlling axial rotation in the knee. Knee Surg Sports Traumatol Arthrosc 1997; 5(3):145–9.
47. Odensten M, Gillquist J. Functional anatomy of the anterior cruciate ligament and a rationale for reconstruction. J Bone Joint Surg Am 1985;67(2):257–62.
48. Ferretti M, Ekdahl M, Shen W, et al. Osseous landmarks of the femoral attachment of the anterior cruciate ligament: an anatomic study. Arthroscopy 2007;23(11): 1218–25.
49. Hutchinson MR, Ash SA. Resident's ridge: assessing the cortical thickness of the lateral wall and roof of the intercondylar notch. Arthroscopy 2003;19(9):931–5.
50. Mochizuki T, Muneta T, Nagase T, et al. Cadaveric knee observation study for describing anatomic femoral tunnel placement for two-bundle anterior cruciate ligament reconstruction. Arthroscopy 2006;22(4):356–61.
51. Kaeding CC, Pedroza AD, Reinke EK, et al, MOON Consortium. Risk factors and predictors of subsequent ACL injury in either knee after ACL reconstruction: prospective analysis of 2488 primary ACL reconstructions From the MOON cohort. Am J Sports Med 2015;43(7):1583–90.
52. Edwards A, Bull AM, Amis AA. The attachments of the anteromedial and posterolateral fibre bundles of the anterior cruciate ligament: Part 1: tibial attachment. Knee Surg Sports Traumatol Arthrosc 2007;15(12):1414–21.
53. Tallay A, Lim MH, Bartlett J. Anatomical study of the human anterior cruciate ligament stump's tibial insertion footprint. Knee Surg Sports Traumatol Arthrosc 2008;16(8):741–6.
54. LaPrade CM, Ellman MB, Rasmussen MT, et al. Anatomy of the anterior root attachments of the medial and lateral menisci: a quantitative analysis. Am J Sports Med 2014;42(10):2386–92.

55. Ferretti M, Doca D, Ingham SM, et al. Bony and soft tissue landmarks of the ACL tibial insertion site: an anatomical study. Knee Surg Sports Traumatol Arthrosc 2012;20(1):62–8.

56. Hara K, Mochizuki T, Sekiya I, et al. Anatomy of normal human anterior cruciate ligament attachments evaluated by divided small bundles. Am J Sports Med 2009;37(12):2386–91.

57. Guenther D, Irrrázaval S, Nishizawa Y, et al. Variation in the shape of the tibial insertion site of the anterior cruciate ligament: classification is required. Knee Surg Sports Traumatol Arthrosc 2015. [Epub ahead of print].

58. Scapinelli R. Vascular anatomy of the human cruciate ligaments and surrounding structures. Clin Anat 1997;10(3):151–62.

59. Kennedy JC, Weinberg HW, Wilson AS. The anatomy and function of the anterior cruciate ligament. As determined by clinical and morphological studies. J Bone Joint Surg Am 1974;56(2):223–35.

60. Schultz RA, Miller DC, Kerr CS, et al. Mechanoreceptors in human cruciate ligaments. A histological study. J Bone Joint Surg Am 1984;66(7):1072–6.

61. Schutte MJ, Dabezies EJ, Zimny ML, et al. Neural anatomy of the human anterior cruciate ligament. J Bone Joint Surg Am 1987;69(2):243–7.

62. Adachi N, Ochi M, Uchio Y, et al. Mechanoreceptors in the anterior cruciate ligament contribute to the joint position sense. Acta Orthop Scand 2002;73(3): 330–4.

63. Georgoulis AD, Pappa L, Moebius U, et al. The presence of proprioceptive mechanoreceptors in the remnants of the ruptured ACL as a possible source of re-innervation of the ACL autograft. Knee Surg Sports Traumatol Arthrosc 2001; 9(6):364–8.

64. Gabriel MT, Wong EK, Woo SL, et al. Distribution of in situ forces in the anterior cruciate ligament in response to rotatory loads. J Orthop Res 2004;22(1):85–9.

65. Hollis JM, Takai S, Adams DJ, et al. The effects of knee motion and external loading on the length of the anterior cruciate ligament (ACL): a kinematic study. J Biomech Eng 1991;113(2):208–14.

66. Takai S, Woo SL, Livesay GA, et al. Determination of the in situ loads on the human anterior cruciate ligament. J Orthop Res 1993;11(5):686–95.

67. Zaffagnini S, Martelli S, Acquaroli F. Computer investigation of ACL orientation during passive range of motion. Comput Biol Med 2004;34(2):153–63.

68. Bach JM, Hull ML, Patterson HA. Direct measurement of strain in the posterolateral bundle of the anterior cruciate ligament. J Biomech 1997;30(3):281–3.

69. Sakane M, Fox RJ, Woo SL, et al. In situ forces in the anterior cruciate ligament and its bundles in response to anterior tibial loads. J Orthop Res 1997;15(2): 285–93.

70. LaPrade RF, Burnett QM 2nd. Femoral intercondylar notch stenosis and correlation to anterior cruciate ligament injuries. A prospective study. Am J Sports Med 1994;22(2):198–202 [discussion: 3].

71. Shelbourne KD, Facibene WA, Hunt JJ. Radiographic and intraoperative intercondylar notch width measurements in men and women with unilateral and bilateral anterior cruciate ligament tears. Knee Surg Sports Traumatol Arthrosc 1997; 5(4):229–33.

72. Pinczewski LA, Salmon LJ, Jackson WF, et al. Radiological landmarks for placement of the tunnels in single-bundle reconstruction of the anterior cruciate ligament. J Bone Joint Surg Br 2008;90(2):172–9.

73. Aglietti P, Zaccherotti G, Menchetti PP, et al. A comparison of clinical and radiological parameters with two arthroscopic techniques for anterior cruciate ligament reconstruction. Knee Surg Sports Traumatol Arthrosc 1995;3(1):2–8.
74. Bernard M, Hertel P, Hornung H, et al. Femoral insertion of the ACL. Radiographic quadrant method. Am J Knee Surg 1997;10(1):14–21 [discussion: 21–2].
75. Amis AA, Beynnon B, Blankevoort L, et al. Proceedings of the ESSKA scientific workshop on reconstruction of the anterior and posterior cruciate ligaments. Knee Surg Sports Traumatol Arthrosc 1994;2:124–32.
76. Järvelä T, Paakkala T, Järvelä K, et al. Graft placement after the anterior cruciate ligament reconstruction: a new method to evaluate the femoral and tibial placements of the graft. Knee 2001;8(3):219–27.
77. Harner CD, Marks PH, Fu FH, et al. Anterior cruciate ligament reconstruction: endoscopic versus two-incision technique. Arthroscopy 1994;10(5):502–12.
78. Zantop T, Wellmann M, Fu FH, et al. Tunnel positioning of anteromedial and posterolateral bundles in anatomic anterior cruciate ligament reconstruction: anatomic and radiographic findings. Am J Sports Med 2008;36(1):65–72.
79. Tashman S, Collon D, Anderson K, et al. Abnormal rotational knee motion during running after anterior cruciate ligament reconstruction. Am J Sports Med 2004; 32(4):975–83.
80. Watanabe S, Satoh T, Sobue T, et al. Three-dimensional evaluation of femoral tunnel position in anterior cruciate ligament reconstruction. Hiza J Japan Knee Soc 2005;30:253–6. [In Japanese].

Graft Selection in Anterior Cruciate Ligament Surgery
Who gets What and Why?

Kyle R. Duchman, MD[a], T. Sean Lynch, MD[b],
Kurt P. Spindler, MD[c],*

KEYWORDS

• ACL • Allograft • Autograft • Anterior cruciate ligament • Graft selection

KEY POINTS

• Rupture of an anterior cruciate ligament graft is a devastating complication.
• Surgeon preference significantly influences graft choice.
• Autograft provides superior outcomes to allograft in the young, active patient population.
• Bone-patella tendon-bone and hamstring tendon autograft provide equivalent outcomes based on the best available evidence.

INTRODUCTION

Anterior cruciate ligament (ACL) tears are a common orthopedic injury, most frequently affecting young and active patients.[1] For those interested in returning to high-level athletic competition, arthroscopic ACL reconstruction has become the standard of care, with nearly 200,000 ACL reconstruction procedures performed annually in the United States.[2] Since the first described report of ACL reconstruction in the early 1900s,[3,4] the amount and quality of research on this topic has expanded exponentially. This research has led to improved understanding of ACL anatomy and function as well as refinement of surgical techniques. Despite the vast amount of research, a great deal of debate still surrounds graft choice during ACL reconstruction and the effect of graft choice on subsequent graft failure.

Disclosures: No relevant commercial or financial conflicts of interest (K.R. Duchman); consultant, Smith & Nephew (T.S. Lynch); National Institute of Arthritis and Musculoskeletal and Skin Diseases of the National Institutes of Health, Donjoy, and Smith & Nephew (K.P. Spindler).
[a] Department of Orthopaedics and Rehabilitation, University of Iowa Hospitals and Clinics, 200 Hawkins Drive, 01008 JPP, Iowa City, IA 52242, USA; [b] Center for Shoulder, Elbow, and Sports Medicine, Columbia University Medical Center, 622 West 168 Street, PH11-Center, New York, NY 10032, USA; [c] Cleveland Clinic Sports Health Center, 5555 Transportation Boulevard, Garfield Heights, OH 44125, USA
* Corresponding author.
E-mail address: spindlk@ccf.org

Recently performed prospective cohort studies have allowed us to recognize patient and surgical factors that predict graft failure following ACL reconstruction.[5–8] Younger patient age, increased activity level, and the use of allograft have all been consistently identified as risk factors for ACL reconstruction graft failure.[5,6,9–11] Of these factors, graft choice is the only modifiable surgical factor for young, active patients who wish to return to competitive sport. As a result, a great deal of time is often spent counseling patients and their families on the risks and benefits associated with various graft options. Given that the surgeon's recommendation remains the primary influence on patients' graft choice,[12] it is imperative that orthopedic surgeons who routinely perform ACL reconstruction not only fully understand graft options but also the goals and nonmodifiable risk factors for patients that can affect their outcomes.

Using the best available evidence, the authors aim to describe the influence of graft choice on outcomes following ACL reconstruction for skeletally mature patients. In doing so, the authors hope to clarify graft options for a diverse patient population, ranging from the competitive high school, college, or professional athlete to the active adult, all of whom have unique goals and risks that must be considered when planning for ACL reconstruction.

MEASURING ANTERIOR CRUCIATE LIGAMENT RECONSTRUCTION OUTCOMES

In order to assess outcomes following ACL reconstruction, it is important to understand the primary end point of interest or, in simpler terms, to understand what is considered a success or failure. The goal of ACL reconstruction is to restore stability of the knee in order to reduce the risk of subsequent articular cartilage and meniscal injury. Throughout the literature, graft failure following ACL reconstruction is the most consistently reported variable; however, this dichotomous outcome fails to address the primary goal of ACL reconstruction. Additionally, this outcome does not acknowledge other outcomes that are important in this active patient population, such as return to sport, activity level, KT-1000 arthrometer laxity measurements, special physical examination tests, and range-of-motion testing.

As health care enters the value-based era, patient-reported outcome measures have become commonplace for a variety of musculoskeletal procedures.[13,14] Although there was initially some thought that these so-called subjective outcome measures were inferior to objective clinician measurements when assessing ACL reconstruction,[15] in reality, the validity of patient-reported outcome measures may better predict return to high-level activity or improved overall health as compared with more objective historical measures.[16] Sorting through the numerous general health and disease-specific outcome measures that have been used to report ACL reconstruction can be arduous,[17,18] and inconsistent reporting of measures can make comparing studies difficult. Additionally, the high frequency of concomitant articular cartilage and meniscal injuries that occur at the time of the ACL injury have been shown to significantly influence outcomes following ACL reconstruction, making it difficult to isolate the effect of ACL reconstruction alone.[19,20] Recent recommendations suggest that a combination of special physical examination tests, activity measures, and patient-reported outcome measures may improve the assessment of ACL reconstruction[21]; but most of the existing literature fails to incorporate all of these recommended measures.

Although the aforementioned issues can make interpretation of the ACL reconstruction literature difficult, it is important to consider when critically analyzing the literature. Although graft failure remains the most consistently reported outcome in high-level studies comparing the influence of graft choice following ACL reconstruction, more recent studies have recognized the importance of including validated patient-reported outcome measures. The following review focuses on the influence of graft choice on ACL reconstruction outcomes using graft failure and patient-reported outcome measures as the outcomes of interest considering what is currently provided by the best-available literature.

GRAFT CHOICE OPTIONS
Autograft

Autograft options for ACL reconstruction most commonly consist of the hamstring tendons (HS) or patellar tendon using the bone-patella tendon-bone (BTB) harvest technique. The BTB autograft has historically served as the gold standard for ACL reconstruction, based not only on its widespread global use but also as the first auto-graft option consistently used for ACL reconstruction. The BTB autograft is typically obtained through harvest of the central one-third of the patellar tendon with adjacent patellar and tibial tuberosity bone blocks at the proximal and distal end of the graft, respectively. HS autografts typically consist of the semitendinosus tendon with or without use of the adjacent gracilis tendon. Although a variety of surgical and graft fixation techniques as well as host graft size may influence graft preparation, a quadrupled, or 4-strand, graft typically yields sufficient graft size for ACL reconstruction. As with any autograft tissue harvest, donor-site morbidity remains a concern for both HS and BTB harvest.[22] Neither graft has shown superior outcomes when evaluating aggregate results from randomized controlled trials.[23] More recently, quadriceps tendon (QT) autograft has been described as a potential autograft option with predictable characteristics that make it a viable option for ACL reconstruction.[24–26] However, as the least used autograft option for ACL reconstruction, further investigation is required in order to determine the efficacy, complications, and donor-site morbidity associated with routine QT autograft use for primary ACL reconstruction.

Allograft

A variety of fresh-frozen allograft options exist for ACL reconstruction, including tibialis anterior and posterior, Achilles, hamstrings, and patellar tendon. Although allograft reconstruction obviates donor-site morbidity issues, potential concerns include disease transmission, immunogenic response, and the effect of allograft processing techniques on failure rates that exist with allograft use for ACL reconstruction.[27–30] There are also concerns about the variability and quality of tissues from country to country as well as between allograft vendors, with the lack of consistency raising concern for some practicing clinicians.

Synthetic Grafts

Although synthetic graft options eliminate both the donor-site morbidity and disease transmission and processing concerns associated with autograft and allograft options, their use today has been significantly limited by consistent failures during their early use. Therefore, their discussion is included primarily for historical perspective. Although newer-generation synthetic graft options have attempted to avoid the general failure associated with their predecessors,[31] the magnitude of the early failures, as well as lack of generalizable results from more recent designs, continues to plague adoption of synthetic grafts for ACL reconstruction.

PATIENT CONSIDERATIONS

Recent results from several large ACL registries with prospectively collected data have made it clear that certain patient factors pose significant independent risks for ACL reconstruction graft failure. From these studies, younger patient age and increased activity level have been consistently identified as patient factors associated with ACL reconstruction graft failures.[10,11,32] Although these patient factors are notably nonmodifiable, they are important to consider for patient counseling. Additionally, and maybe most importantly, these factors should be considered during critical review of the current literature, as these findings suggest that controlling, or at a minimum stratifying by age and activity level, is necessary moving forward.

Given the increased graft failure risk in the young, active population, there is some speculation as to how certain surgical factors, including graft choice, may modify this risk. Data from the Multicenter Orthopedic Outcomes Network (MOON) suggest that the probability of graft failure increases significantly in young patients with allograft ACL reconstructions as opposed to autograft reconstructions before graft failure rates normalize with increasing age (**Fig. 1**).[10] Although defining an absolute age cutoff is admittedly unrealistic for the spectrum of patients that sustain an ACL injury, it is important to consider that both age and activity level are the strongest predictors of graft failure following ACL reconstruction and should be considered during preoperative planning and rehabilitation.[33] Based on these findings, categorizing patients as high school or college athletes and those who are not high school or college athletes may serve as a potential method that takes into account age, activity level, and level of competition, all of which are necessary to consider when assessing and comparing ACL reconstruction outcomes.

EVIDENCE-BASED GUIDELINES FOR GRAFT SELECTION IN PRIMARY ANTERIOR CRUCIATE LIGAMENT RECONSTRUCTION

Despite several randomized comparative studies investigating outcomes between BTB and HS autograft,[34–39] registry data and aggregate data show equivalent results with respect to graft failure following ACL reconstruction, patient-reported outcome measures, and return to sport,[10,23,40] with a single registry study reporting an increased risk of graft failure with HS compared with BTB autograft with minimum 5-year follow-up.[32] This finding has yet to be corroborated by similar well-designed registry studies in other countries.[10,11] In general, the difference in graft failure rates, which are invariably age-dependent across all studies,[10,11,32] and patient-reported outcome measures when comparing HS and BTB autograft have been minimal, with anecdotal differences in anterior knee pain, knee flexion strength, and laxity via

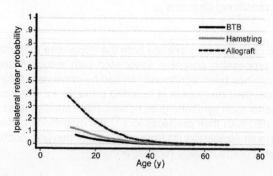

Fig. 1. The probability of graft rupture as a function of age and categorized by graft type. (*From* Kaeding CC, Pedroza AD, Reinke EK, et al. Risk factors and predictors of subsequent ACL injury in either knee after ACL reconstruction: prospective analysis of 2488 primary ACL reconstructions from the MOON cohort. Am J Sports Med 2015;43:1583–90; with permission.)

KT-1000 arthrometer measurements inconsistently reported throughout the litera-ture.[23,41–43] With respect to the use of QT autograft, low utilization, as well as lack of high-quality comparative studies with other autograft options,[44] limit any significant conclusions at this time regarding its use.

When comparing ACL reconstruction outcomes between autograft and allograft, the observed differences are more striking, particularly in the high school– or college-level athlete. Using single surgeon data that were then validated with the MOON consortium data, Kaeding and colleagues[9] described a 4 times increased risk of graft rupture with allograft ACL reconstruction. These findings have been corroborated in subsequent MOON studies with a minimum 6-year follow-up, with allograft ACL reconstruction identified as an independent risk factor for any subse-quent surgery as well as ACL reconstruction graft failure.[6,10] Although acknowledging that return to play is an outcome measure that can be influenced by a variety of extra-neous factors, this is also evidence to suggest that autograft use significantly im-proves return-to-sports rates in young athletes.[45,46] Meanwhile, a recent systematic review focused on allograft versus autograft outcomes for ACL reconstruction in pa-tients less than 25 years of age and reported a 9.6% graft failure rate with autograft compared with 25.0% in this young, active patient population.[8] Interestingly, 19 studies, or nearly one-third of the reviewed studies, for this systematic review had to be excluded because patient age was not appropriately stratified. Given the impor-tance of patient age and activity on outcomes following ACL reconstruction, future studies should aim to improve reporting of these important patient factors in order to better define the roles for different graft types.

Although the literature comparing allograft and autograft for ACL reconstruction in young, active, high school- and college-level athletes would strongly favor the use of autograft, there likely remains a role for allograft use in older, less active patient pop-ulations. Although allograft use eliminates issues with donor-site morbidity, its use must be weighed with the devastating consequence of graft failure. The results following allograft ACL reconstruction remain limited by the quality of the literature. Most notably, several recent systematic reviews investigating outcomes following allograft ACL reconstruction are limited by a lack of adequate age stratification.[47,48] As mentioned previously, age and activity level should always remain a consideration when critically evaluating ACL reconstruction results. However, previous MOON data suggest that graft failure rates normalize as patient age approaches 40 years,[10] which has been corroborated by similar US ACL registry studies.[5] Given the current quality of literature on allograft ACL reconstruction, the purported benefits of allograft use, including decreased donor-site morbidity,[49] must be weighed with the risks associ-ated with allograft use. Based on the best available literature, one of these risks, graft failure, is undoubtedly correlated with patient age. Additionally, surgeons routinely us-ing allografts should be familiar with vendors providing grafts and graft processing techniques, as it is clear that not all allografts are created equal.[27] Although allograft ACL reconstruction may serve as a viable option in older, less active patients, further high-quality research that approaches the quality of research currently available for autograft ACL reconstruction options is necessary in order to better guide treatment decisions.

EVIDENCE-BASED GUIDELINES FOR GRAFT SELECTION IN REVISION ANTERIOR CRUCIATE LIGAMENT RECONSTRUCTION

ACL reconstruction graft failure poses significant challenges for patients with ACL in-juries as well as the treating surgeon. With respect to graft selection, graft options may be limited depending on the graft choice for the primary ACL reconstruction. The Multicenter ACL Revision Study (MARS) cohort provides some of the best data on revision ACL reconstruction, with data collected from a mix a private practice and academic surgeons that makes the information obtained from the study highly generalizable.[50] Although previous graft harvest may limit autograft options, making allograft options enticing, allograft use in revision ACL reconstruction increased the chance of subsequent graft failure nearly 3-fold. Additionally, autograft use in the setting of ACL reconstruction resulted in a significant increase in sports function and patient-reported outcomes.[50] These results are important to understand given that graft choice in revision ACL reconstruction is most strongly driven by the treating surgeon.[51] Based on these data, autograft use during revision ACL reconstruction provides the most favorable results, with graft choice decisions most significantly influenced by the treating surgeon. Therefore, surgeons play a significant role in changing the course of revision ACL reconstruction in the future.

SUMMARY

ACL injuries are common and typically affect a young, active patient population. Rupture of an ACL graft is a devastating complication, and much literature has previously been published on the topic. ACL graft choice remains a topic of interest, with surgeon preference significantly influencing graft choice at the time of primary and revision ACL reconstruction. Because of this, it is important for surgeons to understand the best available evidence on graft choice.

Based on the current literature, autograft seems to be superior to allograft with respect to graft failure, patient-reported outcomes, and return to sport in young, active, high school and college athletes. However, future high-level studies are required to determine if any differences exist between autograft options, including BTB and HS, as current literature does not consistently support one option over the other. Similarly, future high-level studies that consider patient age and activity are required in order to better define the role for allograft in this patient population. Maybe most important to reiterate is the influence surgeons have on graft choice and the consequences associated with those decisions, particularly in young patients who wish to return to sport. Because of this, it is imperative that surgeons not only understand the current literature but also the goals and aspirations of their patients.

REFERENCES

1. Sanders TL, Maradit Kremers H, Bryan AJ, et al. Incidence of anterior cruciate ligament tears and reconstruction: a 21-year population-based study. Am J Sports Med 2016;44:1502–7.
2. Gottlob CA, Baker CL Jr, Pellissier JM, et al. Cost effectiveness of anterior cruciate ligament reconstruction in young adults. Clin Orthop Relat Res 1999;367: 272–82.
3. Hey Groves EW. Operation for repair of the crucial ligaments. Clin Orthop Relat Res 1980;147:4–6.
4. Schindler OS. Surgery for anterior cruciate ligament deficiency: a historical perspective. Knee Surg Sports Traumatol Arthrosc 2012;20(1):5–47.
5. Maletis GB, Chen J, Inacio MC, et al. Age-related risk factors for revision anterior cruciate ligament reconstruction: a cohort study of 21,304 patients from the Kaiser Permanente anterior cruciate ligament registry. Am J Sports Med 2015; 44:331–6.

6. Hettrich CM, Dunn WR, Reinke EK, et al. The rate of subsequent surgery and predictors after anterior cruciate ligament reconstruction two-and 6-year follow-up results from a multicenter cohort. Am J Sports Med 2013;41(7):1534–40.

7. Wasserstein D, Khoshbin A, Dwyer T, et al. Risk factors for recurrent anterior cruciate ligament reconstruction a population study in Ontario, Canada, with 5-year follow-up. Am J Sports Med 2013;41(9):2099–107.

8. Wasserstein D, Sheth U, Cabrera A, et al. A systematic review of failed anterior cruciate ligament reconstruction with autograft compared with allograft in young patients. Sports Health 2015;7:207–16.

9. Kaeding CC, Aros B, Pedroza A, et al. Allograft versus autograft anterior cruciate ligament reconstruction predictors of failure from a MOON prospective longitudinal cohort. Sports Health 2011;3(1):73–81.

10. Kaeding CC, Pedroza AD, Reinke EK, et al. Risk factors and predictors of subsequent ACL injury in either knee after ACL reconstruction: prospective analysis of 2488 primary ACL reconstructions from the MOON cohort. Am J Sports Med 2015;43:1583–90.

11. Andernord D, Desai N, Björnsson H, et al. Patient predictors of early revision surgery after anterior cruciate ligament reconstruction a cohort study of 16,930 patients with 2-year follow-up. Am J Sports Med 2015;43(1):121–7.

12. Cheung SC, Allen CR, Gallo RA, et al. Patients' attitudes and factors in their selection of grafts for anterior cruciate ligament reconstruction. Knee 2012;19(1): 49–54.

13. Keswani A, Uhler LM, Bozic KJ. What quality metrics is my hospital being evaluated on and what are the consequences? J Arthroplasty 2016;31(6):1139–43.

14. Bosco JA, Sachdev R, Shapiro LA, et al. Measuring quality in orthopaedic surgery: the use of metrics in quality management. Instr Course Lect 2014;63:13.

15. Zarins B. Are validated questionnaires valid? J Bone Joint Surg Am 2005;87(8): 1671–2.

16. Sernert N, Kartus J, Köhler K, et al. Analysis of subjective, objective and functional examination tests after anterior cruciate ligament reconstruction: a follow-up of 527 patients. Knee Surg Sports Traumatol Arthrosc 1999;7(3):160–5.

17. Johnson DS, Smith RB. Outcome measurement in the ACL deficient knee–what's the score? Knee 2001;8(1):51–7.

18. Wright RW. Knee injury outcomes measures. J Am Acad Orthop Surg 2009;17(1): 31–9.

19. Cox CL, Huston LJ, Dunn WR, et al. Are articular cartilage lesions and meniscus tears predictive of IKDC, KOOS, and Marx activity level outcomes after anterior cruciate ligament reconstruction? A 6-year multicenter cohort study. Am J Sports Med 2014;42(5):1058–67.

20. Borchers JR, Kaeding CC, Pedroza AD, et al. Intra-articular findings in primary and revision anterior cruciate ligament reconstruction surgery: a comparison of the MOON and MARS study groups. Am J Sports Med 2011;39(9):1889–93.

21. Meuffels DE, Poldervaart MT, Diercks RL, et al. Guideline on anterior cruciate ligament injury: a multidisciplinary review by the Dutch Orthopaedic Association. Acta Orthop 2012;83(4):379–86.

22. Shelton WR, Fagan BC. Autografts commonly used in anterior cruciate ligament reconstruction. J Am Acad Orthop Surg 2011;19(5):259–64.

23. Mohtadi N, Chan DS, Dainty KN, et al. Patellar tendon versus hamstring tendon autograft for anterior cruciate ligament rupture in adults. Cochrane Database Syst Rev 2011;(9):CD005960.

24. Xerogeanes JW, Mitchell PM, Karasev PA, et al. Evaluation of the quadriceps tendon using 3-dimensional magnetic resonance imaging reconstruction applications for anterior cruciate ligament autograft choice and procurement. Am J Sports Med 2013;41:2392–9.
25. Slone HS, Romine SE, Premkumar A, et al. Quadriceps tendon autograft for anterior cruciate ligament reconstruction: a comprehensive review of current literature and systematic review of clinical results. Arthroscopy 2015;31(3):541–54.
26. Shani RH, Umpierez E, Nasert M, et al. Biomechanical comparison of quadriceps and patellar tendon grafts in anterior cruciate ligament reconstruction. Arthroscopy 2016;32(1):71–5.
27. Tejwani SG, Chen J, Funahashi TT, et al. Revision risk after allograft anterior cruciate ligament reconstruction: association with graft processing techniques, patient characteristics, and graft type. Am J Sports Med 2015;43:2696–705.
28. Schmidt T, Hoburg A, Broziat C, et al. Sterilization with electron beam irradiation influences the biomechanical properties and the early remodeling of tendon allografts for reconstruction of the anterior cruciate ligament (ACL). Cell Tissue Bank 2012;13(3):387–400.
29. Cohen SB, Sekiya JK. Allograft safety in anterior cruciate ligament reconstruction. Clin Sports Med 2007;26(4):597–605.
30. Barbour SA, King W. The safe and effective use of allograft tissue—an update. Am J Sports Med 2003;31(5):791–7.
31. Olson EJ, Kang JD, Fu FH, et al. The biochemical and histological effects of artificial ligament wear particles: in vitro and in vivo studies. Am J Sports Med 1988; 16(6):558–70.
32. Persson A, Fjeldsgaard K, Gjertsen J-E, et al. Increased risk of revision with hamstring tendon grafts compared with patellar tendon grafts after anterior cruciate ligament reconstruction: a study of 12,643 patients from the Norwegian Cruciate Ligament Registry, 2004-2012. Am J Sports Med 2014;42(2):285–91.
33. Wiggins AJ, Grandhi RK, Schneider DK, et al. Risk of secondary injury in younger athletes after anterior cruciate ligament reconstruction: a systematic review and meta-analysis. Am J Sports Med 2016;44(7):1861–76.
34. Aglietti P, Giron F, Buzzi R, et al. Anterior cruciate ligament reconstruction: bone-patellar tendon-bone compared with double semitendinosus and gracilis tendon grafts. J Bone Joint Surg Am 2004;86(10):2143–55.
35. Maletis GB, Cameron SL, Tengan JJ, et al. A prospective randomized study of anterior cruciate ligament reconstruction a comparison of patellar tendon and quadruple-strand semitendinosus/gracilis tendons fixed with bioabsorbable interference screws. Am J Sports Med 2007;35(3):384–94.
36. Laxdal G, Kartus J, Hansson L, et al. A prospective randomized comparison of bone-patellar tendon-bone and hamstring grafts for anterior cruciate ligament reconstruction. Arthroscopy 2005;21(1):34–42.
37. Shaieb MD, Kan DM, Chang SK, et al. A prospective randomized comparison of patellar tendon versus semitendinosus and gracilis tendon autografts for anterior cruciate ligament reconstruction. Am J Sports Med 2002;30(2):214–20.
38. Sajovic M, Vengust V, Komadina R, et al. A prospective, randomized comparison of semitendinosus and gracilis tendon versus patellar tendon autografts for anterior cruciate ligament reconstruction: five-year follow-up. Am J Sports Med 2006; 34(12):1933–40.
39. Feller JA, Webster KE. A randomized comparison of patellar tendon and hamstring tendon anterior cruciate ligament reconstruction. Am J Sports Med 2003;31(4):564–73.

40. Gabler CM, Jacobs CA, Howard JS, et al. Comparison of graft failure rate between autografts placed via an anatomic anterior cruciate ligament reconstruction technique a systematic review, meta-analysis, and meta-regression. Am J Sports Med 2016;44(4):1069–79.

41. Ardern CL, Webster KE, Taylor NF, et al. Hamstring strength recovery after hamstring tendon harvest for anterior cruciate ligament reconstruction: a comparison between graft types. Arthroscopy 2010;26(4):462–9.

42. Magnussen RA, Carey JL, Spindler KP. Does autograft choice determine intermediate-term outcome of ACL reconstruction? Knee Surg Sports Traumatol Arthrosc 2011;19(3):462–72.

43. Xergia SA, McClelland JA, Kvist J, et al. The influence of graft choice on isokinetic muscle strength 4–24 months after anterior cruciate ligament reconstruction. Knee Surg Sports Traumatol Arthrosc 2011;19(5):768–80.

44. Han HS, Seong SC, Lee S, et al. Anterior cruciate ligament reconstruction: quadriceps versus patellar autograft. Clin Orthop Relat Res 2008;466(1):198–204.

45. Daruwalla JH, Xerogeanes JW, Greis PE, et al. Rates and determinants of return to play after anterior cruciate ligament reconstruction in division 1 college football athletes: a study of the ACC, SEC, and PAC-12. Orthop J Sports Med 2014; 2(Suppl 1). 2325967114S2325900007.

46. Spindler KP, Huston LJ, Wright RW, et al. The prognosis and predictors of sports function and activity at minimum 6 years after anterior cruciate ligament reconstruction a population cohort study. Am J Sports Med 2011;39(2):348–59.

47. Mascarenhas R, Erickson BJ, Sayegh ET, et al. Is there a higher failure rate of allografts compared with autografts in anterior cruciate ligament reconstruction: a systematic review of overlapping meta-analyses. Arthroscopy 2015;31(2): 364–72.

48. Zeng C, Gao SG, Li H, et al. Autograft versus allograft in anterior cruciate ligament reconstruction: a meta-analysis of randomized controlled trials and systematic review of overlapping systematic reviews. Arthroscopy 2016;32(1):153–63.

49. Brown CA, McAdams TR, Harris AH, et al. ACL reconstruction in patients aged 40 years and older: a systematic review and introduction of a new methodology score for ACL studies. Am J Sports Med 2013;41:2181–90.

50. Wright RW, Huston LJ, Haas AK, et al. Effect of graft choice on the outcome of revision anterior cruciate ligament reconstruction in the Multicenter ACL Revision Study (MARS) cohort. Am J Sports Med 2014;42(10):2301–10.

51. Group M. Factors influencing graft choice in revision anterior cruciate ligament reconstruction in the MARS group. J Knee Surg 2016;29(6):458–63.

Management of the Anterior Cruciate Ligament–Injured Knee in the Skeletally Immature Athlete

Christian N. Anderson, MD, Allen F. Anderson, MD*

KEYWORDS

- ACL • Reconstruction • Skeletally immature • Physeal sparing • Knee • Pediatric

KEY POINTS

- Anterior cruciate ligament (ACL) injuries are being diagnosed with increasing frequency in the skeletally immature population.
- Treatment options for these injuries include nonoperative, early surgical reconstruction, or delayed surgical reconstruction.
- Growing evidence demonstrates that nonoperative/delayed reconstruction results in worse functional outcomes compared with reconstruction within 6 to 12 weeks from the time of injury.
- Clinical and basic science studies have demonstrated risk of limb length discrepancy and angular deformity with transphyseal ACL reconstruction.
- All-epiphyseal ACL reconstruction minimizes the risk of growth disturbance, prevents recurrent instability, restores normal function, and is biomechanically superior to extraarticular and modified physeal-sparing procedures.

INTRODUCTION

Intrasubstance anterior cruciate ligament (ACL) injuries are being reported with increasing frequency in the skeletally immature population. Epidemiologic data from a large integrated health care system demonstrated an overall incidence of 0.11 per 10,000 at 8 years of age that gradually increases to 2.42 per 10,000 by 14 years of age.[1] Although ACL injuries in children and adolescents are relatively rare, a recent

Disclosure Statement: C.N. Anderson has nothing to disclose. A.F. Anderson has the following financial disclosures: Orthopediatrics patent, royalties, and paid consultant. Depuy Mitek paid consultant.
Tennessee Orthopaedic Alliance, 4230 Harding Road, Suite 1000, Nashville, TN 37205, USA
* Corresponding author. Tennessee Orthopaedic Alliance, The Lipscomb Clinic, 4230 Harding Road, St. Thomas Medical Building, Suite 1000, Nashville, TN 37205.
E-mail address: andersonaf@toa.com

study demonstrated a 19% increase in reported ACL tears in patients 10 to 14 years old from 2007 to 2011.[2] The exact reason for the increase in ACL injuries is unclear, but may be attributed to an increase in sports participation combined with improved examination and diagnostic methods. An increased rate of ACL reconstructions in this population has also been observed over the last 20 years.[2,3] This increase in pediatric ACL surgery is thought to be commensurate with increasing injury incidence; however, this phenomenon may also represent a change in management preferences from nonoperative to operative because of improved surgical techniques[4-14] and awareness that increased meniscal and chondral pathology may be associated with nonoperative[15-23] or delayed surgical treatment.[23-31]

Pediatric ACL tears present significant concern because of the detrimental effects they can have on the health, function, and well-being of young athletes. Although the best management strategy is still the subject of significant debate, early ACL reconstruction in skeletally immature patients has been shown to be effective at restoring normal knee function and stability[5,32] and reducing concomitant intraarticular injuries.[23-30] Surgical reconstruction techniques can be categorized into 3 groups: transphyseal, physeal-sparing, and hybrid techniques. The surgical technique most appropriate for reconstruction should be based on the patient's skeletal age at the time of surgery. Appropriate treatment is paramount in avoiding iatrogenic growth disturbance and additional intraarticular injury, and for return to sports participation and overall quality of life.

PATIENT EVALUATION
History and Physical Examination

The evaluation of an ACL tear in skeletally immature patients should begin with a thorough history. Patients often report an audible pop at the time of injury, and up to 65% of individuals can present with an acute hemarthrosis.[33] ACL tears are most likely to occur while children are participating in various sports, with highest injury rates observed during soccer and basketball in females and football and lacrosse in males.[34] The mechanism of injury is comparable to what is observed in adults—a noncontact valgus or rotational force on a relatively extended knee.[24,35] ACL avulsion fractures typically occur with a similar mechanism; however, biomechanical studies have shown intrasubstance ACL injuries are more likely to occur during faster loading rates.[36]

The physical examination should consist of a complete neurologic and vascular evaluation of the lower extremity, as well as a thorough musculoskeletal examination of the knee. Several studies have shown an association between ACL tears and injury to the collateral ligaments, menisci, and articular cartilage.[15,24,37] Surgeons should be cognizant of these associated injuries and treat them appropriately when encountered.

Radiographic Evaluation and Assessment of Skeletal Maturity

The radiographic evaluation begins with anteroposterior and lateral radiographs of the knee to rule out ACL avulsion fracture or other osseous trauma. MRI is the preferred imaging modality to confirm ACL injury and to evaluate associated knee pathology. MRI has a sensitivity of 95% and specificity of 88% for identifying ACL tears, with primary findings including abnormal Blumensaat angle, abnormal ACL signal intensity, and ligamentous discontinuity.[38] Secondary findings for ACL injury include bone bruise, anterior tibial displacement, uncovered posterior horn lateral meniscus, positive posterior cruciate line, and abnormal posterior cruciate angle.[38] Radiographic risk factors associated with ACL injury in pediatric patients include increased patellar tendon length,[39] Insall-Salvati ratio,[39] posterior tibial slope,[40,41] and intercondylar roof inclination angle,[42] as well as a decrease in intercondylar notch volume[43] and the notch width index.[44]

Once the diagnosis is confirmed, bilateral standing anteroposterior long leg radiographs should be obtained both before and after ACL reconstruction to evaluate leg length discrepancy and angular deformity. Skeletal maturity is assessed by comparing hand and wrist radiographs with the Greulich and Pyle atlas.[45] When using this reference, emphasis should be placed on the phalanges and metacarpals, because the maturity of carpal bones vary significantly and often demonstrate a younger bone age than is actually present.[46,47] In determining these factors, the relative risk and potential consequences of iatrogenic physeal injury can be estimated. Subsequently, the appropriate surgical technique can be selected to minimize the chance of leg length discrepancy or angular deformity.

NONSURGICAL AND DELAYED SURGICAL TREATMENT

The technical challenges associated with ACL reconstruction in patients with open growth plates resulted in an historical approach of nonoperative treatment. Nonoperative treatment programs typically consist of functional bracing, physical therapy, and activity modification.[20,48,49] Currently, there are no higher level of evidence (LOE) studies evaluating the efficacy nonoperative treatment compared with surgical reconstruction. Even so, several LOE III and 4 studies have demonstrated poor and "unacceptable" outcomes with conservative management, including high rates of recurrent instability, meniscal damage, early arthritis, and sports-related disability.[15–23] Possible contributing factors to these poor outcomes include both noncompliance[25] and significantly higher activity levels observed in the pediatric population.[50]

Delaying surgical reconstruction until skeletal maturity has the advantage decreasing the risk of iatrogenic growth disturbance from physeal injury and improved compliance with postoperative therapy. Despite these advantages, delayed reconstruction has been associated with recurrent instability and an increased incidence of associated knee pathology in LOE II and III studies.[23–31]

Several studies have evaluated the consequences of delay in surgery greater than 6 to 12 weeks after injury.[24,25,29,30] Millett and colleagues[24] (LOE III) found a highly significant relationship between the time of surgery and medial meniscus tears, with 36% of patients having delay of surgery of more than 6 weeks sustaining medial meniscus tears compared with only 11% with earlier reconstruction. In a retrospective cohort study of 70 patients (LOE III), Lawrence and colleagues[25] found that a delay in surgical reconstruction of more than 12 weeks resulted in a 4-fold increase in medial meniscal injuries, as well as increased medial and lateral compartment chondral injuries (odds ratios of 5.6 and 11.3, respectively). Anderson and Anderson[29] (LOE III) evaluated 135 patients with a median age of 14 years and showed increased time to surgery had a bivariate association with both lateral and medial meniscal tears. Increased time to surgery was also a significant risk factor for sustaining a chondral injury.[29] In patients younger that 14 years old, Newman and coworkers[30] (LOE III) found patients with surgical delay of more than 3 months were 4.8 times more likely to require additional operative procedures.

Other studies have evaluated additional injuries associated with delay in ACL reconstruction for at least 6 months after the initial injury. In a cross-sectional study, Dumont and colleagues[26] (LOE III) demonstrated a statistically significant increase in the rate of medial meniscal tears (53.5% vs 37.8%) and medial tibial cartilage injuries (7.8% vs

2.1%) when reconstruction was delayed more than 150 days. Henry and colleagues[28] (LOE II) determined that delay in reconstruction until skeletal maturity resulted in a higher rate of medial meniscal tears (41% vs 16%) and a higher rate of meniscectomy compared with early reconstruction. In a retrospective review (LOE IV) of 112 adolescents, Guenther and colleagues[31] showed patients with new or worsened medial meniscal tears had waited significantly longer for surgery (445 vs 290 days). Additionally, bucket handle meniscal tears increased steadily in frequency for more than 1 year after ACL injury.[31]

Similar to the observations of Guenther and colleagues, other authors have noted increasing severity of meniscal and chondral pathology with operative delay. Anderson and Anderson[29] determined time to surgery greater than 12 weeks after injury resulted in a 4.0-fold higher odds of medial and a 2.8 times higher odds of lateral meniscal tears severity. Newman and associates[30] found a significant relationship between time to surgery and meniscal injury severity, as well as the development of an irreparable meniscal injury. Both Anderson and Anderson, and Newman and coworkers observed a relationship between increased time to surgery and increasing chondral injury grade as well.[29,30] The higher grade meniscal and chondral injuries associated with operative delay in these studies suggests progressive intraarticular damage with ongoing ACL deficiency.

In contrast with the growing body of evidence demonstrating poor outcomes with conservative or delayed treatment, relatively few studies support the use of nonsurgical treatment algorithms in skeletally immature patients.[48,49,51,52] Even so, a recent metaanalysis overwhelmingly favored early surgical stabilization over conservative treatment or delayed reconstruction.[23] In this study, the aggregate data of nonsurgical or delayed surgical treatment were associated with a 34-fold increase in knee instability.[23] Furthermore, patients treated nonsurgically had a 12-fold increase in the rate of medial meniscal tears, and none were able to return to their preinjury level of play.[23] Given the increasing evidence of poor outcomes with nonsurgical and delayed surgical treatment, our current recommendation is early reconstruction to avoid recurrent instability and associated knee pathology.

RESEARCH ON PHYSEAL INJURY AND GROWTH DISTURBANCE
Basic Science Research

Basic science studies performed on animal models have revealed important findings regarding the risk of growth disturbance after physeal injury. Several studies have shown that the threshold for growth disturbance is destruction between 1% to 7% of the cross-sectional area of the physis.[53–56] Studies in pediatric patients using 3-dimensional MRI demonstrate an 8-mm transphyseal femoral tunnel results in damage to 2.4% to 4.2% of the total physeal volume.[57,58] A 9-mm tunnel corresponds with 2.6% and 2.3% of the cross-sectional area of the tibial and femoral growth plates, respectively.[59] In patients with a mean bone age of 13.2 years, drilling transphyseal tibial tunnels resulted in damage to 5.4% of the physeal area.[60] These anatomic studies demonstrate that transphyseal drilling results in physeal damage within the reported threshold causing growth disturbance in animal models. Consequently, we recommend caution when drilling transphyseal tunnels in skeletally immature patients.

Studies from Guzzanti and colleagues[53] and Houle and colleagues[54] suggest that the proximal tibial physis is more susceptible to growth disturbance compared with the distal femoral physis. Even so, in the human knee, drilling of the tibial tunnel into the anatomic footprint of the ACL places the drill hole central and relatively perpendicular to the physis, which decreases physeal damage[57,61] and theoretically minimizes the chance of growth disturbance. Conversely, placement of an anatomic femoral tunnel requires an oblique tunnel trajectory, resulting in eccentric physeal damage of greater cross-sectional area compared with tibial tunnel reaming.[61,62]

Regarding femoral tunnel drilling techniques, Chudik and colleagues[63] determined that all-epiphyseal tunnels resulted in less angular deformity and more closely maintained the anatomic position of the ACL graft compared with transphyseal tunnels. They also noted that transphyseal tibial tunnels often lead to overgrowth and subsequent deformity.[63] Even so, other studies on large animal models showed no signs of growth disturbance with transphyseal drill tunnels on either the femoral or tibial side during ACL reconstruction with soft tissue grafts.[64,65] The reason for this discrepancy is unclear, but may be related to the use of surgical techniques that avoid growth disturbance, including using small drill tunnel diameters and keeping tunnels perpendicular to the growth plate to minimize physeal damage, as well as not overtensioning the graft.[64,65] Graft overtensioning can cause a growth abnormality by generating compressive forces on the physis that inhibit longitudinal growth via the Hueter–Volkmann principle.[63,66]

Some studies have demonstrated a protective effect of placing a soft tissue graft across the physis in preventing bone bridging and growth arrest,[65,67] although others have not.[54] A recent study by Babb and colleagues[68] demonstrated that empty transphyseal drill holes and those containing soft tissue grafts developed bone bridges and angular deformity; however, the addition of stem cells to the graft was protective against bone bridge formation and subsequent growth arrest.

Clinical Research

Iatrogenic growth disturbance is uncommon after ACL reconstruction in skeletally immature patients, but has been observed in physeal sparing,[69] transphyseal,[59,70–77] and hybrid, physeal-sparing transphyseal, procedures (**Table 1**).[78–81] The most common causes of growth disturbance are technical error,[69,71,79,81,82] from placement of either hardware or a bone plug across the physis, and transphyseal drilling,[70,73–78,82] which account for 28 of the 33 cases of growth disturbance reported in the literature. Drilling across the physis can cause overgrowth, undergrowth, or arrest of the femoral or tibial physis.[70,73–78,82] Transphyseal drilling during ACL reconstruction with soft tissue grafts has also been shown to cause subclinical physeal disturbance.[59,72] Higuchi and colleagues[72] noted physeal narrowing and tunnel corticalization on postoperative MRI and radiographs in 10 of 10 patients with a mean age of 14.5 years undergoing transphyseal ACL reconstruction with hamstring autografts. Yoo and colleagues[59] reported that 5 of 43 patients (11.6%) with a mean bone age of 15.1 years developed MRI evidence of physeal bone bridge formation after transphyseal hamstring ACL reconstruction. The absence of clinically relevant limb growth abnormalities in these studies may be owing to the fact that most patients included were nearing skeletal maturity at the time of surgery. Even so, Shifflett and coworkers[75] identified 4 patients nearing skeletal maturity (mean bone age, 14.4 years; range, 13.5–16) that developed growth arrest and subsequent deformity after transphyseal ACL reconstruction. The aforementioned studies underscore the risk of both clinical and subclinical growth disturbance with transphyseal ACL reconstruction in skeletally immature patients.

In addition to reports of leg length discrepancy and angular deformity after transphyseal reconstruction, 3 cases of growth disturbance have been reported during physeal sparing procedures (see **Table 1**).[69,80,82] A survey study from Kocher and colleagues[82] of The Herodicus Society and The ACL Study Group reported one case of distal femoral valgus deformity from bone-bridge formation after a femoral over-the-top procedure. The femoral over-the-top position is in close proximity to the

Table 1
Review of the literature on reports of growth disturbance after anterior cruciate ligament reconstruction in skeletally immature patients

Procedure Type	Author	Technique	Chronologic Age/Skeletal Age/Tanner Stage	No. of Growth Disturbances	Growth Disturbance	Likely Cause of Deformity
Growth plate sparing	Robert & Casin,[69] 2010	Clocheville Technique	14.5/13.9/Tanner I	1	Femoral, 13° valgus and 9° recurvatum	Tethering effect on physis vs technical error causing damage to femoral physis owing to close proximity of tunnel
Hybrid Technique	Rozbruch et al,[81] 2013	Over-the-top femoral, transphyseal tibial	12/NA/NA	1	4.5 cm limb shortening with complex varus and recurvatum deformity	Tibial physeal arrest from bone block vs transphyseal drilling
	Lawrence et al,[80] 2011	Femoral transepiphyseal, tibial transphyseal	14.0/13.5/NA	1	7.7° femoral valgus 22 mm difference in MAD	Premature lateral femoral physeal closure from indirect physeal damage (no bar or detectable physeal breach)
	Chotel et al,[78] 2010	Over-the-top femoral, transphyseal tibial	Patient 1–7/NA/NA; Patient 2–10/10.5/NA	2	Patient 1–1.5 cm tibial overgrowth; Patient 2–6° tibial valgus	Patient 1 – Transphyseal tibial drilling causing symmetric overgrowth; Patient 2 – Transphyseal tibial drilling causing asymmetric overgrowth
	Lipscomb & Anderson,[79] 1986	Transepiphyseal femoral, transphyseal tibial + extraarticular procedure	Mean 13.5 (range, 12–15)/NA/NA	1	2 cm of limb shortening	Stapling of both tibial and femoral physes

Transphyseal	Shifflett et al,[75] 2016	Transphyseal with hamstring	Mean, 14.2 (range, 13.5–14.8)/mean, 14.4 (range, 13.5–16)/NA	4	Case 1°–8° tibial recurvatum Case 2°–10° tibial recurvatum Case 3°–6.4° genu valgum Case 4°–9° genu valgum	Cases 1 and 2 – premature closure of the tibial apophysis Case 3- central tibial and posterocentral femoral physeal arrest Case 4- physeal arrest around the graft
	Zimmerman et al,[77] 2015	Transphyseal with posterior tibialis tendon	11/NA/Tanner II	1	Symmetric limb length overgrowth of 2.8 cm	Hyperemia associated with transphyseal drilling
	Kohl et al,[73] 2014	Transphyseal with quadriceps tendon (without bone plug), femoral tunnel drilled transtibially	Mean 12.8 (range, 6.2–15.8)/NA/Tanner II-IV	2	Patient – 1°–6° femoral valgus and 1.8 cm shortening Patient – 2–2.0 cm shortening	Patient 1 – Transphyseal femoral drilling Patient 2 – Transphyseal femoral vs tibial drilling
	Lemaitre et al,[76] 2014	Transphyseal hamstring with femoral tunnel drilled through AM portal	NA/mean,13.5 (range, 11–15.5)/NA	2	4° femoral valgus in both cases	Femoral epiphysiodesis in both cases
	Kumar et al,[74] 2013	Transphyseal with quadrupled hamstring, femoral tunnel drilled transtibially	Mean, 11.25 (range, 9.5–14)/NA/Tanner I-III	1	6.2° valgus and 1.6 cm shortening	Transphyseal femoral vs tibial drilling
	McIntosh et al,[70] 2006	Transphyseal with quadrupled (n = 13) or doubled (n = 3) hamstring	Mean 13.8 males, 13.3 females/wide open physes/NA	1	1.5 cm overgrowth	Transphyseal drilling causing symmetric overgrowth
	Koman & Sanders,[71] 1999	Transphyseal with doubled hamstring	14.33/NA/NA	1	14° valgus	Femoral screw crossing the lateral femoral physis

(continued on next page)

Table 1
(continued)

Procedure Type	Author	Technique	Chronologic Age/ Skeletal Age/Tanner Stage	No. of Growth Disturbances	Growth Disturbance	Likely Cause of Deformity
Mixed	Kocher et al,[82] 2002	Several different techniques	NA	15	NA	6 cases hardware across physis 3 cases of bone plug across physis 2 cases of large drill tunnel (12 mm) and bone plug across physis 2 cases lateral extraarticular tenodesis 1 case with femoral over-the-top graft 1 case of tibial overgrowth from transphyseal drilling

Abbreviations: AM, anteromedial; MAD, mechanical axis deviation; NA, not available.

posterolateral distal femoral physis and perichondrial ring of La Croix.[83] Although the details of this case are unknown, damage to the physis at this location may have occurred from graft passage or excessive rasping, resulting in the described deformity. A second case occurred after reconstruction using the Clocheville technique,[69] which requires tensioning of the graft proximal to the femoral physis and may have created a tethering effect on the growth plate. However, the authors also noted a technical error where the extraphyseal transmetaphyseal tunnel was drilled in close proximity to the posterolateral femoral physis, possibly resulting in eccentric physeal damage and eventual valgus deformity.[69] Last, Lawrence and colleagues[80] reported a case of premature lateral femoral physeal closure and subsequent valgus deformity after drilling a revision transepiphyseal femoral tunnel. Because there was no evidence of physeal injury during arthroscopic inspection of the tunnel or with postoperative MRI, they hypothesized the physis was indirectly damaged from thermal injury, vascular insult, or excessive pressure after expanding the existing tunnel by 1.5 mm.[80] Even so, the risk of thermal injury to the physis from transepiphyseal drilling has been shown to be very low in a skeletally immature ovine model.[84]

The sequelae of leg length discrepancy and angular deformity often are severe and can require corrective surgery.[69,71,75,77,78,81] Regardless of technique chosen, surgeons should take great care to avoid technical errors that predispose to growth disturbance.

SURGICAL TREATMENT

Options for surgical treatment in skeletally immature patients include transphyseal, physeal- sparing, and hybrid reconstruction techniques. Both transphyseal and hybrid techniques require drilling through one or both of the growth plates. Most studies (LOE IV) demonstrate favorable results using these techniques, with good subjective outcome scores, objective measures, and low complication rates.[73,74,85–88] In a 10-year follow-up study (LOE IV) on 27 skeletally immature patients (mean age, 13 years; range, 12–16), Calvo and colleagues[88] demonstrated average International Knee Documentation Committee and Lysholm scores of 94 and 92, respectively, after transphyseal hamstring autograft ACL reconstruction. In a case series (LOE IV) of 32 children with a mean age of 13 years (range, 8–16), Goddard and colleagues[85] evaluated the outcomes of "living donor" transphyseal hamstring allograft ACL reconstruction. At the 2-year follow-up, 97% had normal or nearly normal International Knee Documentation Committee scores and 93% were regularly participating in strenuous activities.[85] Even so, a recent study by Schmale and coworkers[89] (LOE IV) demonstrated only 41% of skeletally immature patients maintained their preinjury level of sport 2 years after hamstring autograft or nonirradiated allograft transphyseal ACL reconstruction. Although the studies by Calvo, Goddard, and Schmale their colleagues did not demonstrate any growth disturbances, both basic science[53–56,63,66,68] and clinical research studies[70,73–78,82] indicate a risk of iatrogenic leg length discrepancy or angular deformity with transphyseal drilling. Advocates of transphyseal ACL reconstruction recommend minimizing drill tunnel diameter and placing tunnels as vertically as possible to decrease physeal damage and risk of growth deformity.[73,74,85–89] However, vertical femoral tunnel placement results in a nonanatomic graft position[90] that does not restore the normal kinematics of the knee.[91]

Physeal-sparing techniques can be described as extraphyseal,[7,92] transepiphyseal,[5,6] or all epiphyseal.[8,10–12,14] These techniques theoretically decrease the risk of growth disturbance by avoiding damage to the physis. Micheli and colleagues[7] described a modification of the McIntosh and Darby reconstruction, whereby the iliotibial band is rerouted to an over-the-top femoral position and through the knee (**Fig. 1**). Although favorable clinical results have been observed,[7,92,93] this procedure is not anatomic.

In 2003, Anderson[5] described an anatomic transepiphyseal reconstruction that followed the generally accepted principles of ACL reconstruction in adults but relied on tunnels drilled through the epiphyses, avoiding both the tibial and femoral growth plates (**Fig. 2**). In a biomechanical study by Kennedy and colleagues,[94] the Anderson technique was shown to partially restore rotatory and anteroposterior stability of the knee, whereas the Micheli iliotibial band technique overconstrained these movements. However, a follow-up study demonstrated that the Anderson technique was more effective than the Micheli technique at restoring native knee kinematics during pivot shift loading.[32] The Anderson technique relies on extraphyseal graft fixation on the tibial side, whereas the Micheli technique relies on extraphyseal graft fixation on both the femoral and tibial sides. Because both techniques rely on extraphyseal fixation they theoretically risk a soft tissue tether on the growth plate. The clinical results of these techniques in patients with substantial postoperative growth, however, have not demonstrated growth abnormality.[5,7,92,93]

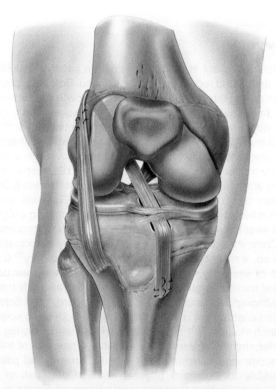

Fig. 1. The Micheli technique is a combined intraarticular and extraarticular physeal sparing reconstruction. The iliotibial band is rerouted in an over-the-top femoral position, through the knee, underneath the intermeniscal ligament, and secured both proximally and distally with sutures. (*From* Anderson AF, Anderson CN. Anterior cruciate ligament reconstruction in skeletally immature patients. In: The anterior cruciate ligament reconstruction and basic science. Prodromos C, editor. Philadelphia: Saunders-Elsevier; 2008. p. 466; with permission.)

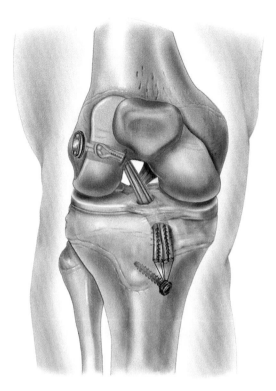

Fig. 2. Anderson's concept of reconstruction of the anterior cruciate ligament (ACL) in skeletally immature patients follows the generally accepted principles of ACL reconstruction in adults but relies on anatomic tunnels drilled completely within the epiphysis. The transepiphyseal technique uses suspensory Endobutton fixation within the epiphysis proximally and an extraphyseal metaphyseal screw and post distally. (*From* Anderson AF, Anderson CN. Anterior cruciate ligament reconstruction in skeletally immature patients. In: The anterior cruciate ligament reconstruction and basic science. Prodromos C, editor. Philadelphia: Saunders-Elsevier; 2008. p. 465; with permission.)

More recently, other authors have described modifications to the Anderson transepiphyseal technique. These so called all-epiphyseal reconstructions eliminate the possibility of soft tissue tethering of the growth plate by fixing the graft completely within the femoral and tibial epiphysis. In 2010, Lawrence and colleagues[8] described the first all-epiphyseal reconstruction, which used intraepiphyseal interference screws for graft fixation. McCarthy and colleagues[11] described a technique using a quadrupled hamstring with suspensory fixation within the proximal and distal epiphyses. Wall and colleagues[10,50] performed reconstructions by looping a doubled hamstring graft through 2 small diameter tibial tunnels over a bony bridge and securing the graft within the femoral epiphysis using an interference screw. We have also recently adopted an all-epiphyseal technique[14] (OrthoPediatrics, Warsaw, IN) with suspensory fixation on the tibial side and shielded screw fixation on the femoral side that prevents the physis from being damaged by the interference screw (**Fig. 3**). Although long-term outcomes are not available, these techniques have significant advantages, are clinically appealing, and have an acceptable safety profile in short-term LOE IV studies.[95]

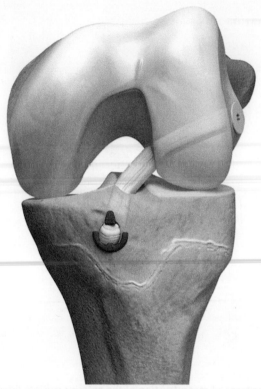

Fig. 3. The all-epiphyseal modification of Anderson's technique relies on anatomic transepiphyseal drill tunnels with suspensory fixation on the tibial side and shielded screw fixation on the femoral side. Suspensory fixation is achieved by looping the graft in the ArmorLink device and pulling tension proximally to seat the implant on the anterior surface of the tibia. A graft shield is placed in the femoral tunnel to prevent physeal compression by the interference screw. (*Courtesy of* OrthoPediatrics, Warsaw, IN; with permission.)

Our algorithm for surgical technique selection involves risk stratifying patients based on skeletal age, a direct indicator of the amount of knee growth remaining.[96] Boys with bone age of less than 13 years and girls with a bone age of less than 12 years have significant knee growth remaining,[96] and consequently, are placed in a high-risk category. Boys with a bone age of 13 to 15 years and girls with a bone age of 12 to 13 years are placed in an intermediate risk category because they have at least 1 to 2 cm of knee growth remaining.[96] The distal femoral and proximal tibial physes contribute 40% and 27% of the overall lower extremity length,[97] respectively, and the effects of physeal growth arrest in patients classified as high and intermediate would be severe.[98] Consequently, we do not recommend transphyseal drilling in high-risk patients (boys with bone age <13 years and girls <12 years) or younger intermediate risk patients (boys with bone age 13–14 years and girls 12–13 years). Boys with a bone age of greater than 15 years and girls with a bone age of greater than 13 years are classified as low risk because they have 1 cm or less of knee growth remaining[96] and iatrogenic physeal damage would likely result in no significant growth disturbance.

For high-risk patients, we recommend an all-epiphyseal reconstruction with hamstring autograft, using suspensory fixation on the tibial side and shielded screw fixation on the femoral side (see **Fig. 3**). Younger patients in the intermediate group also may be treated with an all-epiphyseal reconstruction (boys with bone age 13–14 years and girls 12–13 years). Older patients in the intermediate risk group (boys with bone age of 14–15 years and girls of 13 years) may be treated with either a transphyseal or a hybrid reconstruction using hamstring autografts. Transphyseal reconstruction in this group should be performed with a modified, vertical femoral tunnel, whereas hybrid reconstruction is performed with a more anatomic transepiphyseal femoral tunnel. Low-risk patients can undergo adult-type reconstruction with quadrupled hamstring autografts and anatomic femoral tunnel drilling through the anteromedial portal. Once patients reach skeletal maturity (males bone age of 16 years and females of 14 years), reconstruction can be safely performed with bone–patellar tendon–bone autograft and interference screw fixation.

SUMMARY

Appropriate treatment of ACL injuries in skeletally immature patients is paramount to the restoration of knee function, return to sports participation, and overall quality of life. Surgical treatment type should be dictated based on the skeletal age of the patient at the time of injury. Surgical reconstruction techniques can be categorized into 3 groups—transphyseal, physeal-sparing, and hybrid techniques. Clinical and basic science studies demonstrate that techniques requiring transphyseal drilling have a small risk of growth disturbance. Vertical transphyseal tunnels and modified extraphyseal reconstructions have been shown to be nonanatomic and do not restore normal knee kinematics. To minimize the chance of growth disturbance and to place tunnels anatomically, we recommend reconstruction that relies on tunnels drilled completely within the epiphysis for patients with significant growth remaining.

REFERENCES

1. Funahashi KM, Moksnes H, Maletis GB, et al. Anterior cruciate ligament injuries in adolescents with open physis: effect of recurrent injury and surgical delay on meniscal and cartilage injuries. Am J Sports Med 2014;42(5):1068–73.
2. Werner BC, Yang S, Looney AM, et al. Trends in pediatric and adolescent anterior cruciate ligament injury and reconstruction. J Pediatr Orthop 2016;36(5):447–52.
3. Dodwell ER, LaMont LE, Green DW, et al. 20 Years of pediatric anterior cruciate ligament reconstruction in New York state. Am J Sports Med 2014;42(3):675–80.
4. Kim SH, Ha KI, Ahn JH, et al. Anterior cruciate ligament reconstruction in the young patient without violation of the epiphyseal plate. Arthroscopy 1999;15(7): 792–5.
5. Anderson AF. Transepiphyseal replacement of the anterior cruciate ligament in skeletally immature patients a preliminary report. J Bone Joint Surg Am 2003; 85(7):1255–63.
6. Guzzanti V, Falciglia F, Stanitski CL. Physeal-sparing intraarticular anterior cruciate ligament reconstruction in preadolescents. Am J Sports Med 2003;31(6):949–53.
7. Micheli LJ, Rask B, Gerberg L. Anterior cruciate ligament reconstruction in patients who are prepubescent. Clin Orthop Relat Res 1999;364:40–7.
8. Lawrence JT, Bowers AL, Belding J, et al. All-epiphyseal anterior cruciate ligament reconstruction in skeletally immature patients. Clin Orthop Relat Res 2010;468(7):1971–7.
9. Bonnard C, Fournier J, Babusiaux D, et al. Physeal-sparing reconstruction of anterior cruciate ligament tears in children: results of 57 cases using patellar tendon. J Bone Joint Surg Br 2011;93(4):542.

10. Lykissas MG, Nathan ST, Wall EJ. All-epiphyseal anterior cruciate ligament reconstruction in skeletally immature patients: a surgical technique using a split tibial tunnel. Arthrosc Tech 2012;1(1):e133–9.

11. McCarthy MM, Graziano J, Green DW, et al. All-epiphyseal, all-inside anterior cruciate ligament reconstruction technique for skeletally immature patients. Arthrosc Tech 2012;1(2):e231–9.

12. Makani A, Franklin CC, Kanj WW, et al. All-epiphyseal anterior cruciate ligament reconstruction using fluoroscopic imaging. J Pediatr Orthop B 2013;22(5):445–9.

13. Lemos SE, Keating PM, Scott TP, et al. Physeal-sparing technique for femoral tunnel drilling in pediatric anterior cruciate ligament reconstruction using a posteromedial portal. Arthrosc Tech 2013;2(4):e483–90.

14. Anderson AF, Anderson CN. Technique: Anderson technique. In: Cordasco F, Green D, editors. Pediatric and adolescent knee surgery. Philadelphia: Lippincott; 2015. p. 46–52.

15. Angel KR, Hall DJ. Anterior cruciate ligament injury in children and adolescents. Arthroscopy 1989;5(3):197–200.

16. Streich NA, Barié A, Gotterbarm T, et al. Transphyseal reconstruction of the anterior cruciate ligament in prepubescent athletes. Knee Surg Sports Traumatol Arthrosc 2010;18(11):1481–6.

17. Aichroth PM, Patel DV, Zorrilla P. The natural history and treatment of rupture of the anterior cruciate ligament in children and adolescents. A prospective review. J Bone Joint Surg Br 2002;84(1):38–41.

18. Graf BK, Lange RH, Fujisaki CK, et al. Anterior cruciate ligament tears in skeletally immature patients: meniscal pathology at presentation and after attempted conservative treatment. Arthroscopy 1992;8(2):229–33.

19. Mizuta H, Kubota K, Shiraishi M, et al. The conservative treatment of complete tears of the anterior cruciate ligament in skeletally immature patients. J Bone Joint Surg Br 1995;77(6):890–4.

20. McCarroll JR, Rettig AC, Shelbourne KD. Anterior cruciate ligament injuries in the young athlete with open physes. Am J Sports Med 1988;16(1):44–7.

21. Kannus P, Jarvinen M. Knee ligament injuries in adolescents. Eight year follow-up of conservative management. J Bone Joint Surg Br 1988;70(5):772.

22. Vavken P, Murray MM. Treating anterior cruciate ligament tears in skeletally immature patients. Arthroscopy 2011;27(5):704–16.

23. Ramski DE, Kanj WW, Franklin CC, et al. Anterior cruciate ligament tears in children and adolescents: a meta-analysis of nonoperative versus operative treatment. Am J Sports Med 2014;42(11):2769–76.

24. Millett PJ, Willis AA, Warren RF. Associated injuries in pediatric and adolescent anterior cruciate ligament tears: does a delay in treatment increase the risk of meniscal tear? Arthroscopy 2002;18(9):955–9.

25. Lawrence JT, Argawal N, Ganley TJ. Degeneration of the knee joint in skeletally immature patients with a diagnosis of an anterior cruciate ligament tear: is there harm in delay of treatment? Am J Sports Med 2011;39(12):2582–7.

26. Dumont GD, Hogue GD, Padalecki JR, et al. Meniscal and chondral injuries associated with pediatric anterior cruciate ligament tears: relationship of treatment time and patient-specific factors. Am J Sports Med 2012;40(9):2128–33.

27. McCarroll JR, Shelbourne KD, Porter DA, et al. Patellar tendon graft reconstruction for midsubstance anterior cruciate ligament rupture in junior high school athletes. An algorithm for management. Am J Sports Med 1994;22(4):478–84.

28. Henry J, Chotel F, Chouteau J, et al. Rupture of the anterior cruciate ligament in children: early reconstruction with open physes or delayed reconstruction to skeletal maturity? Knee Surg Sports Traumatol Arthrosc 2009;17(7):748–55.
29. Anderson AF, Anderson CN. Correlation of meniscal and articular cartilage injuries in children and adolescents with timing of anterior cruciate ligament reconstruction. Am J Sports Med 2015;43(2):275–81.
30. Newman JT, Carry PM, Terhune EB, et al. Factors predictive of concomitant injuries among children and adolescents undergoing anterior cruciate ligament surgery. Am J Sports Med 2015;43(2):282–8.
31. Guenther ZD, Swami V, Dhillon SS, et al. Meniscal injury after adolescent anterior cruciate ligament injury: how long are patients at risk? Clin Orthop Relat Res 2013;472(3):990–7.
32. Sena M, Chen J, Dellamaggioria R, et al. Dynamic evaluation of pivot-shift kinematics in physeal-sparing pediatric anterior cruciate ligament reconstruction techniques. Am J Sports Med 2013;41:826–34.
33. Stanitski CL, Harvell JC, Fu F. Observations on acute knee hemarthrosis in children and adolescents. J Pediatr Orthop 1993;13(4):506–10.
34. Gornitzky AL, Lott A, Yellin JL, et al. Sport-specific yearly risk and incidence of anterior cruciate ligament tears in high school athletes: a systematic review and meta-analysis. Am J Sports Med 2015. [Epub ahead of print].
35. Krosshaug T, Slauterbeck JR, Engebretsen L, et al. Biomechanical analysis of anterior cruciate ligament injury mechanisms: three-dimensional motion reconstruction from video sequences. Scand J Med Sci Sports 2006;17(5):508–19.
36. Noyes FR, Delucas JL, Torvik PJ. Biomechanics of anterior cruciate ligament failure: an analysis of strain-rate sensitivity and mechanisms of failure in primates. J Bone Joint Surg Am 1974;56(2):236–53.
37. Samora WP, Palmer R, Klingele KE. Meniscal pathology associated with acute anterior cruciate ligament tears in patients with open physes. J Pediatr Orthop 2011;31(3):272–6.
38. Lee K, Siegel MJ, Lau DM, et al. Anterior cruciate ligament tears: MR imaging-based diagnosis in a pediatric population. Radiology 1999;213(3):697–704.
39. Degnan AJ, Maldjian C, Adam RJ, et al. Comparison of Insall-Salvati ratios in children with an acute anterior cruciate ligament tear and a matched control population. Am J Roentgenol 2015;204(1):161–6.
40. O'Malley MP, Milewski MD, Solomito MJ, et al. The association of tibial slope and anterior cruciate ligament rupture in skeletally immature patients. Arthroscopy 2015;31(1):77–82.
41. Dare DM, Fabricant PD, McCarthy MM, et al. Increased lateral tibial slope is a risk factor for pediatric anterior cruciate ligament injury: an MRI-Based Case-Control Study of 152 Patients. Am J Sports Med 2015;43(7):1632–9.
42. Samora W, Beran MC, Parikh SN. Intercondylar roof inclination angle: is it a risk factor for ACL tears or tibial spine fractures? J Pediatr Orthop 2016;36(6):e71–4.
43. Swami VG, Mabee M, Hui C, et al. Three-dimensional intercondylar notch volumes in a skeletally immature pediatric population: a magnetic resonance imaging. Arthroscopy 2013;29(12):1954–62.
44. Shaw KA, Dunoski B, Mardis N, et al. Knee morphometric risk factors for acute anterior cruciate ligament injury in skeletally immature patients. J Child Orthop 2015;9(2):161–8.
45. Pyle SI, Greulich WW. Radiographic atlas of skeletal development of the hand and wrist. Stanford (CA): Stanford University Press; 1959.

46. Carpenter CT, Lester EL. Skeletal age determination in young children: analysis of three regions of the hand/wrist film. J Pediatr Orthop 1993;13(1):76–9.

47. Sanders JO, Browne RH, McConnell SJ, et al. Maturity assessment and curve progression in girls with idiopathic scoliosis. J Bone Joint Surg Am 2007;89(1): 64–73.

48. Moksnes H, Engebretsen L, Eitzen I, et al. Functional outcomes following a nonoperative treatment algorithm for anterior cruciate ligament injuries in skeletally immature children 12 years and younger. A prospective cohort with 2 years follow-up. Br J Sports Med 2013;47(8):488–94.

49. Moksnes H, Engebretsen L, Risberg MA. Prevalence and incidence of new meniscus and cartilage injuries after a nonoperative treatment algorithm for ACL tears in skeletally immature children: A Prospective MRI Study. Am J Sports Med 2013;41(8):1771–9.

50. Wall EJ, Myer GD, May MM. Anterior cruciate ligament reconstruction timing in children with open growth plates: new surgical techniques including all-epiphyseal. Clin Sports Med 2011;30(4):789–800.

51. Woods GW. Delayed anterior cruciate ligament reconstruction in adolescents with open physes. Am J Sports Med 2004;32(1):201–10.

52. Moksnes H, Engebretsen L, Risberg MA. Performance-based functional outcome for children 12 years or younger following anterior cruciate ligament injury: a two to nine-year follow-up study. Knee Surg Sports Traumatol Arthrosc 2007;16(3): 214–23.

53. Guzzanti V, Falciglia F, Gigante A, et al. The effect of intra-articular ACL reconstruction on the growth plates of rabbits. J Bone Joint Surg Br 1994;76(6):960–3.

54. Houle JB, Letts M, Yang J. Effects of a tensioned tendon graft in a bone tunnel across the rabbit physis. Clin Orthop Relat Res 2001;(391):275.

55. Mäkelä EA, Vainionpää S, Vihtonen K, et al. The effect of trauma to the lower femoral epiphyseal plate. An experimental study in rabbits. J Bone Joint Surg Br 1988;70(2):187–91.

56. Janarv PM, Wikström B, Hirsch G. The influence of transphyseal drilling and tendon grafting on bone growth: an experimental study in the rabbit. J Pediatr Orthop 1998;18(2):149–54.

57. Kercher J, Xerogeanes J, Tannenbaum A, et al. Anterior cruciate ligament reconstruction in the skeletally immature: an anatomical study utilizing 3-dimensional magnetic resonance imaging reconstructions. J Pediatr Orthop 2009;29(2):124–9.

58. Shea KG, Belzer J, Apel PJ, et al. Volumetric injury of the physis during singlebundle anterior cruciate ligament reconstruction in children: a 3-dimensional study using magnetic resonance imaging. Arthroscopy 2009;25(12):1415–22.

59. Yoo WJ, Kocher MS, Micheli LJ. Growth plate disturbance after transphyseal reconstruction of the anterior cruciate ligament in skeletally immature adolescent patients: An MR Imaging Study. J Pediatr Orthop 2011;31(6):691.

60. Nawabi DH, Jones KJ, Lurie B, et al. All-inside, physeal-sparing anterior cruciate ligament reconstruction does not significantly compromise the physis in skeletally immature athletes: a postoperative physeal magnetic resonance imaging analysis. Am J Sports Med 2014;42(12):2933–40.

61. Kopf S, Martin DE, Tashman S, et al. Effect of tibial drill angles on bone tunnel aperture during anterior cruciate ligament reconstruction. J Bone Joint Surg Am 2010;92(4):871–81.

62. Kachmar M, Piazza SJ, Bader DA. Comparison of growth plate violations for transtibial and anteromedial surgical techniques in simulated adolescent anterior cruciate ligament reconstruction. Am J Sports Med 2016;44(2):417–24.

63. Chudik S, Beasley L, Potter H, et al. The influence of femoral technique for graft placement on anterior cruciate ligament reconstruction using a skeletally immature canine model with a rapidly growing physis. Arthroscopy 2007;23(12):1309–19.

64. Meller R, Kendoff D, Hankemeier S, et al. Hindlimb growth after a transphyseal reconstruction of the anterior cruciate ligament: a study in skeletally immature sheep with wide-open physes. Am J Sports Med 2008;36(12):2437–43.

65. Seil R, Pape D, Kohn D. The risk of growth changes during transphyseal drilling in sheep with open physes. Arthroscopy 2008;24(7):824–33.

66. Edwards TB, Greene CC, Baratta RV, et al. The effect of placing a tensioned graft across open growth plates. A gross and histologic analysis. J Bone Joint Surg Am 2001;83(5):725–34.

67. Stadelmaier DM, Arnoczky SP, Dodds J, et al. The effect of drilling and soft tissue grafting across open growth plates. A histologic study. Am J Sports Med 1995; 23(4):431–5.

68. Babb JR, Ahn JI, Azar FM, et al. Transphyseal anterior cruciate ligament reconstruction using mesenchymal stem cells. Am J Sports Med 2008;36(6):1164–70.

69. Robert HE, Casin C. Valgus and flexion deformity after reconstruction of the anterior cruciate ligament in a skeletally immature patient. Knee Surg Sports Traumatol Arthrosc 2009;18(10):1369–73.

70. McIntosh AL, Dahm DL, Stuart MJ. Anterior cruciate ligament reconstruction in the skeletally immature patient. Arthroscopy 2006;22(12):1325–30.

71. Koman JD, Sanders JO. Valgus deformity after reconstruction of the anterior cruciate ligament in a skeletally immature patient. A case report. J Bone Joint Surg Am 1999;81(5):711–5.

72. Higuchi T, Hara K, Tsuji Y, et al. Transepiphyseal reconstruction of the anterior cruciate ligament in skeletally immature athletes: an MRI evaluation for epiphyseal narrowing. J Pediatr Orthop B 2009;18(6):330–4.

73. Kohl S, Stutz C, Decker S, et al. Mid-term results of transphyseal anterior cruciate ligament reconstruction in children and adolescents. Knee 2014;21(1):80–5.

74. Kumar S, Ahearne D, Hunt DM. Transphyseal anterior cruciate ligament reconstruction in the skeletally immature. J Bone Joint Surg Am 2013;95(1):e11.

75. Shifflett GD, Green DW, Widmann RF. Growth arrest following ACL reconstruction with hamstring autograft in skeletally immature patients: a review of 4 cases. J Pediatr Orthop 2016;36(4):355–61.

76. Lemaitre G, de Chou ES, Pineau V, et al. ACL reconstruction in children: a transphyseal technique. Orthop Traumatol Surg Res 2014;100(4):S261–5.

77. Zimmerman LJ, Jauregui JJ, Riis JF, et al. Symmetric limb overgrowth following anterior cruciate ligament reconstruction in a skeletally immature patient. J Pediatr Orthop B 2015;24(6):530–4.

78. Chotel F, Henry J, Seil R, et al. Growth disturbances without growth arrest after ACL reconstruction in children. Knee Surg Sports Traumatol Arthrosc 2010; 18(11):1496–500.

79. Lipscomb AB, Anderson AF. Tears of the anterior cruciate ligament in adolescents. J Bone Joint Surg Am 1986;68(1):19–28.

80. Lawrence JT, West RL, Garrett WE. Growth disturbance following ACL reconstruction with use of an epiphyseal femoral tunnel: a case report. J Bone Joint Surg Am 2011;93(8):e39.

81. Rozbruch SR, Fryman C, Schachter LF, et al. Growth arrest of the tibia after anterior cruciate ligament reconstruction: lengthening and deformity correction with the Taylor spatial frame. Am J Sports Med 2013;41(7):1636–41.

82. Kocher MS, Saxon HS, Hovis WD, et al. Management and complications of anterior cruciate ligament injuries in skeletally immature patients: survey of the Herodicus Society and the ACL Study Group. J Pediatr Orthop 2002;22(4):452–7.

83. Behr CT, Potter HG, Paletta GA. The relationship of the femoral origin of the anterior cruciate ligament and the distal femoral physeal plate in the skeletally immature knee. An anatomic study. Am J Sports Med 2001;29(6):781–7.

84. Tenfelde AM, Esquivel AO, Cracchiolo AM, et al. Temperature change when drilling near the distal femoral physis in a skeletally immature ovine model. J Pediatr Orthop 2016;36(7):762–7.

85. Goddard M, Bowman N, Salmon LJ, et al. Endoscopic anterior cruciate ligament reconstruction in children using living donor hamstring tendon allografts. Am J Sports Med 2013;41(3):567–74.

86. Redler LH, Brafman RT, Trentacosta N, et al. Anterior cruciate ligament reconstruction in skeletally immature patients with transphyseal tunnels. Arthroscopy 2012;28(11):1710–7.

87. Hui C, Roe J, Ferguson D, et al. Outcome of anatomic transphyseal anterior cruciate ligament reconstruction in tanner stage 1 and 2 patients with open physes. Am J Sports Med 2012;40(5):1093–8.

88. Calvo R, Figueroa D, Gili F, et al. Transphyseal anterior cruciate ligament reconstruction in patients with open physes: 10-year follow-up study. Am J Sports Med 2015;43(2):289–94.

89. Schmale GA, Kweon C, Larson RV, et al. High satisfaction yet decreased activity 4 years after transphyseal ACL reconstruction. Clin Orthop Relat Res 2014; 472(7):2168–74.

90. Strauss EJ, Barker JU, McGill K, et al. Can anatomic femoral tunnel placement be achieved using a transtibial technique for hamstring anterior cruciate ligament reconstruction? Am J Sports Med 2011;39(6):1263–9.

91. Wang H, Fleischli JE, Zheng N. Transtibial versus anteromedial portal technique in single-bundle anterior cruciate ligament reconstruction: outcomes of knee joint kinematics during walking. Am J Sports Med 2013;41(8):1847–56.

92. Kocher MS, Garg S, Micheli LJ. Physeal sparing reconstruction of the anterior cruciate ligament in skeletally immature prepubescent children and adolescents. J Bone Joint Surg Am 2005;87(11):2371–9.

93. Willimon SC, Jones CR, Herzog MM, et al. Micheli anterior cruciate ligament reconstruction in skeletally immature youths: a retrospective case series with a mean 3-year follow-up. Am J Sports Med 2015;43(12):2974–81.

94. Kennedy A, Coughlin DG, Metzger MF, et al. Biomechanical evaluation of pediatric anterior cruciate ligament reconstruction techniques. Am J Sports Med 2011; 39(5):964–71.

95. Cruz AI, Fabricant PD, McGraw M, et al. All-epiphyseal ACL reconstruction in children: review of safety and early complications. J Pediatr Orthop 2015. [Epub ahead of print].

96. Green WT, Anderson M. Experiences with epiphyseal arrest in correcting discrepancies in length of the lower extremities in infantile paralysis a method of predicting the effect. J Bone Joint Surg Am 1947;29(A):659–78.

97. Anderson M, Green WT, Messner MB. Growth and predictions of growth in the lower extremities. J Bone Joint Surg Am 1963;45-A:1–14.

98. Wester W, Canale ST, Dutkowsky JP, et al. Prediction of angular deformity and leg-length discrepancy after anterior cruciate ligament reconstruction in skeletally immature patients. J Pediatr Orthop 1994;14(4):516–21.

Single-Bundle Anatomic Anterior Cruciate Ligament Reconstruction
Surgical Technique Pearls and Pitfalls

Chaitu S. Malempati, DO[a], Adam V. Metzler, MD[b],
Darren L. Johnson, MD[a],*

KEYWORDS

• Anterior cruciate ligament • Anatomic • Single-bundle • Reconstruction

KEY POINTS

• Single-bundle anatomic anterior cruciate ligament reconstruction is an important technique to restore knee anatomy, knee kinematics, and ultimately knee function.

• The technique for this procedure relies on proficient arthroscopic visualization and the use of native anatomic landmarks for the accurate placement of femoral and tibial tunnels. Potential complications and pitfalls can also be avoided in a precise and reproducible manner.

• Objective outcomes are improved over transtibial nonanatomic reconstruction and similar to anatomic double-bundle ACL reconstruction.

INTRODUCTION

Anterior cruciate ligament (ACL) ruptures are one of the most frequent orthopedic sports-related injuries, with a yearly incidence of more than 250,000.[1] An ACL injury is potentially devastating for the patient and can result in both acute and long-term clinical sequelae. In young athletes, high-level participation in sports is difficult without surgical reconstruction. Furthermore, the long-term development of knee osteoarthritis (OA) is common and deleterious. One particular study with 12-year follow-up

Disclosures: Consultant: Smith and Nephew Endoscopy; Royalties: Instrument Development; Institution: Research/Education. Smith and Nephew Endoscopy and DJO Orthopedics (D.L. Johnson). No other disclosures, commercial or financial conflicts of interest for any other authors.
[a] Division of Sports Medicine, Department of Orthopaedic Surgery, University of Kentucky School of Medicine, 740 South Limestone Street, Lexington, KY 40536-0284, USA; [b] Division of Sports Medicine, Commonwealth Orthopaedic Centers, 560 South Loop Road, Edgewood, KY 41017, USA
* Corresponding author. Department of Orthopaedic Surgery, Kentucky Clinic, University of Kentucky School of Medicine, K401, 740 South Limestone Street, Lexington, KY 40536-0284.
E-mail address: dljohns@uky.edu

Clin Sports Med 36 (2017) 53–70
http://dx.doi.org/10.1016/j.csm.2016.08.010

after ACL reconstruction found that 50% of patients had radiographic OA at a mean age of 31 years; at this age, there are no good treatment options for a symptomatic osteoarthritic knee.[2–4] Therefore, the ACL continues to be of great interest to orthopedic surgeons and scientists worldwide.

ACL insufficiency leads to joint instability, increases the load on knee compartments during anterior and rotational joint loading, and alters gait and native kinematics.[5–7] Reconstruction can improve knee kinematics, reverse anteroposterior and rotational laxity, and prevent further damage to other knee structures.[8–11] Reconstruction techniques for the ACL have evolved considerably over the last several decades. Today, most of these reconstructions are performed using transtibial, accessory anteromedial portal, and outside-in drilling techniques. Renewed interest in detailed ACL insertional anatomy and recent data that demonstrated suboptimal outcomes for return to play in high-level athletes in whom transtibial techniques were used for ACL reconstruction led to an interest in anatomic femoral and tibial tunnel placement.[12–14] Furthermore, basic science time zero data showed better kinematics and better initial stability using independent femoral drilling techniques to recreate native ACL anatomy.[15]

The goal of anatomic ACL reconstruction is to replicate the native knee's normal anatomy and replicate its normal kinematics. This article emphasizes the native insertional anatomy of the ACL and the appropriate techniques required to reproduce these anatomic footprints reliably and accurately in single-bundle ACL reconstruction.

SURGICAL TECHNIQUE
Preoperative Planning

It is crucial to plan for an anatomic ACL reconstruction in both the primary and revision settings. This planning allows for all of the appropriate equipment and instrumentation to be readily available during the procedure. Furthermore, planning allows for an appropriate and concise stepwise plan to be made before the actual surgery.

The appropriate imaging should be obtained before any surgery scheduling. Imaging typically includes radiographs and a noncontrast MRI scan. Radiographs allow for an accurate representation of the overall knee alignment and any obvious bony abnormalities or deformities. The MRI can be used to evaluate bony anatomy and the soft tissue and ligamentous structures within the knee joint. The ACL injury should be clearly seen on the scan as a femoral-sided avulsion, intrasubstance tear, or tibial-sided avulsion. Furthermore, any concomitant injuries such as cartilage lesions, meniscal injuries, and other ligamentous conditions can be evaluated, and preoperative planning can be performed accordingly.

Another aspect of preoperative planning that is imperative to a successful result is the reduction in swelling and maintenance of adequate range of motion after an acute ACL injury. This injury typically results in a large hemarthrosis and subsequent effusion inside the knee joint leading to pain, decreased motion, and an inhibition of the quadriceps musculature. Cryotherapy to reduce swelling and range of motion should be encouraged preoperatively to ensure adequate motion and appropriately functioning quadriceps before surgical reconstruction. Large joint effusions may be aspirated to allow for appropriate rehabilitation before surgery.

During a primary ACL reconstruction, the anatomic femoral footprint of the native ACL is preserved on the posterior aspect of the lateral femoral condyle. This allows for improved visualization and easier access for femoral tunnel drilling. However, the posterior wall or over the back position must be visualized entirely without any guessing. If the posterior cortex cannot be visualized, then the residual femoral ACL footprint should be debrided. Furthermore, the femoral footprint should be visualized with the knee at 90° of flexion, helping to ensure accurate tunnel placement.

In the revision ACL reconstruction setting, considerations need to be made for the previous tunnel placement and prior hardware. This consideration greatly increases the complexity of the procedure and often distorts the native knee and ACL anatomy. Visualization can be difficult, and preoperative planning is essential. Advanced imaging, such as computed tomography or MRI, is necessary to accurately evaluate the femoral and tibial tunnel placement and to assess the hardware used for femoral and tibial fixation. Furthermore, any tunnel lysis can also be seen on imaging and aids in preoperative planning. Bone grafting and a staged procedure may be necessary if tunnel widening or lysis is greater than 15 mm. For anatomic ACL reconstruction in the revision setting, knowledge of the previous tunnel location and proximity to the desired native location is imperative. This knowledge allows the surgeon to decide if the same tunnel can be used or if a new, more anatomic tunnel is needed. Previous hardware may need to be removed during femoral and tibial tunnel reaming if they are directly in the way. However, if the previous fixation devices do not interfere with revision tunnel location, then they should be left alone to prevent any bone void defects. Previous preoperative and postoperative imaging, operative notes, and arthroscopic pictures are all useful and necessary in planning for anatomic tunnel placement and hardware considerations in the revision setting.

Preparation and Patient Positioning

Patient positioning, more importantly leg position, is crucial to the surgeon for a successful anatomic ACL reconstruction. Also, if concomitant procedures such as cartilage or meniscal work are planned, the patient should be positioned to allow these certain procedures to be performed. A well-padded tourniquet is placed as proximal as possible on the thigh, and an arthroscopic leg holder is used proximal enough on the thigh to allow the surgeon complete access to the knee and distal femur. The leg holder is angled back approximately 45° to allow for hip flexion (**Fig. 1**). Hip flexion in turn allows for knee hyperflexion of a minimum of 130°. The operative table may need to be reflexed so that the long axis of the femur is parallel to the floor. The nonoperative limb is placed and secured in a well leg holder with adequate padding. It is important to ensure that the well leg is out of the way from all members of the surgical team. Furthermore, it is imperative that the knee can be hyperflexed to approximately 130° before any prepping or draping is done. Again, hip flexion allows for knee hyperflexion. Adequate knee hyperflexion allows for all-inside anatomic femoral tunnel drilling. If the knee cannot be hyperflexed to 130°, then the femoral tunnel must be drilled using an outside-in technique or flexible drills. Also, in patients with a large circumference of the thigh and lower leg, where hyperflexion is not possible, femoral tunnels should be drilled from the outside in, also known as *2-incision ACL surgery*.

Another important aspect of the standard preoperative routine is a preoperative examination under anesthesia including side-to-side variation in Lachman and pivot shift testing, which should be performed and documented. Range of motion and joint effusions should also be noted. Once this is done, an alcohol-based preparation can be used for preparing the limb unless an allergy or wound would necessitate a betadine paint with scrub.

Surgical Technique

Step 1

The ACL graft is harvested first using either the central patellar tendon or both the gracilis and semitendinosus hamstring tendons. The hamstring tendons may be augmented with semitendinosus allograft if the autograft size is less than 8 mm in

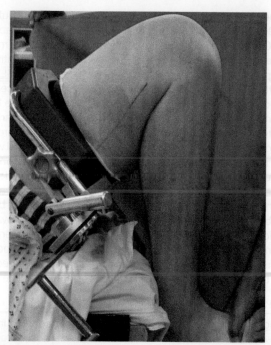

Fig. 1. Arthroscopic leg holder placed at midthigh and angled backward approximately 45°
to allow for hip flexion and knee hyperflexion. Note that the hyperflexion of the knee is
checked intraoperatively before preparing. At least 130° of hyperflexion is necessary for
all-inside femoral tunnel drilling.

diameter. Magnussen and colleagues[16] and Mariscalco and colleagues[17] found
increased revision rates with hamstring graft sizes less than 8 mm in diameter.

Step 2
Three main portals are established during this procedure. First, a high and tight anterolateral portal is created proximal and adjacent to the inferolateral aspect of the patella.
This portal is the primary initial viewing portal. This high and tight portal allows
improved and accurate visualization of the ACL tibial footprint during anatomic tibial
tunnel placement. An anteromedial portal is also created with the aid of a spinal needle
under direct arthroscopic visualization. This portal is directly medial to the patellar
tendon and is in line with the ACL footprint on the tibia. The anteromedial portal is
used for both visualization and instrumentation during the procedure. This portal
should be made vertical to avoid horizontal transection of the medial aspect of the
patellar tendon. These 2 portals are made to do all the notch, meniscal, and articular
cartilage work in the knee. Only when all of this work is done and prior to drilling the
femoral tunnel is the far medial accessory portal made.

Lastly, a far accessory anteromedial portal is created using a spinal needle under
arthroscopic visualization. This is done with the knee position at 90° of flexion. This
portal is typically 2.5 cm from the anteromedial portal and should be low and medial
just above the anterior horn of the medial meniscus (**Fig. 2**). Adequate arthroscopic
visualization is important during this step to avoid injury to the medial meniscus and
the medial femoral condyle. This portal should be made horizontal to allow for

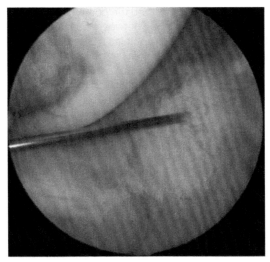

Fig. 2. Accessory anteromedial portal created with the aid of a spinal needle under direct arthroscopic visualization. Note the placement of this portal low and medial just above the anterior horn of the medial meniscus.

side-to-side movement when reaming the tunnel. Also, a low accessory medial portal will allow for anatomic placement of an all-inside long femoral tunnel at the native femoral footprint. Furthermore, this low and medial portal helps avoid breaching the back wall or drilling a short femoral tunnel. Failure to make this portal far medial will lead to a short femoral tunnel or drilling out the back of the knee. It also ensures you are drilling perpendicular to the lateral wall, which ensures an oval tunnel the same size as the drill at the aperture. Drilling an oblique tunnel leads to a larger opening at the aperture. For example, if you are drilling a 10-mm circular drill in an oblique manner, the actual opening at the aperture of the finished tunnel may be 14 mm.

Step 3
After the anterolateral and anteromedial portals are created, any concomitant injuries can be addressed and meniscal and chondral work can be done inside the knee joint. A formal assessment of the entire joint should also be performed.

Step 4
The notchplasty, if needed, should be performed before the far accessory medial portal is created. This process is started with the scope in the anterolateral portal and the shaver in the anteromedial portal. A limited notchplasty of approximately 3 mm is generally performed. The knee is positioned at 90° of flexion, and excess soft tissue is removed from the anterior compartment to allow for appropriate visualization. It is important during the notchplasty to pay careful attention to preserve the bony landmarks and the native ACL fibers, especially the femoral and tibial footprints. No bone should ever be removed from the native footprint on the femur. To complete this step and accurately visualize the entire femoral ACL footprint, the arthroscope is placed in the anteromedial portal and the shaver through the far accessory medial portal. Piefer and colleagues[18] determined that the native anatomic location of the ACL femoral footprint is 43% of the distance from the proximal articular margin to the distal articular margins. Furthermore, they showed that a rim of bone of 2.5 mm

exists between the posterior ACL fibers and the posterior articular cartilage margin. It is imperative to distinguish the difference between the lateral intercondylar ridge and the lateral bifurcate ridge, as the latter separates the 2 anatomic bundles of the native ACL. There are no fibers of the ACL that insert superior to the lateral intercondylar ridge. Additionally, the surgeon should be able to delineate the back wall and the inferior articular cartilage, as this also helps establish the native footprint (**Fig. 3**). Adequate visualization of the inferior articular cartilage and the true back wall is the crucial and necessary step to achieve anatomic femoral tunnel placement. Alternatively, a 70° arthroscope can also be through the anteromedial portal to assess the femoral ACL footprint and the back wall. Leaving the insertional remnants of the femoral and tibial attachments of the ACL during the notchplasty and debridement steps makes it easier to recognize the femoral footprint and the tibial footprint for anatomic tunnel placement.

Step 5
The next step is to create the starting point for the femoral tunnel. The arthroscope is placed in the anteromedial portal and with the knee at 90° of flexion, a femoral guide is placed on the native femoral footprint (**Fig. 4**). A 45° microfracture awl through the far accessory anteromedial portal is then placed in the middle of this guide and malleted into the bone leaving a sufficient hole to reference when inserting the guidewire (**Fig. 5**). Once this is done, good visualization is necessary to gain an overall perspective of the starting point pilot hole in relation to the native femoral ACL footprint, the back wall, and the inferior articular cartilage (**Fig. 6**).

Step 6
Once the starting point is created, the knee is then adequately hyperflexed (minimum 130°) slowly by the surgical assistant, and the guide pin is drilled for the femoral tunnel under arthroscopic visualization using the previous starting point created in the previous step. The guide pin is aimed toward the lateral epicondyle of the femur and is drilled out the skin on the lateral aspect of femur. This method ensures exit at the appropriate site and tunnel lengths of 30 to 40 mm in all patients. Hyperflexion is

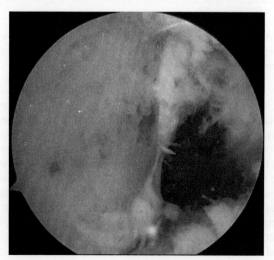

Fig. 3. Adequate visualization of the back wall and inferior articular cartilage is shown here after notchplasty.

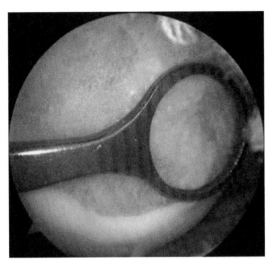

Fig. 4. Femoral guide placed over the remnant native femoral ACL footprint. Leaving this remnant footprint aids in anatomic femoral tunnel placement.

held by the assistant for the entire time that the guide pin is placed to avoid bending or breaking the pin inside the knee joint. Once the guide pin is placed and is thought to be in good position under arthroscopic visualization, reaming is performed sequentially using a single-fluted reamer to not damage the articular cartilage of the medial femoral condyle. A smaller-size reamer is used initially in creating the tunnel, and the back wall is checked periodically to ensure there is no penetration out the back. Sequential reaming is performed up to the desired femoral tunnel size, and the guide pin is then removed. If there is any doubt as to the location of the tunnel during the reaming

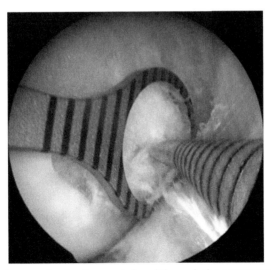

Fig. 5. Forty-five–degree microfracture awl placed through the accessory anteromedial portal and into the center of the femoral guide is used to create a starting point pilot hole for the femoral tunnel.

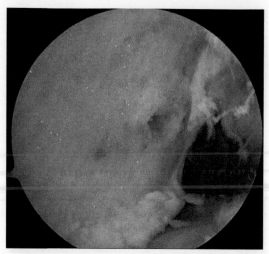

Fig. 6. A broad and adequate perspective of the starting point for the femoral tunnel in relation to the back wall and the inferior articular cartilage.

process, the guide pin can be pulled out and moved in any direction to achieve a more anatomic tunnel after the initial smaller reamer is used. Single fluted reamers are beneficial with accessory anteromedial portal drilling to prevent medial femoral condyle cartilage injury. The medial femoral condyle should be viewed when inserting the reamer through this accessory anteromedial portal.

Once reaming is completed, hyperflexion is no longer necessary until the graft is passed later in the procedure. It is important to achieve an adequate perspective of the femoral tunnel created to ensure that it is reamed to an adequate depth and that there is at least 2 mm of back wall preserved (**Figs. 7** and **8**). The most common error seen in the last 5 years is to leave too large a back wall, which will overconstrain

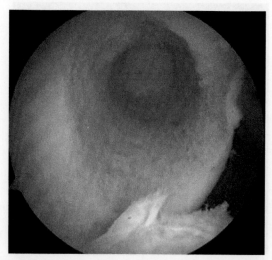

Fig. 7. Representation of the depth of the femoral tunnel created. With an accurate accessory anteromedial portal and adequate hyperflexion of the knee, a 30- to 40-mm femoral tunnel is created in all patients.

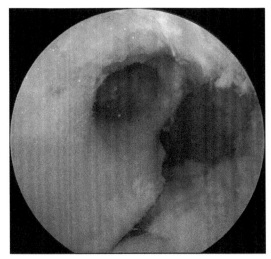

Fig. 8. Arthroscopic visualization of the femoral tunnel after reaming. Note the adequate 2 mm of back wall preserved.

the knee, and the patient will either lose flexion or stretch out the graft. The shaver can then be used to debride the anterior aperture of the femoral tunnel to aid in graft passage later in the procedure.

Step 7
In this next step, attention is turned to anatomic tibial tunnel placement. The scope is placed in the high and tight anterolateral portal to again give an accurate perspective of the entire tibial ACL footprint. This placement requires some debridement of the fat pad to ensure one sees the entire anterior fibers of the native footprint. The tibial guide used is placed through the far accessory medial portal at the center of the remnant ACL tibial attachment (**Fig. 9**). It is helpful to leave some of the tibial footprint fibers intact during notchplasty and debridement to get a good idea of the native tibial attachment and to preserve proprioceptive fibers from the native ACL. Hwang and colleagues[19] showed that the ACL tibial footprint is 15 mm anterior to the posterior cruciate ligament and two-fifths of the medial-lateral width of the interspinous distance with most of the ACL fibers attaching anterior to the posterior margin of the anterior horn of the lateral meniscus. Landmarks to aid in finding anatomic tibial tunnel placement include being in line with the body of the anterior horn of the lateral meniscus and just adjacent to the medial articular cartilage (**Fig. 10**). The tibial guide should, therefore, be placed keeping these important anatomic structures in mind. Alternatively, a Trukor gauge or malleable ruler can be used to measure the length and width of the tibial ACL footprint under arthroscopic visualization. Using this method, the tibial guide is placed in the center of the native ACL stump or anatomic footprint. Once the guide is placed in an appropriate position, a guide pin is drilled under arthroscopic visualization. The guide pin is then docked into the femur to avoid movement during the reaming process. Similar to femoral tunnel reaming, sequential reaming is performed for the tibial tunnel using standard reamers and starting with a smaller-sized reamer. Once the first smaller reamer is placed, the guide pin can be moved in any direction to achieve a more desired or anatomic tunnel and is again docked into the femur. Reaming is performed sequentially up to the desired tibial tunnel size. Once reaming is

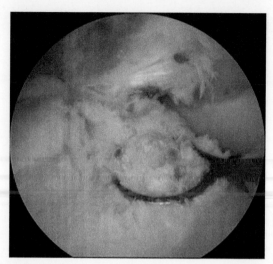

Fig. 9. Tibial guide placed at the center of the native tibial ACL footprint. Leaving this tibial stump intact aids in anatomic tibial tunnel placement and preserves proprioceptive fibers from the native ACL.

completed, a shaver is introduced into the tunnel to remove any entrapped soft tissue ensuring that there is a complete bone tunnel (**Fig. 11**).

Step 8
At this point during the procedure, it is important to take a moment and gain an accurate perspective of both the femoral and tibial tunnels to ensure that there is anatomic positioning, and no further changes are necessary before graft passage (**Fig. 12**). Before graft passage, the graft is soaked in mineral oil after preparation, which aids

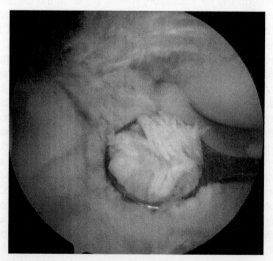

Fig. 10. Tibial guide in relation to important anatomic landmarks for tibial tunnel drilling. Note the location of the guide in relation to the body of the anterior horn of the lateral meniscus and the medial articular cartilage.

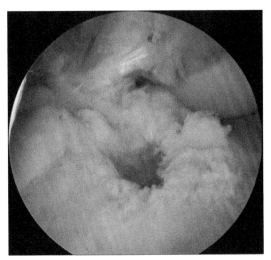

Fig. 11. Arthroscopic view of the tibial tunnel created. Note the good visualization made possible by a high and tight anterolateral portal.

in passing the graft. While passing the graft, the arthroscope is placed in the antero-medial portal, and the knee is hyperflexed to pass a beath pin through the far accessory medial portal and through the femoral tunnel out the skin on the lateral aspect of the femur. This places a looped suture into the notch, which is then retrieved through the tibial tunnel with an arthroscopic grasper or pituitary. The graft is then passed under arthroscopic visualization, and a trochar or hemostat can be used through the accessory medial portal as a lever to aid the graft passage as tension is pulled on the femoral side by the surgical assistant. Using this method, the graft is pulled into final position (**Fig. 13**).

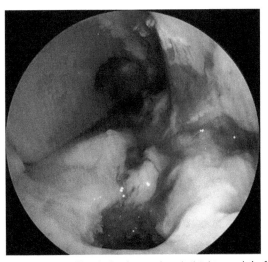

Fig. 12. Good arthroscopic view of both the femoral and tibial tunnels before graft passage.

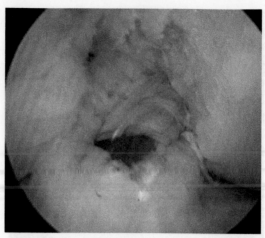

Fig. 13. Graft pulled into final position. Note the marking on the graft 10 mm longer than the femoral tunnel length to allow assessment of the suspensory device in relation to the lateral femoral cortex.

Step 9

The fixation used depends on the graft that is chosen. There are multiple options available for both hamstring and patellar tendon grafts. For hamstring grafts, cortical suspensory buttons can be used with or without an extension depending on the size of the tunnel or whether the femoral tunnel is drilled outside in or all inside. For the all-inside technique, the cortical suspensory device is used without the extension. The graft is marked from the femoral side 10 mm longer than the length of the femoral tunnel drilled. This mark aids in graft passage because as the mark nears the femoral aperture, it can be inferred that the cortical suspensory device has penetrated through the lateral cortex of the femur and, therefore, only needs to be flipped. The graft should then be pulled back down toward the tibia to ensure that the suspensory device is seated on the lateral femoral cortex. If one is unsure if the device is flipped on the lateral distal femoral cortex, fluoroscopy should be used to confirm that the device is, in fact, flipped and in good position on the femoral cortex before proceeding. Tibial fixation can be achieved using a biocomposite interference screw, and back-up fixation can be achieved using a post, such as a large fragment bicortical screw and washer or a staple. Back-up fixation is more important on the tibial side, as this side is the weak point of fixation in an ACL reconstruction.

For patellar tendon grafts, interference screws can be placed in both the femoral and tibial tunnels. It is important to use a guidewire when placing these screws to avoid screw migration. When placing the femoral screw, a notcher or trochar should be used to make room for the screw superior to the graft to avoid increased tension and breaking the femoral bone block. Additionally, tension should be placed proximally and distally on the graft when placing the femoral screw. Furthermore, the guidewire should be removed before fully seating either screw to avoid the wire bending or breaking.

Regardless of the type of graft used, the knee should be cycled at least 10 times from 0° to 120° after femoral-sided fixation and before tibial-sided fixation. During tibial fixation, a posterior drawer is placed on the tibia, and the tibia is externally rotated to ensure tight fixation. Also, tension is pulled on the tibial sutures to ensure a taut graft. Finally, the arthroscope is reintroduced into the knee joint to check final positioning of the graft, ensure that the graft is taut, and visualize that there is no hardware inside the joint (**Fig. 14**). It is also important to ensure that the knee can achieve full extension without any impingement on the graft.

For pediatric ACL reconstruction with open growth plates, the femoral tunnel is drilled extraphyseal (distal to the physis) using an outside-in technique. Fluoroscopy can be valuable in this setting to ensure that the physis is avoided. The femoral guide is closed to the shortest angle possible, which aids in drilling an extraphyseal tunnel. The tibial tunnel is drilled perpendicular to the physis and medial to avoid the tibial apophysis. For the tibial tunnel, the tibial guide is opened up to create a wider angle and longer tibial tunnel that is perpendicular and medial. In pediatric patients, soft tissue grafts should be used, and interference screws are avoided. Additionally, the cortical suspensory device on the femoral side should be flipped vertically on the lateral femoral cortex as opposed to horizontally, which helps avoid the distal femoral physis. Using an outside-in technique helps with this issue. Tibial fixation can be performed using a post or a staple.

PITFALLS
Tunnel Malposition

The most common error in ACL reconstructive surgery is tunnel malposition, more specifically, a femoral tunnel that is too anterior or shallow in the notch.[20–22] This error can commonly occur when there is inadequate visualization or an inadequate notchplasty is performed. As mentioned earlier, excellent visualization of the back wall and the inferior articular cartilage and a thorough understanding of the anatomy are necessary to achieve anatomic femoral tunnel placement. If an inadequate notchplasty is performed or the back wall is not visualized before reaming, it is possible to place the femoral tunnel too anterior or shallow. Furthermore, suboptimal visualization can cause confusion between the lateral intercondylar ridge (resident's ridge) and lateral bifurcate ridge, which is the actual anatomic location between the anteromedial and posterolateral bundles of the native ACL. This suboptimal visualization can also lead

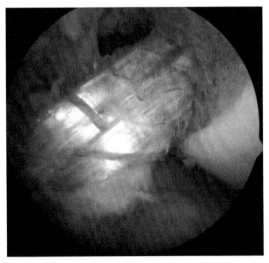

Fig. 14. Final arthroscopic picture of the ACL graft placed anatomically.

to a femoral tunnel that is too anterior. Furthermore, improper placement of the accessory anteromedial portal can lead to a malpositioned femoral tunnel. To avoid this pitfall, it is imperative to achieve optimal visualization of the back wall and the inferior articular cartilage before creating a femoral tunnel. The arthroscope should be placed in the anteromedial portal for best visualization, and a 70° scope can also be used if improved visualization is necessary. Additionally, it is important to perform a notchplasty so that the ACL femoral footprint is adequately visualized.

Another possible type of tunnel malposition involves creating a short femoral tunnel or a tunnel that blows out the back wall. Again, adequate visualization during the entire procedure is crucial to accurate anatomic tunnel placement. A low and far medial accessory medial portal will also help avoid a short femoral tunnel or a malpositioned femoral tunnel that could breach the back wall. As mentioned earlier, this portal needs to be as low and medial as possible just above the medial meniscus and needs to be performed under adequate arthroscopic visualization. This visualization will also help avoid a vertical femoral tunnel. Furthermore, inadequate hyperflexion of the knee (<130°) during femoral tunnel drilling can lead to a short or posterior femoral tunnel. The aiming point for the femoral pin once the knee is in hyperflexion is the attachment site of the fibular collateral ligament on the femur, not the back wall. For this reason, it is imperative to have an adequate surgical assistant during the procedure that is able to perform hyperflexion in the appropriate manner. Also, it is important to ensure that the knee can be hyperflexed to approximately 130° before preparing or draping the patient. As mentioned earlier, hip flexion created by the leg holder helps achieve knee hyperflexion. If the knee cannot be hyperflexed, then outside-in femoral tunnel reaming should be performed.

Tibial tunnel malposition can be avoided by paying close attention to the anatomic landmarks as previously discussed: the body of the entire anterior horn of the lateral meniscus and the medial articular cartilage. Additionally, an arthroscopic ruler can be used to measure the tibial footprint and accurately depict the center of the native ACL tibial stump.

Poor Graft Fixation

Another potential pitfall is the placement of a loose graft that is not taut and prone to failure because of inadequate femoral or tibial fixation. When passing a hamstring graft, it is important to pull retrograde distally to ensure that the suspensory device is flush with the cortex. Additionally, it is imperative to pull tension on the tibial side during tibial fixation. As previously mentioned, a posterior drawer and external rotation needs to be placed on the tibia during tibial fixation.

With respect to a patellar tendon graft, tension needs to be placed on both ends of the graft while performing femoral fixation, and tension needs to be pulled toward the tibial side during tibial fixation. Additionally, it is crucial to create a space for the femoral interference screw so as to not break the femoral bone plug, which would increase the risk of graft failure.

POSTOPERATIVE CARE AND PHYSICAL THERAPY

Postoperative x-rays should be taken at the initial postoperative visit and 6-month and 1-year time points to ensure good hardware positioning and no bony abnormalities and to assess tunnel placement for education (**Figs. 15** and **16**).

The ultimate goal of rehabilitation after reconstructive ACL surgery is to return the patient or athlete to preinjury performance level, including motion and strength, without injuring or elongating the graft. Each athlete is unique; thus, safe return to play should be individualized rather than follow a rigid postoperative timeline.[23]

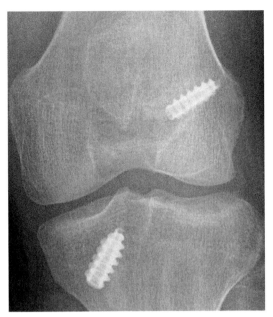

Fig. 15. Postoperative anteroposterior radiograph shows femoral and tibial interference screws in good position.

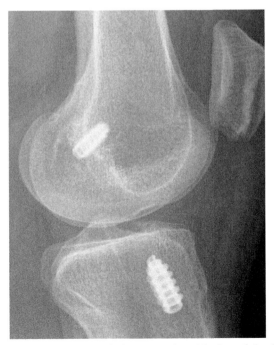

Fig. 16. Postoperative lateral radiograph shows good positioning of the femoral and tibial tunnels.

Early Postoperative Phase (0–4 Weeks)

The goals during this period are to minimize pain and swelling, establish a normal gait pattern and eventually discontinue crutch use, achieve 90° of flexion and full extension, and promote good quadriceps function and good quadriceps control. Physical therapy should be started within the first 3 days, and the patient can ambulate with the postoperative brace locked straight and with crutches unless additional concomitant surgery would preclude immediate weight bearing.

Strengthening Phase (1–6+ Months)

The brace can be shortened and unlocked at the 1-month postoperative point. Crutches should be discontinued at 1 month as a normal gait pattern is established. At 2 months postoperatively, the brace can be exchanged for a hinged knee sleeve. There is a specific emphasis on quadriceps strengthening during this phase. The advancement of strengthening is dictated by the patient's response. There must be no increase in either swelling or articular pain. Specific exercises that should be stressed during strengthening of the limb include mini-squats, mini-lunges, leg press, hamstring curls, step downs, wall sits, and hack squats. Additionally, light in-line jogging can be initiated at approximately 3 to 4 months postoperatively. Furthermore, neuromuscular and cardiopulmonary training are important aspects of this phase.

Return-to-Activity Phase

This phase starts at 3 months postoperatively and continues to return to sport or return to preinjury level. Activity is progressed via patient response. Neuromuscular training should continue to promote neuromuscular control and proprioception. Sport-specific drills can begin at 5 to 6 months postoperatively. Late in this phase, cutting and pivoting training should be introduced as well as advanced plyometrics and team participation without contact. The end of this phase involves the return to sport aspect of ACL rehabilitation at approximately 7 to 9 months postoperatively. A functional limb assessment is often useful to ensure a safe return to play in which strength assessment should be greater than 90% of the opposite limb using either dynamometry or clinical tests.

Outcomes

Numerous studies found the efficacy of anatomic ACL reconstruction in restoring native knee kinematics.[2,15,24,25] Furthermore, several articles showed good results with anatomic single-bundle ACL reconstruction. Iliopoulos and colleagues[5] concluded that anatomic single-bundle reconstruction provided good results and improved locomotion. Also, Kilinc and colleagues[26] found better results with single-bundle anatomic ACL reconstruction than the transtibial nonanatomic technique with respect to clinical, functional, and laboratory results. The investigators concluded that anatomic reconstruction of the ACL could restore native knee kinematics. Furthermore, Herbort and colleagues[27] found equally successful results comparing anatomic single-bundle ACL reconstruction with anatomic double-bundle ACL reconstruction. Therefore, it was shown that anatomic ACL reconstruction is superior to nonanatomic techniques clinically and kinematically. However, debate continues over the efficacy of single-bundle versus double-bundle ACL reconstruction. Future studies with long-term follow-up and patient-reported outcomes are necessary to establish any conclusions with respect to this question.

SUMMARY

Single-bundle anatomic ACL reconstruction is an accurate and reproducible technique that has successful results when the appropriate technique and landmarks are used. Adequate arthroscopic visualization and a thorough understanding of the anatomy and native ACL femoral and tibial footprints are essential in using this technique. This method of ACL reconstruction can restore native knee ACL anatomy and normal knee kinematics and allow a successful return to sport or preinjury level. Consequently, overall function is improved and long-term degenerative changes are avoided.

REFERENCES

1. Gianotti SM, Marshall SW, Hume PA, et al. Incidence of anterior cruciate ligament injury and other knee ligament injuries: a national population-based study. J Sci Med Sport 2009;12:622–7.
2. Fu FH, van Eck CF, Tashman S, et al. Anatomic anterior cruciate ligament reconstruction: a changing paradigm. Knee Surg Sports Traumatol Arthrosc 2015;23: 640–8.
3. Li RT, Lorenz S, Xu Y, et al. Predictors of radiographic knee osteoarthritis after anterior cruciate ligament reconstruction. Am J Sports Med 2011;39:2595–603.
4. Lohmander LS, Ostenberg A, Englund M, et al. High prevalence of knee osteoarthritis, pain, and functional limitations in female soccer players twelve years after anterior cruciate ligament injury. Arthritis Rheum 2004;50:3145–52.
5. Iliopoulos E, Galanis N, Zafeiridis A, et al. Anatomic single-bundle anterior cruciate ligament reconstruction improves walking economy: hamstrings tendon versus patellar tendon grafts. Knee Surg Sports Traumatol Arthrosc 2016;7: 4229–4.
6. Simon D, Mascarenhas R, Saltzman BM, et al. The relationship between anterior cruciate ligament injury and osteoarthritis of the knee. Adv Orthop 2015;2015: 928301.
7. Berchuck M, Andriacchi TP, Bach BR, et al. Gait adaptations by patients who have a deficient anterior cruciate ligament. J Bone Joint Surg Am 1990;72:871–7.
8. Ferber R, Osternig LR, Woollacott MH, et al. Gait mechanics in chronic ACL deficiency and subsequent repair. Clin Biomech 2002;17:274–85.
9. Georgoulis AD, Ristanis S, Chouliaras V, et al. Tibial rotation is not restored after ACL reconstruction with a hamstring graft. Clin Orthop Relat Res 2007;454:89–94.
10. Schurz M, Tiefenboeck TM, Winnisch M, et al. Clinical and functional outcome of all-inside anterior cruciate ligament reconstruction at a minimum of 2 years' follow-up. Arthroscopy 2015;32(2):332–7.
11. Steckel H, Murtha PE, Costic RS, et al. Computer evaluation of kinematics of anterior cruciate ligament reconstructions. Clin Orthop Relat Res 2007;463:37–42.
12. Duffee A, Magnussen RA, Pedroza AD, et al. MOON group: transtibial ACL femoral tunnel preparation increases odds of repeat ipsilateral knee surgery. J Bone Joint Surg Am 2013;95(22):2035–42.
13. McCullough KA, Phelps KD, Spindler KP, et al. MOON Group: return to high school- and college-level football after anterior cruciate ligament reconstruction: a multicenter orthopaedic outcomes network (MOON) cohort study. Am J Sports Med 2012;40(11):2523–9.
14. Shah VM, Andrews JR, Fleisig GS, et al. Return to play after anterior cruciate ligament reconstruction in National Football League athletes. Am J Sports Med 2010;38(11):2233–9.

15. Dhawan A, Gallo RA, Lynch SA. Anatomic tunnel placement in anterior cruciate ligament reconstruction. J Am Acad Orthop Surg 2016;25(7):443–54.
16. Magnussen RA, Lawrence JT, West RL, et al. Graft size and patient age are predictors of early revision after anterior cruciate ligament reconstruction with hamstring autograft. Arthroscopy 2012;28:526–31.
17. Mariscalco MW, Flanigan DC, Mitchell J, et al. The influence of hamstring autograft size on patient-reported outcomes and risk of revision after anterior cruciate ligament reconstruction: a multicenter orthopaedic outcomes network (MOON) cohort study. Arthroscopy 2013;29:1948–53.
18. Piefer JW, Pflugner TR, Hwang MD, et al. Anterior cruciate ligament femoral footprint anatomy: systematic review of the 21st century literature. Arthroscopy 2012; 20(0).072–01.
19. Hwang MD, Piefer JW, Lubowitz JH. Anterior cruciate ligament tibial footprint anatomy: systematic review of the 21st century literature. Arthroscopy 2012;28: 728–34.
20. Uribe JW, Hechtman KS, Zvijac JE, et al. Revision anterior cruciate ligament surgery: experience from Miami. Clin Orthop Relat Res 1996;(325):91–9.
21. Harner CD, Giffin JR, Dunteman RC, et al. Evaluation and treatment of recurrent instability after anterior cruciate ligament reconstruction. Instr Course Lect 2001; 50:463–74.
22. Kato Y, Ingham SJ, Kramer S, et al. Effect of tunnel position for anatomic single-bundle ACL reconstruction on knee biomechanics in a porcine model. Knee Surg Sports Traumatol Arthrosc 2010;18(1):2–10.
23. Malempati C, Jurjans J, Noehren B, et al. Current rehabilitation concepts for anterior cruciate ligament surgery in athletes. Orthopedics 2015;38(11):689–96.
24. Musahl V, Plakseychuk A, VanScyoc A, et al. Varying femoral tunnels between the anatomical footprint and isometric positions: effect on kinematics of the anterior cruciate ligament-reconstructed knee. Am J Sports Med 2005;33(5):712–8.
25. Bedi A, Maak T, Musahl V, et al. Effect of tunnel position and graft size in single-bundle anterior cruciate ligament reconstruction: an evaluation of time-zero knee stability. Arthroscopy 2011;27(11):1543–51.
26. Kilinc BE, Kara A, Oc Y, et al. Transtibial vs anatomical single bundle technique for anterior cruciate ligament reconstruction: a retrospective cohort study. Int J Surg 2016;29:62–9.
27. Herbort M, Domnick C, Raschke MJ, et al. Comparison of knee kinematics after single-bundle anterior cruciate ligament reconstruction via the medial portal technique with a central femoral tunnel and an eccentric femoral tunnel and after anatomic double-bundle reconstruction. Am J Sports Med 2016;44(1):126–32.

Indications for Two-Incision (Outside-In) Anterior Cruciate Ligament Reconstruction

Barton R. Branam, MD*, Christopher J. Utz, MD

KEYWORDS

- Anterior cruciate ligament • Reconstruction • Two-incision • Knee instability
- Outside-in

KEY POINTS

- Two-incision reconstruction of the anterior cruciate ligament (ACL) is a skill that should be mastered by knee reconstructive surgeons.
- Indications include revision surgery, reconstruction in a skeletally immature patient, and when a patient is unable to hyperflex the knee or a long patellar tendon graft would likely result in graft tunnel mismatch.
- The outcomes and complications are similar for single-incision and 2-incision ACL reconstruction.

INTRODUCTION: NATURE OF THE PROBLEM

Anterior cruciate ligament (ACL) reconstruction has experienced numerous changes in the past 30 years evolving from an open technique to primarily arthroscopic techniques. One of the initial arthroscopic assisted techniques was performed with separate incisions for outside-in drilling of both the tibial and femoral tunnels. Over time, inside-out arthroscopic techniques for drilling the femoral tunnel were developed and refined. This advance eliminated the need for a second proximal incision in most ACL reconstruction techniques.[1] Although some surgeons continue to use an outside-in technique for primary ACL reconstructions, the majority of ACL reconstructions are performed using either a transtibial technique or some form of medial portal drilling.[2] There are some cases, however, where use of a 2-incision, outside-in technique can be beneficial and the skilled surgeon should be familiar with its application.

Commercial or Financial Conflicts of Interest for Authors: None.
Division of Sports Medicine, Department of Orthopaedic Surgery, College of Medicine, University of Cincinnati, 1103 Holmes Hospital, Mail Loc-0212, Cincinnati, OH 45267, USA
* Corresponding author.
E-mail address: branambr@ucmail.uc.edu

0278-5919/17/© 2016 Elsevier Inc. All rights reserved.

This article reviews the indications and technical pearls for performing a 2-incision, outside-in ACL reconstruction.

INDICATIONS AND CONTRAINDICATIONS

The 2-incision approach for femoral tunnel creation is a reproducible method that can be used with standard primary ACL reconstructions.[1] There are some unique situations, however, where this technique is advantageous and may be considered as the procedure of choice to address specific technical challenges associated with ACL reconstruction. **Box 1** lists the indications and contraindications for this approach.

Skeletally Immature Patients

ACL injuries are diagnosed with increasing frequency in skeletally immature athletes. This is likely owing to a combination of increased participation, increased competitiveness at younger ages, and improved recognition by pediatricians and athletic trainers.[3,4] Owing to the transphyseal nature of traditional ACL reconstruction techniques, there is an increased risk of growth disturbances in pediatric patients with significant remaining growth and ACL ruptures. Thus, these injuries were historically treated nonoperatively to avoid the potential for iatrogenic growth arrest. Natural history studies, however, have documented poor outcomes from nonoperative treatment.[3,5] As a result, pediatric ACL injuries are increasingly being treated operatively. Traditional endoscopic techniques for pediatric ACL reconstruction are often modified to minimize physeal injury, and can result in nonanatomic tunnel placement.[3,6] With the use of fluoroscopy, an outside-in technique allows the surgeon to create a femoral tunnel from the anatomic ACL footprint that remains completely within the femoral epiphysis, thus sparing the physis.[3,4,7] This minimizes the risk of growth disturbances owing to ACL reconstruction in the young adolescent patient with open physes and significant remaining growth.

Patients with Long Bone–Patella Tendon–Bone Autografts

One of the theoretic benefits of bone–patella tendon–bone autografts is the improved fixation achieved with bone-to-bone healing through the use of interference fixation. Long bone–patella tendon–bone autografts (tendon length >45 mm) can result in problems with graft tunnel mismatch, which creates technical difficulties for tibial fixation of

---

Box 1
Indications and contraindications for 2-incision (outside-in) ACL reconstruction

Indications

- Skeletally immature patients
- Patients with long bone-patella tendon-bone autografts
- Revision ACL reconstructions
- Patients unable to achieve knee hyperflexion.[1,3]

Contraindications

- Significant previous femoral tunnel osteolysis requiring bone grafting in revisions

Abbreviation: ACL, anterior cruciate ligament.

the graft. This is usually managed with the use of staple fixation outside the tibial tunnel. The outside-in femoral tunnel technique results in the ability to pull the graft deeper into the femoral tunnel away from the intraarticular aperture and fix it closer to the lateral cortex. This prevents the graft from protruding outside the tibial tunnel and permits the use of interference screw fixation on both sides.[1,7] Preoperatively, the length of the patella tendon can be measured on MRI to assess for the possibility of graft tunnel mismatch.

Revision Reconstruction of the Anterior Cruciate Ligament

Revision ACL reconstructions pose technical challenges based on the presence of previous tunnels. These tunnels can be nonanatomic, partially anatomic, or enlarged owing to tunnel osteolysis. Significant tunnel osteolysis may require a staged technique with bone grafting followed by later reconstruction once the grafted tunnels have healed.[8] Use of an outside-in technique for femoral tunnel drilling, however, may allow the creation of a virgin or near virgin tunnel located in the anatomic footprint. This technique enables the surgeon to vary the trajectory of the femoral tunnel while maintaining anatomic placement. Therefore, previous tunnels or fixation hardware may be avoided and a single surgery revision can be performed.[1,7] Furthermore, the lateral incision and distal femur exposure presents the surgeon with additional fixation options such as lateral interference screw or post and washer fixation outside the femoral tunnel. This technique can be particularly helpful if the revision tunnel is partially confluent with an old primary tunnel.

Inability to Hyperflex the Knee

Knee hyperflexion is necessary to create an anatomic femoral tunnel when using an accessory medial portal. Occasionally, knee hyperflexion is not possible owing to body habitus or some other constraint. This limits the ability to create an anatomic tunnel using traditional endoscopic techniques. The outside-in technique offers a reproducible method to create an anatomic femoral tunnel without the need for knee hyperflexion.[7]

SURGICAL TECHNIQUE
Preoperative Planning

The preoperative plan is imperative for success with any procedure but critical for the 2-incision ACL reconstruction. The indication for 2-incision ACL reconstruction should be defined during the preoperative planning phase to allow for potential modifications in positioning and/or necessary equipment.

During a primary ACL reconstruction, the patient's anatomy and the bone stock of the lateral femoral condyle is in its native state increasing the predictability of tunnel creation. In this situation, preoperative planning includes ensuring that the necessary equipment is available. The 2-incision ACL is performed with an outside-in guide and standard arthroscopy equipment. Many companies have acceptable equipment for outside-in drilling. The surgeon can use standard reamers as the low-profile reamers used in anteromedial drilling are not imperative because injury to the medial-sided structures is largely obviated with this technique.

In the revision setting, previous tunnel and fixation hardware increase the complexity of the case, further validating the need for meticulous preoperative planning. Knowledge of the previous femoral tunnel(s) is imperative because at least a portion of the tunnel may be in proximity to the desired location of the anatomically located femoral tunnel ideal for revision reconstruction. Additionally, if metal screws or fixation devices are embedded in the condyle, they may need to be removed if they are impeding anatomic femoral socket creation. This may be done more easily from the lateral incision, or alternatively, arthroscopically through standard portals. Current radiographs are imperative and more advanced imaging studies (computed tomography scan and/or MRI) may be helpful as well in anticipating the location of the initial tunnel and hardware. Previous operative notes and arthroscopic pictures if available aid in ensuring equipment is available to remove the previous fixation devices if necessary. If the previous tunnel or fixation devices do not impede outside-in anatomic femoral tunnel creation or fixation, then they should be ignored. Sometimes it is difficult to tell in the revision settings to what degree the index tunnel will be a problem. If the tunnel is nearly anatomic, but not in the ideal location, it can be very difficult to revise the knee in a single-stage procedure. This may be true with arthroscopic transtibial or accessory medial portal drilling, as well as with an outside-in technique. The critical tunnel location is at the aperture. If there is any concern that single stage surgery may be a problem, it is important to consent the patient for a possible 2-stage revision and also to have the necessary bone graft available to bone graft the index tunnel. Despite these concerns, the 2-incision technique should decrease the likelihood of having to do a staged revision owing to the ability to start the tunnel laterally in unaltered bone. It is not recommended, however, that a suboptimal tunnel location be accepted to avoid a 2-stage revision. Meticulous preoperative planning, review of the radiographic studies, and a detailed discussion with the patient regarding mutual expectations increases the likelihood of obtaining the desired outcome in what many surgeons consider a salvage situation.

For a pediatric ACL reconstruction, preoperative planning is imperative. An estimate of the size of the patient is helpful to ensure that appropriately sized reamers are available, including smaller sizes in the very young population. Also, in this situation, fluoroscopy is used to ensure the tunnel does not violate the growth plate or articular cartilage. This may necessitate a change in positioning as described elsewhere in this paper.

In the case of a long patellar tendon, a 2-incision technique may be optimal. The length of the tendon can be measured on preoperative MRI. Other than ensuring outside-in equipment is available, no other specific preoperative planning is necessary beyond that of standard ACL reconstruction.

Perhaps the most common setting for using a 2-incision technique in the nonrevision setting is the inability to hyperflex the knee. This is owing to patient soft tissue factors—most commonly obesity or exceedingly large muscular legs (**Fig. 1**). In addition, performing femoral socket drilling from an anteromedial approach with the knee in hyperflexion is technically demanding and requires a skilled assistant.[9] If the preoperative plan dictates that the knee cannot be hyperflexed or an adequate assistant is unavailable, the 2-incision technique is preferred. This can usually be determined before surgery or at the very latest during positioning before preparation and draping.

Independent of the indication for 2-incision ACL reconstruction, a detailed preoperative plan increases the chances of a successful operation and outcome. Ensuring the availability of instrumentation, assistants, and radiologic equipment is most appropriately done during preoperative planning to diminish the likelihood of surprises during the procedure.

Preparation and Patient Positioning

Patient positioning is important in 2-incision ACL reconstruction. Often concomitant meniscal and articular cartilage procedures are performed and it is imperative to position the patient such that the surgeon has complete access to the knee. Care must be

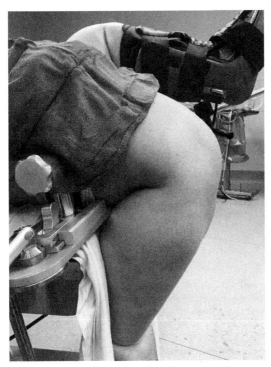

Fig. 1. A large knee that cannot be hyperflexed owing to soft tissue constraints is an indication for use of the 2-incision technique.

taken to place the tourniquet and arthroscopic leg holder proximal enough on the thigh such that complete access to the distal lateral femur is not impeded. The leg is placed in a standard leg holder such that the femur is parallel to the floor. This is in contrast with anteromedial femoral tunnel drilling where the hip is flexed such that the knee can be easily hyperflexed to move the tibia out of the way. The nonoperative limb is placed in the well leg holder with both the hip and knee flexed to move the entire leg out of the way (**Fig. 2**). This is important; often, an assistant is sitting on the medial side of the knee to retrieve sutures from a medial sided incision during an inside-out medial meniscal repair. Also, moving the nonoperative limb as far as possible from the operative knee is helpful in the revision or pediatric setting because frequently intraoperative fluoroscopy is needed to either localize hardware or ensure that the pediatric physis is not violated. In cases where fluoroscopy is used, abducting the bilateral hips is extremely helpful in positioning to avoid crowding of the surgeon, assistants, and equipment (**Fig. 3**). After positioning the patient and ensuring that there is adequate room for personnel and equipment, an alcohol-based preparation is used unless there is an allergy or wound that would necessitate a betadine paint and scrub preparation.

Surgical Approach

The 2-incision technique for femoral tunnel drilling uses an outside-in approach on the lateral femoral condyle. The specific instrumentation and fixation used dictates the size of the incision; however, the approach is the same. A longitudinal incision is made in line with the shaft of the femur over the lateral femoral condyle. A split in the iliotibial band is created in line with the skin incision. The starting point can then

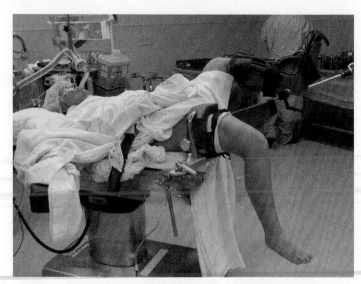

Fig. 2. The operative limb is placed in the arthroscopic leg holder with the femur parallel to the floor. The tourniquet is placed high on the thigh to allow access to the distal femur for femoral tunnel drilling. The nonoperative limb is well out of the way to allow complete access to the knee.

be determined either with direct visualization or with the assistance of fluoroscopy in the setting of pediatric ACL reconstruction.

Surgical Technique/Procedure

Step 1
Unless there is a question of the integrity of the ACL, the graft is harvested first.

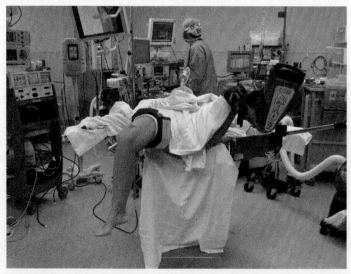

Fig. 3. If fluoroscopy use is anticipated, abducting the bilateral limbs is helpful such that there is room for the surgical team, and the arthroscopy and fluoroscopic equipment without limiting access to any portion of the knee.

Step 2

Three portals should be established to effectively perform the procedure (**Fig. 4**). An anterolateral portal is established that is just lateral to the patellar tendon and as prox-imal as possible. Creating the anterolateral portal just lateral to the patellar tendon al-lows for some visualization of the back wall of the lateral femoral condyle and the proximal location allows for excellent depth perception when choosing the location for the tibial tunnel in the central portion of the native tibial stump. The central portal is created just medial to the patellar tendon and is used for both instrumentation and viewing. The accessory inferomedial portal is created as far medial and inferior as possible with the posterior limit being the medial femoral condyle and the inferior limit being the meniscus.

Step 3

After creating the anterolateral portal and central portal, the meniscal and articular cartilage treatment is performed.

Step 4

Next, the remnant ACL is debrided and the lateral femoral condyle is prepared. The central portal is used for visualization and the accessory inferomedial portal is used as the working portal. Using the central portal for visualization obviates the need for a significant notchplasty and provides outstanding ability to view the entire lateral femoral condyle, removing ambiguity regarding the location of the femoral tunnel rela-tive to its native footprint, the back wall and the inferior articular cartilage. Drilling the femoral tunnel with the 30° arthroscope in the lateral portal results in poor depth perception and landmarks are not well visualized (**Fig. 5**). If the lateral portal is the preferred viewing portal, a 70° arthroscope results in better visualization. The native ACL is debrided, leaving only the insertional remnant on the lateral femoral condyle if desired. In the revision setting, the previous tunnel and fixation is assessed.

Step 5

The femoral tunnel is created next. The arthroscope is placed in the central portal and the knee is flexed to 90°. This is a reproducible position for selecting the location for

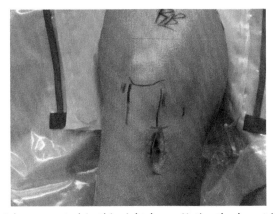

Fig. 4. Three portals are created in this right knee. Notice the hamstring autograft has already been harvested through the anteromedial incision. The anterolateral portal is created just lateral to the patellar tendon as proximal as possible. The central portal is created adjacent to the medial side of the patellar tendon and the inferomedial working portal is created as inferior and posterior as possible.

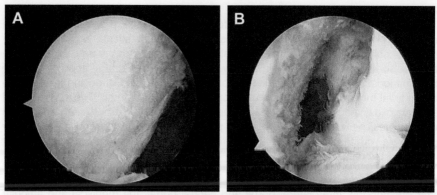

Fig. 5. Viewing the lateral femoral condyle from the central portal (*A*) allows for outstanding visualization of the lateral femoral condyle. The back wall and inferior articular cartilage are well visualized. Viewing from the lateral portal with a 30° arthroscope (*B*) makes depth perception much more challenging and limits the surgeon's ability to properly position the femoral tunnel.

the femoral tunnel and also visualizing the lateral femoral condyle. A microfracture awl is used to create a shallow pilot hole in the lateral femoral condyle in the desired location of the central portion of the femoral tunnel aperture in the notch (**Fig. 6**). The pilot hole should be assessed critically because this determines the location of the femoral tunnel and the ideal location must be chosen (**Fig. 7**). Next, an incision is created in line with the distal femur over the desired location for the guide pin insertion on the extra-articular lateral femoral condyle (**Fig. 8**). The iliotibial band is divided in line with the skin incision. The tip of the outside-in guide is then placed through the lateral portal and into the pilot hole (**Fig. 9**). The starting point for the pin on the lateral side of the femur in the skeletally mature patient is just anterior and proximal to the lateral epicondyle. The guide pin is placed through the guide until it contacts the intraarticular tip of the guide, which is in the previously created pilot hole. The guide is removed and the desired diameter barrel reamer is then used to drill the femoral tunnel over the guide pin. If the pin is noted to be simultaneously advancing into the joint, it can be held in

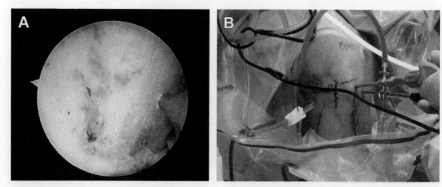

Fig. 6. Viewing from the central portal and working from the accessory inferomedial portal allows for excellent visualization of the lateral femoral condyle (*A*). A microfracture awl can be used to make a pilot hole for the tip of the outside-in guide in the central portion of the anticipated femoral tunnel (*B*).

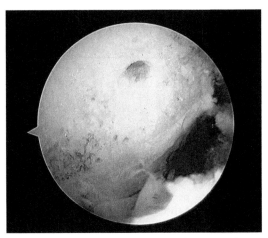

Fig. 7. The pilot hole is evaluated before the insertion of the outside-in guide. If it is suboptimal, it can be manipulated to the correct location.

place with a grasper placed through the accessory inferomedial portal. Alternatively, a retrograde reaming device can be used, which results in creation of the appropriate diameter tunnel by withdrawing the reamer until the reamer creates the desired depth tunnel (**Fig. 10**). Retaining the scope in the central portal allows for evaluation of the femoral tunnel to ensure the back and lateral wall remain intact and there is bone surrounding the tunnel. The femoral tunnel drilling is complete and the tunnel can be assessed (**Fig. 11**).

In a pediatric ACL reconstruction, the starting point must be distal to the femoral physis. In smaller patients, the margin for error can be relatively small as an incorrect starting point or trajectory can result in iatrogenic injury to the physis or articular cartilage. Intraoperative fluoroscopy should be used to select the starting point. A perfect lateral of the knee is obtained and the tip of a guide pin is evaluated to ensure the starting point is ideal to create the desired diameter tunnel distal and parallel to the physis (**Fig. 12**). The tunnel position is limited by the physis proximally and the articular

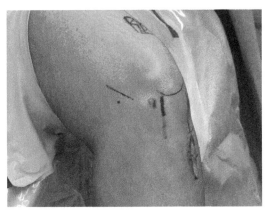

Fig. 8. A small incision is created on the lateral side of the thigh (*straight line*) in line with the distal femur, just anterior to the lateral epicondyle (*dot*).

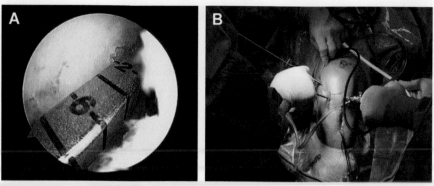

Fig. 9. Viewing from the central portal (*A*), the outside-in guide is placed through the lateral portal and the pin inserted through the guide until it contacts the intraarticular tip, which has been placed in the previously created pilot hole (*B*).

cartilage posteriorly and inferiorly. A retrograde reaming device is then placed through the 2-incision guide. After appropriate placement is confirmed, it is withdrawn to the desired depth leaving the lateral cortex intact. The arthroscope in the central portal confirms the tunnel is entirely intraepiphyseal.

In the revision setting, previous hardware may be encountered. If it is obstructing the creation of the desired tunnel, then it should be removed from either side of the joint. Fluoroscopy is available to assist if necessary. If previous hardware will not obstruct anatomic tunnel creation, then it should be ignored.

If the violation of the lateral cortex is greater than the diameter of the guide pin then a plug must be placed into the femoral tunnel from the outside. This maneuver will inhibit excessive fluid extravasation into the soft tissues and allow for visualization during the remainder of the case.

Step 6
The tibial tunnel is created in the standard fashion.

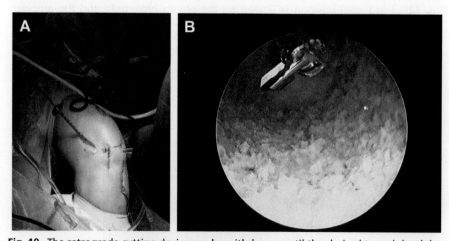

Fig. 10. The retrograde cutting device can be withdrawn until the desired tunnel depth has been obtained (*A*). With the arthroscope still in the central portal, the tunnel can be evaluated to ensure the back wall and lateral cortex have not been violated (*B*).

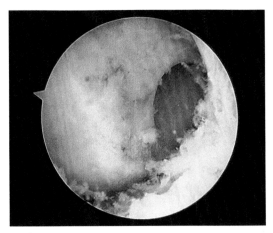

Fig. 11. Femoral tunnel.

Step 7

Fixation depends on the graft that is chosen. In many, situations there are several viable options. For hamstring grafts, a cortical suspensory button can be used with or without an extension depending on the size of the hole in the cortical bone. A passing suture can be passed into the knee in a retrograde fashion and retrieved from inside the knee through the tibial tunnel. The graft is pulled into the knee and suspensory button can be directly visualized through the lateral incision (**Fig. 13**). Once it is seated on the lateral femoral cortex, the knee can be cycled and the graft can be fixed on the tibial side using the desired technique.

For patellar tendon grafts, an interference screw can be placed laterally in a retrograde fashion. This technique can be particularly useful in cases with a longer patellar tendon

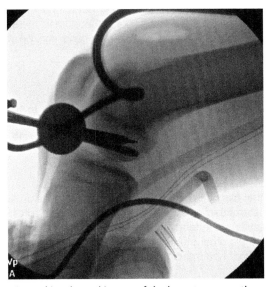

Fig. 12. Fluoroscopy is used in a lateral image of the knee to ensure the appropriate starting point for the all intraepiphyseal femoral tunnel in the pediatric patient. The tunnel must be positioned such that it does not violate the physis.

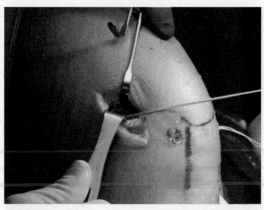

Fig. 13. If a hamstring graft has been used, the flipped endobutton can be visualized to be seated directly on the bone.

when fixing the graft at the aperture would result in graft tunnel mismatch and the tibial bone plug being left outside the tunnel. The graft can be pulled into the knee until the inferior end of the tibial bone plug is at the desired depth. The femoral bone plug can then be fixed on the femoral side. The guidewire for the interference screw is placed retrograde and an interference screw is placed collinearly to the bone plug while tension is placed on the both sides of the graft. The knee is then cycled several times just as with a hamstring graft and then fixed with the device of choice on the tibial side.

If there is any doubt that cortical button or interference screw fixation is tenuous, a post and washer system on the femoral side is an outstanding choice. This is also the preferred fixation choice on the femoral side for violation of the back wall or even the lateral wall when traditional cortical suspensory devices are tenuous. The larger buttons can be bulky and irritate the iliotibial band. The post and washer is placed just proximal to the tunnel on the lateral cortex. Given that the post is placed at the metaphyseal flare, it is significantly deep to the iliotibial band and therefore rarely irritates the iliotibial band. Furthermore, it is extraarticular and can be placed bicortically providing rigid fixation.

COMPLICATIONS AND THEIR MANAGEMENT

Complications of outside-in ACL reconstruction are similar to those for traditional endoscopic techniques and include arthrofibrosis, graft failure, infection, autograft harvest complications, hardware complications, tunnel malposition, and deep vein thrombosis.

Heterotopic Ossification

One complication that has been described that is unique to the outside-in approach is the possibility of heterotopic ossification in the periarticular soft tissues around the lateral femoral condyle by the femoral tunnel. This has been described in a case series[10]; however, multiple other studies of outside-in versus inside-out methods have not noted any significant heterotopic ossification formation.[11–14]

Tunnel Malposition

Two-incision ACL reconstruction allows for creation of a femoral tunnel independent of the tibial tunnel. Also, the technique is advantageous in creating a tunnel with circumferential bone in the revision setting when previous tunnels or fixation make endoscopic femoral tunnel drilling difficult. However, meticulous attention to detail should still be used to ensure ideal tunnel positioning because the tunnel can still be placed improperly. As mentioned, viewing from the lateral portal without a significant notchplasty makes depth perception on the lateral femoral condyle very difficult and could lead to a tunnel placed too anteriorly or too posteriorly with resultant back wall blowout. Thus, medial portal viewing is highly recommended to maximize the advantage in 2-incision femoral tunnel drilling. Also, ensuring the starting point is more distal the starting point on the cortex of the lateral femoral condyle the less collinear the tunnel and intraarticular graft trajectory become creating a "killer turn" analogous to the tibial tunnel in endoscopic posterior cruciate ligament reconstruction should minimize the chance of back wall blowout. In the situation of back wall blowout a post and washer system should be used for fixation.

Infection

A second incision can theoretically increase the likelihood of infection. If an infection occurs at the lateral incision, suspicion for intraarticular involvement should be entertained because, until the graft incorporates, there is communication between the lateral incision and the joint. Furthermore, especially when a soft tissue graft is used, heavy braided nonabsorbable suture is often woven through the graft, which can make eradication of infection difficult. Wound infection from the lateral wound should be treated aggressively with irrigation and debridement, antibiotics, and ensuring no intraarticular involvement. Sometimes the lateral fixation device and heavy suture need to be removed after graft incorporation to successfully eradicate the infection.

Iliotibial Band Irritation

Prominent hardware on the lateral side of the thigh can lead to irritation of the iliotibial band. Cortical buttons are typically lower profile and rarely irritate the soft tissues. If a post and washer is used, it can be placed just proximal to the tunnel. At this location, at the metaphyseal flare, the iliotibial band is not in direct contact with the bone. Thus, the post and washer is rarely symptomatic. As mentioned, if there is any question about fixation, the post and washer system is a predictable option.

POSTOPERATIVE CARE

The rehabilitation protocol for 2-incision ACL reconstruction is the same as for single-incision ACL reconstruction.

Immediate Postoperatively

A patient is allowed to bear weight as tolerated in a postoperative brace locked in full extension, unless meniscal or articular cartilage surgery or collateral ligament surgery preclude immediate weight bearing. Physical therapy should be started within the first 3 to 5 days and focus on working on range of motion and returning quadriceps function.

One Month Postoperatively

The postoperative brace should be unlocked as quadriceps function improves with continued range of motion and quadriceps exercises. The patient should expect nearly full range of motion.

Two Months Postoperatively

If the goals of full range of motion and no limp are achieved, the patient can begin more aggressive closed chain quadriceps strengthening exercises at 0° to 90° and use a hinged knee sleeve when active.

Three Months Postoperatively

Light jogging can be initiated in a straight line in a controlled environment. Continued quadriceps strengthening is emphasized.

Five to Six Months Postoperatively

Sport-specific exercises are emphasized.

Six to Nine Months Postoperatively

Patient is allowed to return to sport. A functional brace is used if requested by the athlete.

OUTCOMES

There have been numerous clinical studies in the literature comparing outside-in femoral drilling with single-incision ACL reconstruction (**Table 1**). The majority of these studies show no difference in outcomes with regard to patient reported outcomes scores, return to sport rate, or rerupture rate.[11–19] Additionally, a metaanalysis performed by Riboh and colleagues[20] in 2013 showed no statistical difference with

Table 1
Outcome studies of single-incision versus 2-incision ACL reconstruction

Author	Patients	Follow-up (mo)	Graft	Outcomes	Results
Brandsson et al,[17] 1999	59	24	BPTB	KT-1000, Lysholm, Tegner, IKDC, 1-leg hop test	NS
Gerich et al,[18] 1997	40	12		KT-1000, Lysholm, Tegner, IKDC, 1-leg hop test	S-I better 1-leg hop test
Reat & Lintner,[19] 1997	30	30		KT-1000, IKDC, 1-leg hop test	NS
O'Neill,[13] 1996	85	42	BPTB	KT-1000, Lysholm, return to sport, IKDC, 1-leg hop test	Return to sport favors T-I (95% vs 89%)
Howell & Deutsch,[12] 1999	108	24	4-S Ham	IKDC, activity level, Lachman, pivot shift, thigh girth, single leg hop	NS
Panni et al,[11] 2001	141	79	BPTB	IKDC, KT-1000, ROM, activity level	NS

Abbreviations: ACL, anterior cruciate ligament; 4-S Ham, 4-strand hamstring graft of semitendinosus and gracilis; BPTB, bone–patella tendon–bone; IKDC, International Knee Documentation Committee; NS, no significant difference; ROM, range of motion; S-I, single-incision group; T-I, 2-incision group.

regards to International Knee Documentation Committee scores, Tegner scores, or failure rates.

SUMMARY

Outside-in femoral tunnel drilling is a well-studied, reproducible technique for ACL reconstruction. Although largely replaced by single-incision endoscopic techniques, there are some specific instances where use of the outside-in, 2-incision technique is beneficial and may be the preferred technique for femoral tunnel drilling. Use of this technique allows the creation of an anatomic femoral tunnel and avoids some of the technical problems with ACL reconstruction in the skeletally immature patient, revision ACL patient, patient with long bone–patella tendon–bone autograft, and obese patient with inability to hyperflex the knee.

REFERENCES

1. Wright RW. Two-incision anterior cruciate ligament reconstruction. J Knee Surg 2014;27(5):343–6.
2. MARS Group, Wright RW, Huston LJ, Spindler KP, et al. Descriptive epidemiology of the Multicenter ACL Revision Study (MARS) cohort. Am J Sports Med 2010; 38(10):1979–86.
3. Breland R, Metzler A, Johnson DL. Indications for 2-incision anterior cruciate ligament surgery. Orthopedics 2013;36(9):708–11.
4. Lawrence JT, Bowers AL, Belding J, et al. All-epiphyseal anterior cruciate ligament reconstruction in skeletally immature patients. Clin Orthop Relat Res 2010;468(7):1971–7.
5. McCarthy MM, Graziano J, Green DW, et al. All-epiphyseal, all-inside anterior cruciate ligament reconstruction technique for skeletally immature patients. Arthrosc Tech 2012;1(2):e231–9.
6. Aichroth PM, Patel DV, Zorrilla P. The natural history and treatment of rupture of the anterior cruciate ligament in children and adolescents. A prospective review. J Bone Joint Surg Br 2002;84(1):38–41.
7. Frosch KH, Stengel D, Brodhun T, et al. Outcomes and risks of operative treatment of rupture of the anterior cruciate ligament in children and adolescents. Arthroscopy 2010;26(11):1539–50.
8. Coats AC, Johnson DL. Two-stage revision anterior cruciate ligament reconstruction: indications, review, and technique demonstration. Orthopedics 2012;35(11): 958–60.
9. Branam BR, Hasselfeld KA. Retrograde technique for drilling the femoral tunnel in an anterior cruciate ligament reconstruction. Arthrosc Tech 2013;2(4):e395–9.
10. Ogilvie-Harris DJ, Sekyi-Otu A. Periarticular heterotopic ossification: a complication of arthroscopic anterior cruciate ligament reconstruction using a two-incision technique. Arthroscopy 1995;11(6):676–9.
11. Panni AS, Milano G, Tartarone M, et al. Clinical and radiographic results of ACL reconstruction: a 5- to 7-year follow-up study of outside-in versus inside-out reconstruction techniques. Knee Surg Sports Traumatol Arthrosc 2001;9(2):77–85.
12. Howell SM, Deutsch ML. Comparison of endoscopic and two-incision techniques for reconstructing a torn anterior cruciate ligament using hamstring tendons. Arthroscopy 1999;15(6):594–606.
13. O'Neill DB. Arthroscopically assisted reconstruction of the anterior cruciate ligament. A prospective randomized analysis of three techniques. J Bone Joint Surg Am 1996;78(6):803–13.

14. O'Neill DB. Arthroscopically assisted reconstruction of the anterior cruciate ligament. A follow-up report. J Bone Joint Surg Am 2001;83-A(9):1329–32.
15. Sgaglione NA, Schwartz RE. Arthroscopically assisted reconstruction of the anterior cruciate ligament: initial clinical experience and minimal 2-year follow-up comparing endoscopic transtibial and two-incision techniques. Arthroscopy 1997;13(2):156–65.
16. George MS, Huston LJ, Spindler KP. Endoscopic versus rear-entry ACL reconstruction: a systematic review. Clin Orthop Relat Res 2007;455:158–61.
17. Brandsson S, Faxén E, Eriksson BI, et al. Reconstruction of the anterior cruciate ligament: comparison of outside-in and all-inside techniques. Br J Sports Med 1999;33(1):42–5.
10. Oerich TO, Lattermann C, Fremerey RW, et al. One- versus two-incision technique for anterior cruciate ligament reconstruction with patellar tendon graft. Results on early rehabilitation and stability. Knee Surg Sports Traumatol Arthrosc 1997;5(4):213–6.
19. Reat JF, Lintner DM. One-versus two-incision ACL reconstruction. A prospective, randomized study. Am J Knee Surg 1997;10(4):198–208.
20. Riboh JC, Hasselblad V, Godin JA, et al. Transtibial versus independent drilling techniques for anterior cruciate ligament reconstruction: a systematic review, meta-analysis, and meta-regression. Am J Sports Med 2013;41(11):2693–702.

Surgical Management and Treatment of the Anterior Cruciate Ligament/Medial Collateral Ligament Injured Knee

 CrossMark

Kevin M. Dale, MD[a],*, James R. Bailey, MD[a],
Claude T. Moorman III, MD[b]

KEYWORDS

- Anterior cruciate ligament • Medial collateral ligament • Surgical technique

KEY POINTS

- Diagnosis should start with physical examination and can be confirmed with MRI and radiographs.
- Anterior cruciate ligament (ACL) reconstruction should be done in a delayed fashion after swelling has gone down and range of motion has returned. This will allow time for the medial collateral ligament (MCL) to potentially heal.
- Proximal MCL injuries have an excellent chance of healing, and distal MCL injuries should be ruled out for a "Stener"-like lesion of the MCL over the pes anserinus.
- Grade 1 and 2 MCL injuries can be treated nonoperatively, and increased scrutiny should be given to grade 3 MCL injuries at the time of surgery.
- After ACL reconstruction, the MCL should be tested with valgus stress testing at 0° and 30° of flexion to evaluate for medial-sided opening of the knee joint necessitating MCL repair or reconstruction.

▶ Video content accompanies this article at http://www.sportsmed.theclinics.com.

Disclosure Statement: See last page of article.
[a] Department of Orthopaedics, Duke University Medical Center, Box 3615, Durham, NC 27710, USA; [b] Department of Orthopaedics, Duke University Medical Center, Box 3639, Durham, NC 27710, USA
* Corresponding author.
E-mail address: Kevin.dale@duke.edu

Clin Sports Med 36 (2017) 87–103
http://dx.doi.org/10.1016/j.csm.2016.08.005
0278-5919/17/© 2016 Elsevier Inc. All rights reserved.

INTRODUCTION
Nature of the Problem

Of knee ligament injuries, the medial collateral ligament (MCL) is the most commonly injured.[1] When there is a severe grade III MCL injury, the risk of associated ligament injury is 78%, and 95% of the time the anterior cruciate ligament (ACL) is involved.[2] ACL injuries alone usually result from a noncontact mechanism, whereas an ACL-MCL injury will result from a contact mechanism that involves a valgus stress with external tibial rotation.

Histologically, the ACL resembles fibrocartilage with poor healing capability.[3] Also, most ACL tears pull apart, leaving frayed tissue with poor healing potential. Therefore, ACL reconstruction is often recommended to allow patients to return to activities that involve change of direction.[4] Histologically, the MCL resembles fibroblast-type cells with good healing capability.[3] Unlike ACL tears, most MCL tears are either proximal or distal with good blood supply for healing.[5] Patients are usually able to return to competitive activities with nonoperative treatment of the MCL.[6]

Controversy arises when dealing with combined ACL-MCL knee injuries. A canine model has shown that when there is transection of the MCL and ACL, the MCL healing was negatively affected by the injured ACL.[7] A recent systematic review confirmed the recommendation for ACL reconstruction, but there is no one recommendation for treatment of the MCL.[8] The treatment of the MCL injury is usually driven by the severity and location of the injury.

Evaluation

A thorough history is the first part of the patient evaluation. This history should include the mechanism of the injury and any treatment that has occurred up to the presenting visit. As with any multiligamentous knee injury, neurologic and vascular status should be evaluated to rule out limb-threatening injury.

A comprehensive knee examination should be performed. This examination should be done with the affected knee joint visible for inspection. Inspection will usually show a medial-sided hematoma or bruising. A knee effusion is usually absent because of the capsular disruption. The contralateral knee should be evaluated as well. With any medial-sided knee injury, the hamstrings, meniscus, medial patellofemoral ligament, posterior cruciate ligament, MCL, and ACL should all be tested (**Table 1**). During the

Table 1	
Physical examination of the medial collateral ligament and anterior cruciate ligament	
Ligament	**Examination**
MCL	Palpation: Tenderness along medial side of the knee: proximal for a tear at MCL origin and distal for a tear at MCL insertion
	Valgus stress at 30° extension: Isolates sMCL, tear if gapping compared with opposite side
	Valgus stress at 0° extension: Medial laxity associated with cruciate or posteromedial capsular injury
	Anterior drawer in external rotation: Increased anteromedial translation occurs with injury to the posteromedial capsule (POL, dMCL, semimembranous attachment)
ACL	Lachman: Increased forward translation of the tibia with the knee at 30° of flexion
	Pivot shift: With the tibia internally rotated and valgus stress applied, the tibia will reduce under the femur as the knee is brought from extension into flexion

gait examination after a combined ACL and MCL injury, the knee may demonstrate a medial thrust.

Classification

The clinical classification of MCL injuries is based on the amount of opening on the medial side of the knee with a valgus force applied at 0° and 30° of flexion (**Table 2**).[9] Laxity with valgus stress at 30°, but not at 0°, is associated with a primary MCL injury, whereas laxity at 0° and 30° is associated with an MCL and posterior oblique ligament (POL) or cruciate injury, usually the ACL. The ACL acts as a secondary restraint to valgus stress of the knee.

Imaging

First-line imaging is weight bearing if tolerated plain radiographs (anteroposterior/ sagittal plane [AP] weight bearing, 45° flexion weight bearing, lateral, and sunrise views). Initial imaging may show a Segond fracture signaling the likelihood of an ACL injury.

Valgus stress radiographs are usually too painful during the initial visit. They may be helpful in assessing chronic MCL laxity (**Fig. 1**) and determining an MCL versus physeal injury in a patient with open growth plates.

When concern arises for multiple ligament injuries around the knee, MRI is used for identifying the soft tissue injuries. The MRI will provide information on the location of the MCL injury (femoral or tibial) (**Fig. 2**A), an ACL tear (**Fig. 2**B), and associated injuries, for example, meniscal tear, POL, bone bruise.

SURGICAL INDICATIONS/CONTRAINDICATIONS

The authors' preferred method of treatment of ACL tears associated with MCL injury is bracing and range-of-motion (ROM) rehabilitation of the MCL for 6 weeks followed by ACL reconstruction. Contraindication for MCL repair or reconstruction is a knee stable to valgus stress after the ACL reconstruction is performed. Indications for MCL repair is a "Stener"-like tear of the distal MCL because of concern the MCL will not heal due to the interposed pes anserinus, an MCL entrapped in the joint, and meniscal tear requiring repair.[10,11] In cases where there is still an opening of the medial joint space with valgus stress under fluoroscopic imaging after ACL reconstruction, MCL repair or reconstruction is performed. Chronic MCL injuries resulting in valgus instability require an MCL reconstruction at the time of ACL reconstruction (**Table 3**).

SURGICAL TECHNIQUE/PROCEDURE
Preoperative Planning

- Graft choices are discussed with patient before day of surgery:
  - ACL graft preference: Patella bone-tendon-bone (BTB) autograft for high-level athletes
  - MCL graft preference: Repair if possible or semitendinosus (Semi-T) autograft reconstruction/augmentation for high-level athletes

Table 2
Medial collateral ligament injury

Grade	Amount of Opening (mm)	Clinical Severity
I	0–5	Mild
II	5–10	Moderate
III	>10	Severe

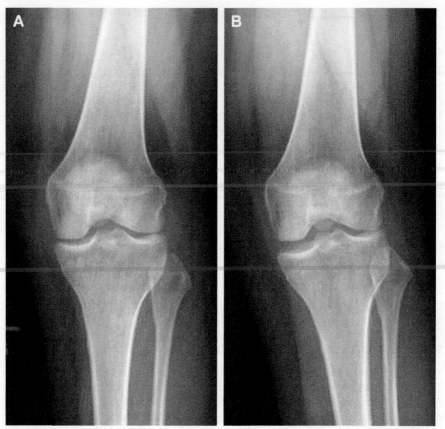

Fig. 1. (A) Neutral AP radiograph of the knee. (B) Valgus stress radiograph of the knee.

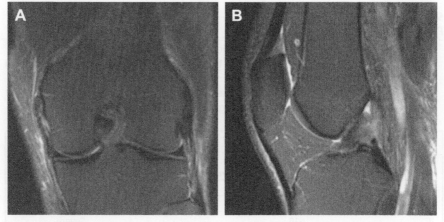

Fig. 2. (A) T2 MRI sequence of grade 2 MCL injury. (B) T2 MRI sequence of ACL tear.

Table 3 Treatment of anterior cruciate ligament and medial collateral ligament injuries based on grade of medial collateral ligament injury	
MCL Injury	**Treatment of Combined ACL and MCL Injuries**
Grade I	MCL: Rehabilitation for 6 wk ACL: Reconstruction after MCL rehabilitation
Grade II	MCL: Rehabilitation for 6 wk; early surgical repair for Stener-like distal tear ACL: Reconstruction after MCL rehabilitation
Grade III	MCL: Rehabilitation for 6 wk; repair or reconstruction if valgus instability on examination after ACL reconstruction; reconstruction for chronic MCL tears ACL: Reconstruction after MCL rehabilitation

- ○ There are various combinations to consider based on the activity level of the patient. For recreational athletes, a common combination is autograft of choice for ACL and direct repair versus Semi-T allograft for MCL.
- Images are reviewed before surgery, and key slices posted or pulled up on the computer at the time of surgery.
- Examination under anesthesia (Video 1) should be performed before surgical draping. This examination should include an ROM assessment and full ligamentous examination of both knees (eg, Lachman test, anterior and posterior drawer tests, pivot shift test, varus/valgus stress test at 30° and 0°, anterior drawer in external rotation, and supine dial test).

Preparation and Patient Positioning

- The patient is positioned in the supine position on a regular operating room table.
- A bump in placed under the knee with a lateral post.
- Patient is prepared and draped in usual fashion with appropriate antibiotics.

SURGICAL APPROACH

- ACL
  - ○ An approximately 6- to 8-cm midline incision from the inferior pole of patella to the tibial tubercle.
  - ○ TIP: This incision should be cheated just medial to midline. It potentially is more comfortable with kneeling in the future. Furthermore, this will allow easier access to hamstring harvesting (if needed), tibial tunnel drilling, and extension of dissection to the MCL (if desired).
- MCL
  - ○ An approximately 6- to 8-cm medial incision from just proximal to the medial epicondyle of the femur to the MCL insertion on the tibia.
  - ○ TIP: It is the senior author's preference to perform a combined ACL/MCL surgery through a single incision. This surgery is accomplished by extending the BTB harvest incision both proximally and distally by a centimeter or 2 to allow for dissection over to the medial part of the knee (**Fig. 3**).

Surgical Procedure

- ACL
  - ○ The incision is just medial to the midline of the knee. With the knee in full extension, the incision starts right at the inferior pole of the patella and goes to just medial to the tibial tubercle.

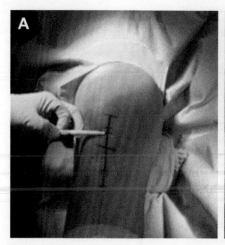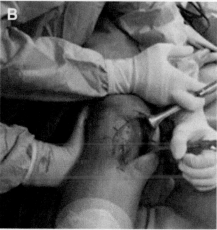

Fig. 3. (*A*) The incision is marked out before the procedure for single incision ACL and MCL reconstruction. The marking pin points to the normal proximal extent of the ACL reconstruction only incision. (*B*) Exposure for MCL reconstruction.

- o The incision is made sharply down to the paratenon. The paratenon is split vertically over the mid portion of the patellar tendon. It is important to develop the paratenon both medially and laterally for a layered closure.
- o The central one-third of the patellar tendon is then harvested with the appropriately sized bone plugs.
  - ■ TIP: Make the cuts deeper in the tibia when harvesting the bone plug so you can use that excess cancellous bone to back fill the patellar defect.
- o Perform diagnostic arthroscopy at this time while the graft is being prepared.
  - ■ TIP: If the examination under anesthesia clearly confirms an ACL tear, the graft should be harvested before the arthroscopic portion of the case.
- o At this point, the notch is debrided of any remnant ACL, and a notchplasty is performed only if needed for visualization or a V-shaped notch.
- o Next, tibial and femoral tunnels are drilled in the anatomic position using either a flexible reamer or a retro-cutting device.
- o The graft is then passed and secured based on surgeon preference.
  - ■ TIP: At this point, the authors recommend reexamining the MCL. Occasionally, by performing the ACL reconstruction, the knee is adequately stabilized to treat the MCL nonoperatively.
- o Pack the patellar defect with cancellous bone from the tibial harvest and close the paratenon with 0 absorbable sutures in a running fashion.
- o Final closure can be performed now or at the end of the case with interrupted buried 2-0 absorbable suture followed by a running subcutaneous 3-0 suture and Steri-Strips.
- • MCL repair
  - o A longitudinal incision just posterior to the superficial MCL (sMCL) is now performed unless the decision is made to perform both ACL reconstruction and MCL repair through a single anterior just medial to midline incision.
  - o The Sartorius facia and medial retinaculum (layer 1) is incised in line with its fibers while taking care to protect the saphenous nerve.
  - o At this point, the sMCL (layer 2) should be fully evaluated at the proximal femoral origin, midbody, and distal tibial insertion.

○ Structural evaluation of both the POL/posteromedial capsule and deep MCL (dMCL) should be performed.
○ If there is an acute tear of the sMCL or underlying dMCL (so the joint line is visible), these can be repaired and reefed directly with nonabsorbable suture.
○ If the sMCL is torn off the femoral origin, the senior author prefers to place a Krackow stitch with nonabsorbable no. 2 suture through the torn end of the sMCL, advance the ligament proximally, and tie the suture around a screw and spiked washer. Another option is to advance/reef the ligament over a 5.5-mm knotless anchor placed in the anatomic position of the femur.
  ▪ TIP: The anatomic origin of the MCL is 3.2 mm proximal and 4.8 mm posterior to the medial epicondyle.[12]
○ The sMCL is tightened with the knee at 30° of flexion and in slight varus to maximally tighten the sMCL.
○ If needed, the POL/posteromedial capsule is also reefed/plicated to the more anterior sMCL with nonabsorbable no. 2 suture. This is done in effort to enhance rotational stability of the knee.
○ Layered closure is performed with 0 absorbable suture for the retinaculum followed by interrupted buried 2-0 absorbable sutures and a running subcutaneous 3-0 suture with Steri-Strips.
• MCL reconstruction (modified Bosworth procedure, the senior author's preferred technique)
○ The anterior incision made for the BTB harvest is extended both superiorly and inferiorly by 1 to 2 cm. This allows one to perform both ACL and MCL reconstruction through a single anterior just medial to midline incision (the senior author's preference). If desired, a separate longitudinal incision just posterior to the sMCL can be made instead.
○ The Sartorius facia and medial retinaculum (layer 1) is incised in line with its fibers while taking care to protect the saphenous nerve.
○ At this point, the residual sMCL (layer 2) should be fully evaluated.
○ Structural evaluation of both the POL/posteromedial capsule and the dMCL should be performed.
○ If there is a tear of the underlying dMCL (so the joint line is visible), it can be repaired and reefed directly with nonabsorbable suture.
○ Any tears of the POL should be repaired directly at this time. The POL will later be reefed to the sMCL reconstruction graft.
○ At this point, the Semi-T tendon is harvested with an open-ended tendon stripper, leaving the tibial insertion intact.
○ The free end of the tendon is removed from the wound, stripped of its muscle, and whip-stitched with suture.
○ The Semi-T autograft is then taken posterior and anchored first to screw and spiked washer on the tibia just posterior to the pes anserinus insertion at a distance of approximately 6 cm distal to the joint line[13] (**Fig. 4**).
○ The graft is then tunneled deep to the Sartorius fascia and looped around a second screw and spiked washer from posterior to anterior. This screw is placed in the anatomic femoral attachment of the sMCL 3.2 mm proximal and 4.8 mm posterior to the medial epicondyle.[12]
○ The remaining tendon is then brought back distally and secured over the tibial screw in washer, completing the double-strand reconstruction (**Fig. 5**).
○ This graft construct is tightened with the knee at 30° of flexion and in slight varus to maximally tighten the sMCL (**Fig. 6**).
○ Any residual native sMCL can be sewn/repaired to the allograft.

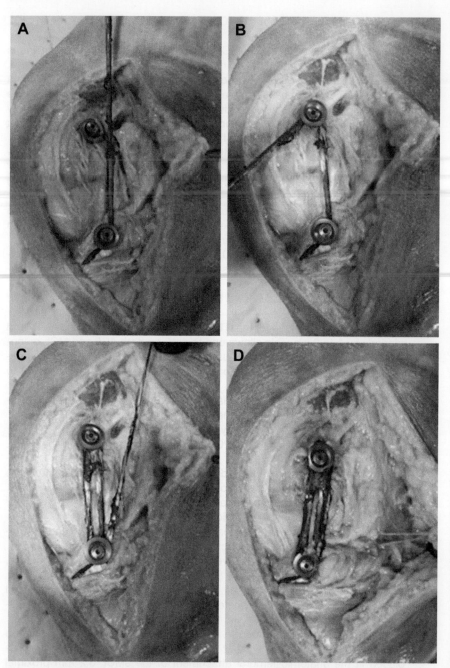

Fig. 4. Modified Bosworth MCL reconstruction steps performed in a cadaver. Autograft tendon marked with blue dye. (*A*) Graft taken posterior around tibial screw. (*B*) Graft is looped from posterior to anterior around femoral screw. (*C*) Remaining graft is looped once again around tibial screw from anterior to posterior and tensioned while the screws are secured. (*D*) Completed modified Bosworth reconstruction.

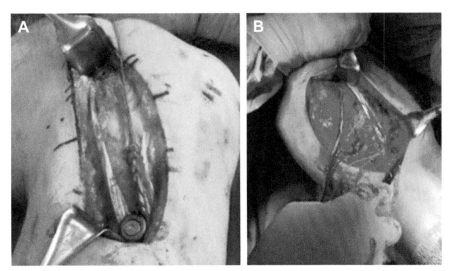

Fig. 5. Completed modified Bosworth MCL reconstruction through MCL-only incision (*A*) and combined ACL/MCL incision (*B*). In **Fig. 4A**, the graft was first taken proximally over the femoral screw and then distally around the tibial screw. This is an alternate method for shorter grafts.

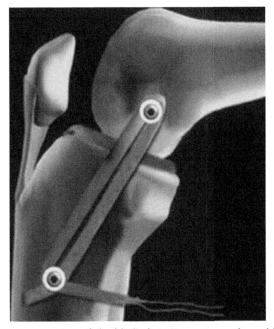

Fig. 6. Computer representation of double-limb MCL reconstruction with semitendinosus graft. Anterior limb of graft secured in flexion. (*From* Lonergan KT, Taylor DC. Medial collateral ligament injuries of the knee: an evolution of surgical reconstruction. Tech Knee Surg 2002;1:143; with permission.)

Table 4
Postoperative rehabilitation protocol

Phase 1 (0–6 wk)	Phase 2 (6–8 wk)	Phase 3 (2–6 mo)	Phase 4 (6–9 mo)	Phase 5 (9+ mo)
• Active assist ROM	• Discontinue brace and crutches	• Stair stepper and/or elliptical	Progress strength, power, and proprioception to prepare for sports-specific retraining	Sports-specific retraining including jumping, cutting, endurance
• Quad sets	• Wall slides 0–45°	• Advance closed kinetic chain activities (leg press, one-leg mini squats, step-ups)		
• Straight leg raise exercises in all planes (with brace locked in full extension until quad is strong enough to prevent extension lag)	• Stationary bike with high seat	• Progress proprioceptive activities		
• Patellar mobilization	• Closed chain terminal knee extension	• Progress aquatic program to include pool running and swimming (no breaststroke)		
• Prone knee flexion	• Balance exercises			
• Hamstring stretching	• Aquatic therapy with emphasis on gait normalization			
	• Continued hamstring stretching			

Criteria to advance to phase 2: full extension to 90° of flexion, no signs of active inflammation, and straight leg raise without extension lag.

Table 5
Outcomes of treatment of combined complete tears of the anterior cruciate and medial collateral ligaments

Author, Year	Level of Evidence and Type of Study[a]	Groups	Patients	Outcome Measure	Results
Halinen et al,[16] 2006[b]	Level I RCT	1. ACLR + MCL repair 2. ACLR + MCL NSx	1. 23 2. 24	ROM, laxity, Telos (Weiterstadt, Germany), quadriceps peak torque, 1-leg hop, IKDC knee evaluation, Lysholm, activity level	No difference in any outcomes
Halinen et al,[17] 2009[b]	Level I RCT	1. ACLR + MCL repair 2. ACLR + MCL NSx	1. 23 2. 24	Knee ROM, quadriceps peak torque, 1-leg hop	No difference in extension ROM; less flexion early in MCL repair, equal long-term; early increased quadriceps deficit in MCL repair, equal long-term
Andersson & Gillquist,[18] 1992	Level II Quasi-RCT	1. ACL/MCL repair 2. NSx ACL + MCL repair	1. 21 2. 24	AP laxity, functional tests, quadriceps and hamstrings strength, Tegner, Lysholm	Increased AP laxity in group 2; better hop test and figure-8 run in group 1; no difference in strength; group 1 returned to higher activity level; Lysholm, 92 vs 87
Petersen and Laprell,[19] 1999	Level II Prospective cohort	1. Early ACLR + NSx MCL 2. Late ACLR + NSx MCL	1. 27 2. 37	Quadriceps and hamstring isokinetic torque, ROM, need for second arthroscopy, AP/valgus instability, Lysholm, Tegner	No difference in strength, instability, and Tegner; more ROM problems and more second arthroscopies in early ACLR; Lysholm higher in late ACLR (89.9 vs 85.3)

(continued on next page)

Table 5
(*continued*)

Author, Year	Level of Evidence and Type of Study[a]	Groups	Patients	Outcome Measure	Results
Nakamura et al,[20] 2003	Level II Prospective cohort	1. ACLR + NSx MCL 2. ACLR + MCLR	1. 11 2. 6	MRI, IKDC knee evaluation, AP laxity, valgus laxity	MRI classification correlated with resolution of valgus stability; once instability fixed, no difference in outcomes
Robins et al,[5] 1993	Level III Retrospective cohort	All had ACLR and MCL repair 1. Proximal MCL injury 2. Distal MCL injury	1. 13 2. 7	Time to recovery of extension and flexion ROM	Distal tears had faster return of flexion and extension ROM, better maximum flexion, fewer additional procedures required to regain ROM
Aglietti et al,[21] 1991	Level IV Case series	Augmented ACL repair + MCL repair	31	ROM, pain, strength, AP and valgus laxity, second operation	19% had MUA, 29% had motion problems, 1-leg hop >90% in 81% of patients, pivot absent, Lachman 1+ in 35%, valgus 1+ in 29%
Ballmer et al,[22] 1991	Level IV Case series	BPTB ACLR and NSx MCL	14	ROM, clinical and stress radiograph laxity	All returned to preinjury activity; FROM in 12 patients; 2 patients had medial opening of 3–5 mm at 30° flexion; 5 patients had >2 mm AP laxity
Frölke et al,[23] 1998	Level IV Case series	NSx ACL + MCL repair	22	IKDC knee evaluation, clinical examination	100% FROM, improvements in valgus and AP laxity, improvements in IKDC subjective and symptom report
Hughston,[24] 1994	Level IV Case series	ACL debridement or repair of avulsion + repair of MCL and POL	24	Valgus laxity, AP laxity, pivot shift	Valgus: 11 patients had 0, 13 patients had 1+; AP laxity: 12 patients had 0, 7 patients had 1+, 5 patients had 2+; pivot: 18 patients had 0, 4 patients had 1+, 1 patient had 2+

Study	Level of evidence	Treatment	N	Outcome measures	Results
Jokl et al,[15] 1984	Level IV Case series	NSx ACL + NSx MCL	28	Return to activity, HSS knee score	68% returned to previous activity level; HSS, 71% good to excellent
Millett et al,[25] 2004	Level IV Case series	ACLR + MCL NSx	12	Clinical examination, Lysholm, Tegner	No valgus instability; no pivot; Lysholm, 94.6; Tegner, 8.4
Noyes & Barber-Westin,[26] 1995	Level IV Case series	ACLR + MCL repair, 2 patients had MCLR	34	AP and valgus laxity, strength, return to sport	59% had AP laxity <3 mm at 134 N, strength deficits up to 20%, 50% had decreased level of sports
Sankar et al,[27] 2006	Level IV Case series	ACLR + MCL NSx	3	Lysholm, reoperation	96.3 (94–100), 1 patient had arthrofibrosis
Shelbourne and Porter,[28] 1992	Level IV Case series	ACLR + NSx MCL	68	Clinical valgus laxity, AP laxity, ROM, subjective instability, secondary procedures	All had firm valgus endpoint, 2-mm side-side difference in AP laxity, FROM, 9 patients required MUA for flexion, 5 patients required debridement for extension, 96% had no instability episodes
Shirakura et al,[29] 2000	Level IV Case series	ACL NSx + MCL repair	14	Valgus stress, Lysholm, Tegner	1 patient (+) valgus at 0°; 9 patients (+) valgus at 30°; Lysholm, 98.5; Tegner, 5.2
Yoshiya et al,[14] 2005	Level IV Case series	ACLR + MCLR	12	AP and medial laxity, IKDC knee evaluation	AP laxity, 0.3 mm; medial laxity, 2.5 mm; IKDC symptoms, 92% normal/nearly normal; IKDC ROM, 100% normal/nearly normal

Abbreviations: ACLR, anterior cruciate ligament reconstruction; BPTB, bone–patellar tendon–bone graft; FROM, full range of motion; HSS, hospital for special surgery; IKDC, International Knee Documentation Committee; MCLR, medial collateral ligament reconstruction; MCL, medial collateral ligaments; MUA, manipulation under anesthesia; NSx, nonsurgical.

[a] Levels of evidence according to *Journal of Bone and Joint Surgery.*[30]

[b] These 2 studies by Halinen and colleagues[16,17] report on the same group of patients from the same RCT.

From Grant JA, Tannenbaum E, Miller BS, et al. Treatment of combined complete tears of the anterior cruciate and medial collateral ligaments. Arthroscopy 2012;28(1):113–4; with permission.

- ○ The dMCL and POL can also be sewn/reefed to the allograft.
- ○ Layered closure is performed with 0 absorbable suture for the retinaculum followed by interrupted buried 2-0 absorbable sutures and a running subcutaneous 3-0 suture with Steri-Strips.

Postoperative Care

- • Patients are usually kept overnight in observation for pain control and antibiotics.
- • The authors usually use a continuous nerve block catheter, which is removed by the patient within 3 days.
- • Once the catheter has been removed, the authors allow the patient to be full weight bearing with crutches for support as long as the brace is locked in full extension for 6 weeks.
- • The patient should sleep with the brace locked in extension for 4 weeks.
- • The patient should avoid open kinetic chain hamstring work for 6 weeks.
- • Supervised physical therapy typically for 3 to 9 months (**Table 4**).

Complications and Management

- • Arthrofibrosis: This is debatable. Historically, there has been a concern for loss of motion with combined ACL/MCL reconstruction but that has not been proven with recent literature.
- • Saphenous nerve injury: This should be identified and protected during medial exposure.
- • Postoperative laxity: The ACL and MCL exhibit load-sharing properties on both valgus and anterior-posterior stability; therefore, these combined injuries are inherently less stable and subject to laxity and failure if not protected postoperatively.

OUTCOMES

Grant and colleagues[8] performed an excellent systematic review looking at the treatment of combined injuries of the ACL and the MCL (**Table 5**). In patients that underwent an ACL reconstruction with MCL repair, they concluded that distal MCL injuries regain ROM sooner than proximal injuries; 38% of cases required a second operation to regain ROM, and valgus stability is usually achieved, but sagittal-plane laxity will remain in a substantial number of patients.[8] When ACL reconstruction was done with nonoperative MCL treatment, flexion deficits were found more often than extension deficits, and patients generally regain both sagittal and valgus stability.[8] Yoshiya and colleagues[14] looked at patients with chronic instability that underwent both ACL and MCL reconstructions and found normal or near normal ROM and sagittal laxity of 2.5 mm and medial opening of 0.3 mm on valgus stress radiographs. Jokl and colleagues[15] treated combined tears of the ACL and MCL, and at a mean of 3 years, only 68% of people had returned to their previous activity levels with worse results in older patients and recreational athletes.

SUMMARY

1. Diagnosis should start with physical examination and can be confirmed with MRI and radiographs.
2. ACL reconstruction should be done in a delayed fashion after swelling has gone down and ROM has returned. This will allow time for the MCL to potentially heal.
3. Proximal MCL injuries have an excellent chance of healing, and distal MCL injuries should be ruled out for a "Stener"-like lesion of the MCL over the pes anserinus.

4. Grade 1 and 2 MCL injuries can be treated nonoperatively, and increased scrutiny should be given to grade 3 MCL injuries at the time of surgery.
5. After ACL reconstruction, the MCL should be tested with valgus stress testing at 0° and 30° of flexion to evaluate for medial-sided opening of the knee joint necessitating MCL repair or reconstruction.
6. A good rehabilitation protocol is necessary for regaining ROM, strength, and avoiding arthrofibrosis.

DISCLOSURE STATEMENT

The author has nothing to disclose (K.M. Dale). The views expressed in this article are those of the authors and do not necessarily reflect the official policy or position of the Department of the Navy, Department of Defense, or the US Government. "I am a military service member (or employee of the US Government). This work was prepared as part of my official duties. Title 17, USC, §105 provides that 'Copyright protection under this title is not available for any work of the US Government.' Title 17, USC, §101 defines a US Government work as a work prepared by a military service member or employee of the US Government as part of that person's official duties. The study protocol was approved by the Duke University Institutional Review Board in compliance with all applicable Federal regulations governing the protection of human subjects" (J.R. Bailey). Enlyten Sports Strips (stockholder, advisor), Breg (fellowship support), Smith-Nephew (fellowship support), DJO (fellowship support), Mitek (fellowship support), Arthrex (fellowship support), PrivIT (stockholder, advisory board), Regado Biosciences (stockholder), Regenerative Medicine (advisory board), Head Trainer (consultant) (C.T. Moorman).

SUPPLEMENTARY DATA

Supplementary data related to this article can be found at http://dx.doi.org/10.1016/j.csm.2016.08.005.

REFERENCES

1. Miyasaka K, Daniel D, Stone M, et al. The incidence of knee ligament injuries in the general population. Am J Knee Surg 1991;4:3–8.
2. Fetto JF, Marshall JL. Medial collateral ligament injuries of the knee: a rationale for treatment. Clin Orthop Relat Res 1978;(132):206–18.
3. Lyon RM, Akeson WH, Amiel D, et al. Ultrastructural differences between the cells of the medical collateral and the anterior cruciate ligaments. Clin Orthop Relat Res 1991;(272):279–86.
4. Strehl A, Eggli S. The value of conservative treatment in ruptures of the anterior cruciate ligament (ACL). J Trauma 2007;62(5):1159–62.
5. Robins AJ, Newman AP, Burks RT. Postoperative return of motion in anterior cruciate ligament and medial collateral ligament injuries. The effect of medial collateral ligament rupture location. Am J Sports Med 1993;21(1):20–5.
6. Indelicato PA, Hermansdorfer J, Huegel M. Nonoperative management of complete tears of the medial collateral ligament of the knee in intercollegiate football players. Clin Orthop Relat Res 1990;(256):174–7.
7. Woo SL, Young EP, Ohland KJ, et al. The effects of transection of the anterior cruciate ligament on healing of the medial collateral ligament. A biomechanical study of the knee in dogs. J Bone Joint Surg Am 1990;72(3):382–92.

8. Grant JA, Tannenbaum E, Miller BS, et al. Treatment of combined complete tears of the anterior cruciate and medial collateral ligaments. Arthroscopy 2012;28(1): 110–22.

9. Hughston JC, Andrews JR, Cross MJ, et al. Classification of knee ligament instabilities. Part I. The medial compartment and cruciate ligaments. J Bone Joint Surg Am 1976;58(2):159–72.

10. Corten K, Hoser C, Fink C, et al. Case reports: a Stener-like lesion of the medial collateral ligament of the knee. Clin Orthop Relat Res 2010;468(1):289–93.

11. Azar FM. Evaluation and treatment of chronic medial collateral ligament injuries of the knee. Sports Med Arthrosc 2006;14(2):84–90.

12. LaPrade RF, Engebretsen AH, Ly TV, et al. The anatomy of the medial part of the knee. J Bone Joint Surg Am 2007;89(9):2000–10.

13. Wijdicks CA, Michalski MP, Rasmussen MT, et al. Superficial medial collateral ligament anatomic augmented repair versus anatomic reconstruction: an in vitro biomechanical analysis. Am J Sports Med 2013;41(12):2858–66.

14. Yoshiya S, Kuroda R, Mizuno K, et al. Medial collateral ligament reconstruction using autogenous hamstring tendons: technique and results in initial cases. Am J Sports Med 2005;33(9):1380–5.

15. Jokl P, Kaplan N, Stovell P, et al. Non-operative treatment of severe injuries to the medial and anterior cruciate ligaments of the knee. J Bone Joint Surg Am 1984; 66(5):741–4.

16. Halinen J, Lindahl J, Hirvensalo E, et al. Operative and nonoperative treatments of medial collateral ligament rupture with early anterior cruciate ligament reconstruction: a prospective randomized study. Am J Sports Med 2006;34(7): 1134–40.

17. Halinen J, Lindahl J, Hirvensalo E. Range of motion and quadriceps muscle power after early surgical treatment of acute combined anterior cruciate and grade-III medial collateral ligament injuries. A prospective randomized study. J Bone Joint Surg Am 2009;91(6):1305–12.

18. Andersson C, Gillquist J. Treatment of acute isolated and combined ruptures of the anterior cruciate ligament. A long-term follow-up study. Am J Sports Med 1992;20(1):7–12.

19. Petersen W, Laprell H. Combined injuries of the medial collateral ligament and the anterior cruciate ligament. Early ACL reconstruction versus late ACL reconstruction. Arch Orthop Trauma Surg 1999;119(5–6):258–62.

20. Nakamura N, Horibe S, Toritsuka Y, et al. Acute grade III medial collateral ligament injury of the knee associated with anterior cruciate ligament tear. The usefulness of magnetic resonance imaging in determining a treatment regimen. Am J Sports Med 2003;31(2):261–7.

21. Aglietti P, Buzzi R, Zaccherotti G, et al. Operative treatment of acute complete lesions of the anterior cruciate and medial collateral ligaments: a 4- to 7-year follow-up study. Am J Knee Surg 1991;4:186–94.

22. Ballmer PM, Ballmer FT, Jakob RP. Reconstruction of the anterior cruciate ligament alone in the treatment of a combined instability with complete rupture of the medial collateral ligament. A prospective study. Arch Orthop Trauma Surg 1991;110(3):139–41.

23. Frölke JP, Oskam J, Vierhout PA. Primary reconstruction of the medial collateral ligament in combined injury of the medial collateral and anterior cruciate ligaments. Short-term results. Knee Surg Sports Traumatol Arthrosc 1998;6(2):103–6.

24. Hughston JC. The importance of the posterior oblique ligament in repairs of acute tears of the medial ligaments in knees with and without an associated rupture of

the anterior cruciate ligament. Results of long-term follow-up. J Bone Joint Surg Am 1994;76(9):1328–44.

25. Millett PJ, Pennock AT, Sterett WI, et al. Early ACL reconstruction in combined ACL-MCL injuries. J Knee Surg 2004;17(2):94–8.

26. Noyes FR, Barber-Westin SD. The treatment of acute combined ruptures of the anterior cruciate and medial ligaments of the knee. Am J Sports Med 1995; 23(4):380–9.

27. Sankar WN, Wells L, Sennett BJ, et al. Combined anterior cruciate ligament and medial collateral ligament injuries in adolescents. J Pediatr Orthop 2006;26(6): 733–6.

28. Shelbourne KD, Porter DA. Anterior cruciate ligament-medial collateral ligament injury: nonoperative management of medial collateral ligament tears with anterior cruciate ligament reconstruction. A preliminary report. Am J Sports Med 1992; 20(3):283–6.

29. Shirakura K, Terauchi M, Katayama M, et al. The management of medial ligament tears in patients with combined anterior cruciate and medial ligament lesions. Int Orthop 2000;24(2):108–11.

30. Wright JG, Swiontkowski MF, Heckman JD. Introducing levels of evidence to the journal. J Bone Joint Surg Am 2003;85-A(1):1–3.

Surgical Management and Treatment of the Anterior Cruciate Ligament/Posterolateral Corner Injured Knee

⊕ CrossMark

Nicholas I. Kennedy, BA[a,b], Christopher M. LaPrade, BS[c],
Robert F. LaPrade, MD, PhD[b,*]

KEYWORDS

- Posterolateral corner (PLC) • Anterior cruciate ligament (ACL) • Multistaged
- Single stage • Peroneal nerve

KEY POINTS

- Early and accurate diagnosis is of the upmost importance, and an established and verified method for coming to said diagnosis has been adequately described.
- Reconstruction of the posterolateral corner (PLC) is integral to overall function and stability of the tibiofemoral joint and is of particular importance in the native and reconstructed anterior cruciate ligament (ACL).
- Anatomic single-staged reconstruction aimed at most completely replicating the native location and function of the PLC through utilization of definable anatomic landmarks is crucial to postoperative stability.
- With proper surgical technique and appropriate postoperative care, patients with combined PLC/ACL injuries can achieve significantly improved subjective and objective assessment scores.

INTRODUCTION

Assessing overall stability of the anterior cruciate ligament (ACL) deficient knee can often be difficult because of overall instability and tenderness. However, as the understanding of the biomechanics and interdependence of individual stabilizers of the knee evolves, it has become apparent how integral this stability assessment is. Each year, the diagnosis of multiligamentous knee injuries increases because of increased awareness more so than because of increased prevalence. Of those multiligamentous injuries, most involve the ACL and posterolateral corner (PLC).[1]

Disclosure Statement: Dr R.F. LaPrade is a consultant for and receives royalties from Arthrex, Ossur, and Smith & Nephew.
[a] Oregon Health and Science University, 3601 Southwest River Parkway, Unit 519, Portland, OR 97239, USA; [b] Steadman Philippon Research Institute, Vail, CO 81657, USA; [c] Medical College of Wisconsin, 8701 West Watertown Plank Road, Milwaukee, WI 53226, USA
* Corresponding author. Steadman Clinic, 181 West Meadow Drive, Suite 400, Vail, CO 81657.
E-mail address: rlaprade@thesteadmanclinic.com

Clin Sports Med 36 (2017) 105–117
http://dx.doi.org/10.1016/j.csm.2016.08.011
0278-5919/17/© 2016 Elsevier Inc. All rights reserved.

The PLC of the knee has gained more attention in recent years because of increased understanding regarding its anatomy and biomechanical function. The stability of the PLC is of particular importance in regards to ACL reconstruction because it has been shown to be a leading cause of ACL graft failure. LaPrade and colleagues[2] showed the difference in ACL graft forces between deficient and intact PLC structures and found PLC-deficient knees to confer significantly increased forces in comparison to the reconstructed ACL graft. With this in mind, it is important not only to be aware of possible combined ACL and PLC injuries but also to have a standardized approach to the diagnosis and surgical management of said injury.

Standardized Diagnostic Approach

A standardized diagnostic approach to ACL and PLC injured knees is essential. The physical examination is always important and should include the Lachman, pivot shift, dial test at 30° and 90°, posterolateral drawer test with knee at 90° of flexion and 15° of external rotation, and varus stress examination[3] at 0° and 30°. Two additional important examinations, especially in the setting of a multiligamentous knee injury, are the external recurvatum test[4] and the reverse pivot shift. Studies have shown that increased recurvatum in a PLC injured knee suggests a combined ACL injury. The reverse pivot shift is essentially opposite to the pivot shift test and is performed with knee flexed and the foot in external rotation. As the knee is extended, the iliotibial band will reduce the posteriorly subluxed tibia.[3]

However, as previously stated, inflammation, pain, and overall instability make a definitive diagnosis difficult to obtain from physical examination alone. MRI is also helpful and has been shown to be effective in the diagnosis of multiligament injuries.[3,5] However, the gold standard for PLC injuries remains varus stress radiographs. Varus stress radiographs have been validated as a reliable and repeatable objective examination for both isolated fibular collateral ligament (FCL) injuries and combined PLC injuries. LaPrade and colleagues[6] reported that isolated FCL injuries increased varus opening by approximately 2.7 mm; a complete PLC injury led to 4.0 mm of increased gapping, and a combined ACL injury resulted in 5.3 mm of gapping compared with the intact state (**Fig. 1**).

Indications and Contraindications

Once a definitive diagnosis has been made, focus can be turned to surgical reconstruction of the injured structures. Historically, controversy existed on whether to

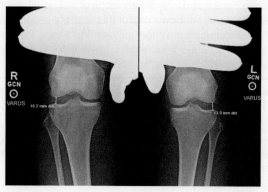

Fig. 1. Varus stress examinations are proven diagnostic techniques for providing quantitative data for PLC injuries.

address the PLC as part of the surgical reconstruction. The reasoning was that mild to moderate medial-sided knee injuries had shown good results with conservative management, with the assumption that PLC injuries should show similar results. However, more recent anatomic studies on the PLC anatomy[7–13] have explained why this is not the case. The PLC of the knee has a unique osseous anatomic structure with a convex lateral tibial plateau articulating with a convex lateral femoral condyle. Therefore, this area of the knee is inherently unstable, preventing the healing of the ligaments. In other words, although PLC structures will undergo scarring down or healing, the knee essentially heals with increased laxity of PLC structures when compared with a native uninjured knee. Other studies have also shown the importance of the PLC structures in regards to forces and stability on ACL reconstructions.[1] These more recent studies have led to a consensus that reconstructing the PLC is necessary not only for the long-term success of an ACL reconstruction but also for restoring native biomechanics and overall stability of the tibiofemoral joint.

SURGICAL TECHNIQUE
Preoperative Planning

In regards to controversies on the surgical technique itself, many still remain. One question that remains prominent is whether to stage the reconstructive technique or address both the ACL and the PLC injuries in a single-stage reconstruction. Advantages to single-stage surgeries are the ability to address all stability issues with the knee in one operation. As mentioned before, failure to address PLC injuries causes increased forces on ACL grafts. Thus, a single-stage surgery allows for stability of the knee to be further restored acutely and should allow for a more aggressive postoperative rehabilitation, which should help to prevent knee motion deficits. Disadvantages to single-stage surgeries are the technical difficulty of the surgery, graft availability, and a slight risk of significant arthrofibrosis, although this last risk can be somewhat combated with early aggressive rehabilitation focused on passive knee motion.

Multistaged surgical technique advantages are simpler individual surgeries, with fewer tunnels and fewer grafts for each individual procedure. Disadvantages include a severely increased treatment and total recovery time, and also increased individual procedures increases risk for surgical complications such as infection and iatrogenic injury.

The investigators suggest a single-staged approach within 3 weeks of injury. The reason for this is 3-fold. First, failure to address the PLC immediately leaves ACL reconstruction at increased risk of failure. Second, acute reconstruction allows for the native anatomic landmarks to be best identified for most anatomic reconstructions. Last, one surgery allows for all issues to be addressed in one operation, leading to a decreased risk of iatrogenic injury with multistaged surgeries and also allows the patient/athlete to initiate their rehabilitation and resume activities faster. Also, a rehabilitation program focused on early knee motion can help to prevent the arthrofibrosis sometimes associated with single-staged procedures.

One pathologic finding, which does argue for a multistaged reconstructive technique in chronic ACL/PLC injuries, is genu varus. Genu varus misalignment in the face of a chronic PLC injury leads to increased forces on the PLC and is associated with a significant risk of graft failure if not corrected.[3,10,14,15] In these cases, a multistaged procedure has been recommended, with the first stage being a proximal tibial osteotomy. It is also worth noting that 38% of the time the proximal tibial osteotomy alone will address the PLC laxity. In most other cases, the osteotomy can be followed after 6 months by a combined ACL/PLC reconstruction.

Preparation and Patient Positioning

First and foremost, it is of the utmost importance to perform an examination under anesthesia. Sometimes, even with the prior physical examination, MRI, and stress radiographs, little subtleties about the injury are missed that can be further ascertained from an examination under anesthesia. At the very least, this examination helps to confirm the diagnosis.

The patient should be in the supine position on the operating table. The foot of the operating table is flexed down, allowing the surgical leg to hang freely at approximately a 70° angle. A well-padded tourniquet is placed around the proximal thigh, and the distal thigh is secured in a leg holder. The nonoperative leg is secured in a leg holder away from the operating field. The operating bed can then be raised to a proper height for the attending surgeon. Once these measures are implemented, proper sterilization and draping can be performed; prophylactic antibiotics can be administered, and the procedure is ready to begin.

Surgical approach and graft preparation

The first order of business is harvest of the graft of choice, a patellar tendon graft, for the ACL reconstruction. Early harvest allows for an assistant to be preparing the graft simultaneous to other operative procedures so time is not wasted later in the procedure. Patellar tendon landmarks are assessed and traced, and a midline incision is made along the superficial skin covering the patellar tendon. Once the incision is made, retraction is done so as to expose the tendon in its entirety. A flexible ruler is then used to measure the width of the tendon at the inferior pole of the patella and the insertion on the tibial tubercle and at a midpoint on tendon. Ideally, the middle 10 mm are measured and marked with a marking pen from proximal to distal.

A surgical blade is then used to dissect out the middle 10 mm of tendon, and a bone saw is used to harvest bone blocks from the patella and tibial tubercle of at least 10 × 1025-mm dimensions. Once the tendon is harvested, it is moved to the preparationtable where an assistant begins to prepare both the patellar tendon graft and an Achilles allograft tendon, which will be needed for the PLC reconstruction.

A split Achilles allograft is the senior author's graft of choice for PLC reconstructions. The calcaneal portion of the graft is split down the middle and the calcaneal bone blocks are shaped to be 9 × 25 mm in dimension. The distal aspects of the Achilles tendon are tubularized for graft passing. The distal ends of the graft, which need to fit through the bone tunnels, should be able to pass easily through a 7-mm-diameter tunnel sizer. However, the more proximal aspect of the graft should be left thicker to restore strength of the popliteus tendon and FCL that they are meant to replace. Passing sutures are placed on both the soft tissue end and the bone block end. The grafts should then be placed under tension and covered with a saline-dampened paper.

The patellar tendon, which has been harvested from the patient, should also be prepared at this point for the ACL reconstruction. The ideal size for this graft is a 10-mm width with bone blocks on either end being sized to 10 × 25-mm dimensions. Passing sutures should again be placed in both ends of the graft. Graft should also be placed under tension and covered with saline-dampened paper to ensure it does not dry out.

With a marking pen, the fibular head, Gerdy tubercle, tibial tubercle, lateral epicondyle, and the best-estimated path of the peroneal nerve should be marked before any PLC incision.[16] The initial superficial hockey-stick incision is made from the posterior midportion of the iliotibial band and extended distally across the knee to the anterior compartment with the incision crossing the knee at the level of Gerdy tubercle.[17] The incision is taken to the depth of the iliotibial band.

The next aspect of the approach is proper identification of the short and long heads of the biceps femoris (**Fig. 2**). These landmarks are of upmost importance in locating the peroneal nerve for the peroneal neurolysis. The peroneal neurolysis is integral to preventing a postoperative foot drop due to increased inflammation present around the peroneal nerve causing compression of the nerve. The neurolysis is important not only for maintaining proper neurologic function of the peroneal nerve and the distal extremity as a whole but also in gaining posteromedial access to the fibular head.

Once the long head of biceps femoris is found, the peroneal nerve can be localized 2 to 3 cm distally (**Fig. 3**). If it is not readily identifiable, it can be palpated 2 cm distal to the fibular head. An extensive decompression, up to 8 cm in length, is necessary to minimize the risk of compression following postoperative swelling and also to ensure gentle retraction during the procedure will not cause iatrogenic injury.

The posteromedial aspect of the fibular head is then exposed via blunt dissection of the soleus. It is here where the popliteofibular ligament inserts and also where the musculotendinous junction of the popliteus tendon can be readily identified.

Next, the distal aspect of the FCL is identified. This identification is done via an incision in the anterior arm of the long head of the biceps femoris proximal to the fibular head (**Fig. 4**), which is extended into the biceps bursa. A traction stitch is placed in the remnant substance of the FCL. This stitch can later be used, by applying distally directed traction, in identifying the femoral attachment of the FCL. The fibular attachment of the FCL can now be subperiosteally resected, and a saddle on the posteromedial aspect of the fibular styloid can be identified, which denotes the insertion of the popliteofibular ligament.

Surgical Procedure

Step 1: drill the transfibular tunnel
With important landmarks of the fibular head identified, the transfibular tunnel can now be drilled. The tunnel should be centered on the attachment of the FCL and drilled in a posteromedial direction so as to exit through the posteromedial downslope of the fibular styloid. It makes sense due to the aim of using this tunnel for both the FCL graft and the reconstructed popliteofibular ligament.

A guide pin is carefully directed along this path using a cruciate aiming device. Protection of the posterior neurovascular structures should be ensured by use of a retractor posterior and medial to fibular head. After proper placement has been confirmed, a 7-mm reamer can be used to overream the tunnel. Again, care should

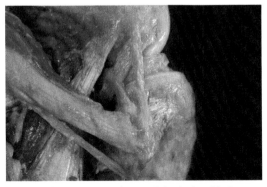

Fig. 2. Anatomic dissection demonstrates the spatial relationship between the structures of the PLC.

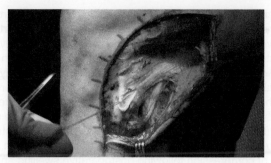

Fig. 3. Left knee shows a suture in the FCL within the biceps bursa and the common peroneal nerve after a neurolysis.

be made to ensure the integrity of the neurovascular structures. Once the fibular tunnel is reamed, a passing suture should be placed in the tunnel to facilitate future graft passage.

Step 2: drill the transtibial tunnel

The next part of the procedure is that which many surgeons deem most unnerving or difficult, and that is the reaming of the transtibial tunnel. Further dissection of the distal attachment of the iliotibial band is needed in order to identify Gerdy tubercle. Posterior and medial to Gerdy tubercle and also adjacent to the lateral aspect of the tibial tubercle is a small flat area. Sharp dissection including rongeur shearing is used to clean soft tissue structures off of the bone. The anterior aperture of the tibial tunnel will be centered on this site.

Attention is then turned to the posterior aspect of this tibial tunnel. Again, the musculotendinous junction of the popliteus tendon is identified, which can be located through the interval between the gastrocnemius and soleus complex. It is at this level approximately 1 cm medial and 1 cm proximal to medial exit of the fibular tunnel that the posterior aspect of the tibial tunnel will exit. An obturator from the arthroscopy set can be placed through the fibular head tunnel to assist in identifying this tibial tunnel posterior exit site.

Before drilling the tibial tunnel, the neurovascular structures of the posterior aspect of the tibia must be protected with a retractor to prevent iatrogenic injury. An ACL

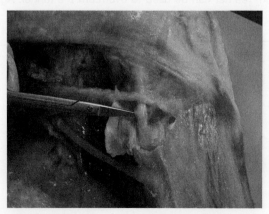

Fig. 4. Dissection shows the distal aspect of the FCL and its relation to the other structures of the PLC.

aiming device is then used to direct a guide pin from the flat area, which has been cleared on the anterior aspect of the tibia to the musculotendinous junction of the popliteus on the posterior tibia. When proper placement of the drill pin has been confirmed, the guide pin can then be overreamed with a 9-mm-diameter reamer (**Fig. 5**).

Step 3: localize and drill the posterolateral corner femoral tunnels

Attention is now turned to the femoral attachments of the structures of the PLC. The authors use the traction sutures previously placed in the midsubstance of the FCL to identify the femoral attachment of the FCL. Although applying posterior traction on the FCL, the superficial fibers of the iliotibial band are split in line with their fibers just anterior to the attachment of the FCL; this provides optimal exposure. The femoral attachment of the popliteus tendon is 18.5 mm anterior and distal to the femoral attachment of the FCL (**Fig. 6**).[16] The femoral attachment of the popliteus tendon is located on the anterior fifth and proximal half of the popliteal sulcus, and a vertical incision through the lateral capsule of the knee allows the femoral attachment of the popliteus to be visualized. If the attachment is not readily identifiable, the knee can be flexed to 70° and the fibular shaft can be followed across the knee. At this angle of knee flexion, the FCL courses parallel to the fibular shaft, and the femoral attachment of the popliteus tendon will be approximately 2 cm anterior to the FCL attachment.

After the femoral attachments have been identified, the femoral tunnels can be reamed. The FCL femoral tunnel is addressed first and the guide pin is directed anteromedially to avoid the intercondylar notch and the saphenous nerve. A second guide pin is placed parallel to the FCL guide pin with the distance between the guide pins being measured at 18.5 mm, with the popliteus guide pin being slightly anterior and distal on the femur. This spacing is very important because proper spacing is needed not only for proper anatomic location of the tunnels but also to ensure a sufficient bone bridge exists between the 2 femoral tunnels. When proper guide pin placement has been confirmed, the tunnels can be overreamed by a 9-mm reamer to the depth of 25 mm for both tunnels. Passing sutures are then passed into both tunnels to facilitate later graft passage.

Step 4: intra-articular phase

Once the PLC femoral tunnels have been prepared, attention can be turned to the intra-articular aspect of the surgery and the ACL abnormality. Two portals are created,

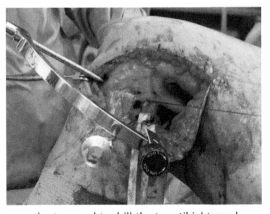

Fig. 5. The technique and setup used to drill the transtibial tunnel.

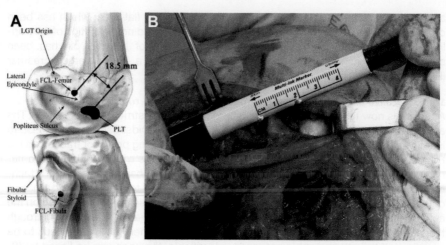

Fig. 6. (*A*) Portrayal of the anatomic location of the femoral attachments of the popliteus tendon and FCL. (*B*) Location of the femoral tunnels of both the popliteus tendon and the FCL. LGT, lateral gastrocnemius tendon; PLT, popliteus tendon.

one anteromedial and one anterolateral. Using the anteromedial portal, the tibial and femoral attachments of the ACL are identified as well as the overall integrity of the ACL. Once that has been established, the meniscal bodies and root attachments as well as overall meniscal integrity are assessed. When meniscus integrity has been confirmed, attention can be turned back to the ACL. An anteromedial portal is now created. The anteromedial portal is used to drill a guide pin between the anteromedial and posterolateral footprints of the ACL. Once guide pin location has been confirmed, a 10-mm reamer can be used to drill a closed socket tunnel to the depth of at least 25 mm to accommodate the femoral ACL bone block. A passing stitch is then placed to allow for later passing of the ACL graft.

The tibial tunnel guide is now positioned just medial to the distal aspect of the tibial tubercle. The ACL tibial guide is used, through the anteromedial portal, and is set at a 65° angle with the guide centered on the tibial footprint of the ACL. The location of the guide pin is important because more recent anatomic studies regarding the tibial footprint and tibial tunnel reaming have shown that any deviation of the tunnel anterior leads to a possibility of iatrogenic injury of the meniscal roots, particularly the anterior root of the lateral meniscus (**Fig. 7**).[18] When the guide is properly positioned and a guide pin has been placed, the pin can then be overreamed with a 10-mm reamer.

The previously placed passing stitch is then pulled down the tibial tunnel. The passing stitch is then used to pull one end of the patellar tendon graft into the femoral tunnel. Fixation in the femoral end is then performed using a 7 × 20-mm titanium screw, while tension is applied to the passing suture.

Step 5: fixation of posterolateral corner grafts

After femoral fixation, attention is turned back to the PLC because tibial fixation of the ACL graft at this stage would lead to increased risk of external rotation deformity. The Achilles PLC grafts can be passed in a femoral-to-tibial direction. Similar to the ACL graft, femoral fixation of the PLC grafts is performed first. The passing sutures that form the bone plugs are placed in the looped passing sutures and pulled into the femoral tunnels. Once a tight fit for both grafts is confirmed, two 7 × 20-mm cannulated screws are fitted to a handheld drill chuck. A guide pin is used protruding past

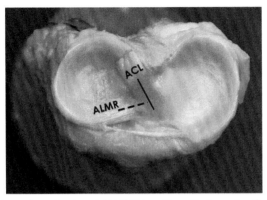

Fig. 7. The anterolateral meniscal root (ALMR) has fibers that overlay the tibial attachment of the ACL.

the screw and is positioned at the margin between the bone plug and the tunnel edge for optimal location of screw fixation.

After femoral fixation, the popliteus tendon is passed distally along the popliteal hiatus and exits the knee in the interval between the lateral gastrocnemius and the soleus. The FCL is then passed toward the fibular head coursing medial or deep to the superficial iliotibial band and lateral aponeurosis of the long head of the biceps femoris. Passage of the FCL graft through the fibular tunnel is achieved with a suture or suture passer. If further graft trimming is needed to ease graft passage, that can be performed at this juncture.

Fixation of the FCL graft is now performed with the knee positioned at 20° of knee flexion, and neutral rotation while a valgus force is being applied.[17] The distal end of the graft is then pulled in a proximal direction and the graft is fixed with a 7-mm bio-absorbable screw in the fibular head tunnel. Following fixation of the FCL graft, a physical examination should be performed to ensure varus stability has been restored. The distal end of the popliteus graft and the distal-most aspect of the FCL graft, which will now be used to reconstruct the popliteofibular ligament, are now passed posterior to anterior through the tibial tunnel. Each graft needs to be cycled individually to ensure no residual laxity and so that proper tension is applied. The posterior entry site of the tunnel should also be palpated to ensure smooth entry of grafts into the tunnel and no graft bunching.

The knee is then taken to 60° of flexion and neutral rotation. Both grafts are individually tensioned while they are fixed with a 9-mm bioabsorbable screw at the anterior tibial tunnel aperture. Again, a physical examination, including both posterolateral drawer and dial tests, is performed to ensure rotational stability is restored. If thought necessary, a backup screw and washer or staple can be used for maximal fixation in patients with concerns of osteopenic bone (**Fig. 8**).

Step 6: tibial fixation of anterior cruciate ligament graft
With rotational stability restored, tibial fixation of the ACL graft can now occur. The ACL graft is then tensioned in the tibial tunnel and fixed with a 9 × 20-mm titanium interference screw while distal traction was being applied to the graft.

The subcutaneous tissues can be repaired with absorbable sutures in the fashion of attending surgeon's choice. A running absorbable suture is then also used for skin closure of the larger incisions, while portals can be closed with absorbable sutures and a simple subcuticular stitch. Loose skin taping is a secondary measure to ensure

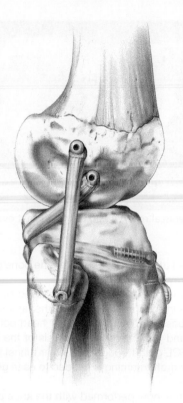

Fig. 8. The correct anatomic location of the PLC grafts.

adequate closure. The incisions should also be sterilely dressed and the knee placed in an immobilizer before termination of anesthesia; this minimizes stress on the reconstruction when the patient awakens.

COMPLICATIONS AND MANAGEMENT

Infection and wound dehiscence remain potential risks as they are with any invasive procedure. Foot drop from common peroneal nerve laceration or compression remains a reported complication, although the steps outlined for peroneal neurolysis should help to minimize this risk. Graft stretching and failure also remain reported risks. This potential of graft stretching or failure is what makes the rehabilitation protocol of utmost importance with objective stepping stones and goals laid out along the way. With new data suggesting increased collagen density of grafts at 1 year versus 6 months,[19] the authors of this segment are beginning to prolong the rehabilitation duration and delay a return to sport to ensure complete healing for long-term restoration of knee stability.

POSTOPERATIVE CARE

Rehabilitation instructions should be explicitly explained to the patient and their physical therapist.[20] Rehabilitation includes 6 weeks of non-weight-bearing with the patient wearing an immobilizer while ambulating. Early knee motion exercises are key, and the first 2 weeks should be focused on regaining passive knee motion from 0 to 90 with passive motion exercises being done up to 4 times per day. Regaining quadriceps function should be another goal of the first 2 weeks with quadriceps contraction sets and straight leg raises, in the knee immobilizer, also being done 4 times daily. If the patient can perform straight leg raises without an extensor lag at 2 weeks, then they can perform quad sets and straight leg raises without the knee immobilizer.

After 2 weeks, knee motion can be gradually advanced with a goal of attaining full knee motion by 6 weeks. After 6 weeks, patients can slowly be weaned off of crutches with weight bearing as tolerated if limping is absent. When knee flexion reaches greater than 110° to 115°, then a stationary bike and low-resistance exercises can be initiated.

At 12 weeks postoperatively, low-impact exercises, such as swimming, cycling, walking, and using an elliptical machine, are permissible, with the goal of attaining full strength and range of motion in activities by 6 months. After 6 months, varus stress radiographs are performed to assess stability. Return to play varies depending on the individual and the sport of choice, but goal of return to competition by 1 year is usually attainable.

OUTCOMES

There is some paucity regarding long-term follow-up on these combined injuries, because of both the relative rarity of the injury and the age of the surgical techniques. That being said, outcomes studies that have been done are very encouraging. LaPrade and colleagues[21] looked at 64 patients with chronic PLC injuries, including 22 with concurrent ACL injuries. Objective scores such as varus opening at 20°, external rotation at 30°, reverse pivot shift, and single leg hop were all shown to have significant postoperative improvement. In 2011, Geeslin and LaPrade[22] evaluated outcomes following acute PLC injuries. In their study, 29 patients, including 10 with concurrent ACL tears, were followed. Patients were found to have significantly improved mean Cincinnati (21.9 initial to 81.4 follow-up), mean International Knee Documentation Committee score (29.1–81.5), and varus stress radiograph gapping side-to-side difference (6.2–0.1 mm). These studies would suggest that the ligaments do not heal as well in chronic injuries, which seem to be more detrimental to the long-term success of chronic PLC reconstructions. The investigators recommend early PLC reconstruction, within the first 3 weeks and preferably by day 14,[23,24] with an early preoperative focus on reducing inflammation and regaining knee motion with an aim of 0° to 130° by postoperative week 6.

SUMMARY

Because of the devastating affects ACL/PLC injuries have on joint stability and subjective measures, it is imperative to have a definitive diagnostic and treatment approach. In this article, the authors have outlined both a reproducible and an accurate means of diagnosis and an anatomically derived reconstructive technique. With this template in place, the task of addressing combined ACL/PLC injured knees need not be so daunting.

REFERENCES

1. LaPrade RF, Wentorf FA, Fritts H, et al. A prospective magnetic resonance imaging study of the incidence of posterolateral and multiple ligament injuries in acute knee injuries presenting with a hemarthrosis. Arthroscopy 2007;23(12):1341–7.

2. LaPrade RF, Resig S, Wentorf F, et al. The effects of grade III posterolateral knee complex injuries on anterior cruciate ligament graft forces. Am J Sports Med 1999;27(4):469–75.
3. LaPrade RF, Wentorf F. Diagnosis and treatment of posterolateral knee injuries. Clin Orthop Relat Res 2002;402:110–21.
4. LaPrade RF, Ly TV, Griffith C. The external rotation recurvatum test revisited: reevaluation of the sagittal plane tibiofemoral relationship. Am J Sports Med 2008;36(4):709–12.
5. LaPrade RF, Gilbert TJ, Bollom TS, et al. The magnetic resonance imaging appearance of individual structures of the posterolateral knee. A prospective study of normal knees and knees with surgically verified grade III injuries. Am J Sports Med 2000,20(2).191–9.
6. LaPrade RF, Heikes C, Bakker AJ, et al. The reproducibility and repeatability of varus stress radiographs in the assessment of isolated fibular collateral ligament and grade-III posterolateral knee injuries. An in vitro biomechanical study. J Bone Joint Surg Am 2008;90(10):2069–76.
7. LaPrade RF. Arthroscopic evaluation of the lateral compartment of knees with grade 3 posterolateral knee complex injuries. Am J Sports Med 1997;25: 596–602.
8. LaPrade RF, Hamilton CD. The fibular collateral ligament-biceps femoris bursa. An anatomic study. Am J Sports Med 1997;25:439–43.
9. LaPrade RF, Hamilton CD, Engebretsen L. Treatment of acute and chronic combined anterior cruciate ligament and posterolateral knee ligament injuries. Sports Med Arthrosc Rev 1997;5:91–9.
10. LaPrade RF, Terry GC. Injuries to the posterolateral aspect of the knee: association of anatomic injury patterns with clinical instability. Am J Sports Med 1997;25: 433–8.
11. Stäubli HU, Birrer S. The popliteus tendon and its fascicles at the popliteal hiatus: gross anatomy and functional arthroscopic evaluation with and without anterior cruciate ligament deficiency. Arthroscopy 1990;6:209–20.
12. Terry GC, LaPrade RF. The posterolateral aspect of the knee: anatomy and surgical approach. Am J Sports Med 1996;24:732–9.
13. Terry GC, LaPrade RF. The biceps femoris muscle complex at the knee: its anatomy and injury patterns associated with acute anterolateral-anteromedial rotatory instability. Am J Sports Med 1996;24:2–8.
14. Harner CD, Vogrin TM, Höher J, et al. Biomechanical analysis of a posterior cruciate ligament reconstruction: deficiency of the posterolateral structures as a cause of graft failure. Am J Sports Med 2000;28:32–9.
15. Neuschwander DC, Drez D, Paine RM. Simultaneous high tibial osteotomy and ACL reconstruction for combined genu varus and symptomatic ACL tear. Orthopedics 1993;16:679–84.
16. LaPrade RF, Ly TV, Wentorf FA, et al. The posterolateral attachments of the knee: a qualitative and quantitative morphologic analysis of the fibular collateral ligament, popliteus tendon, popliteofibular ligament, and lateral gastrocnemius tendon. Am J Sports Med 2003;31(6):854–60.
17. LaPrade RF, Spiridonov SI, Coobs PR, et al. Fibular collateral ligament anatomical reconstructions: a prospective outcomes study. Am J Sports Med 2010;38(10): 2005–11.
18. Watson JN, Wilson KJ, LaPrade CM, et al. Iatrogenic injury of the anterior meniscal root attachments following anterior cruciate ligament reconstruction tunnel reaming. Knee Surg Sports Traumatol Arthrosc 2015;23(8):2360–6.

19. Rabuck SJ, Baraga MG, Fu FH. Anterior cruciate ligament healing and advances in imaging. Clin Sports Med 2013;32(1):13–20.
20. Lunden JB, Bzdusek PJ, Monson JK, et al. Current concepts in the recognition and treatment of posterolateral corner injuries of the knee. J Orthop Sports Phys Ther 2010;40(8):502–16.
21. LaPrade RF, Johansen S, Agel J, et al. Outcomes of an anatomic posterolateral knee reconstruction. J Bone Joint Surg Am 2010;92:16–22.
22. Geeslin AG, LaPrade RF. Outcomes of treatment of acute grade-III isolated and combined posterolateral knee injuries: a prospective case series and surgical technique. J Bone Joint Surg Am 2011;93(18):1672–83.
23. Harner CD, Waltrip RL, Bennett CH, et al. Surgical management of knee dislocations. J Bone Joint Surg Am 2004;86-A(2):262–73.
24. Ibrahim SA, Ahmad FH, Salah M, et al. Surgical management of traumatic knee dislocation. Arthroscopy 2008;24(2):178–87.

Surgical Management and Treatment of the Anterior Cruciate Ligament–Deficient Knee with Malalignment

Matthew D. Crawford, MD*, Lee H. Diehl, MD, Annunziato Amendola, MD

KEYWORDS

- ACL deficiency • Varus malalignment • Tibial slope • HTO

KEY POINTS

- Malalignment can increase stress on anterior cruciate ligament (ACL) reconstruction, contributing to recurrent instability.
- Varus malalignment can lead to overload of the medial compartment and symptomatic arthritis.
- Realignment osteotomy can reduce symptoms of ACL instability and unload or reduce mechanical wear of the medial compartment.
- Correction of varus malalignment can improve outcomes of revision ACL reconstruction.
- Changes of tibial slope can affect symptomatic ACL laxity.

INTRODUCTION

In all patients with knee instability, arthritis, or combined instability and arthritis, a thorough evaluation of coronal (varus or valgus) and sagittal alignment (tibial slope) should be performed. Individuals with ligamentous injury compounded by predisposing malalignment have a higher failure rate with soft tissue reconstruction alone. Malalignment can be a cause of recurrent instability following anterior cruciate ligament (ACL) reconstruction. There are 2 common forms of malalignment that can exacerbate instability and arthritis in an ACL-deficient knee: varus malalignment with early

Disclosures: M.D. Crawford and L.H. Diehl have nothing to disclose. A. Amendola has associations with Arthrex (consultant, royalties), Smith and Nephew (royalties), Arthrosurface (royalties, stock), First Ray (Scientific Advisory Board [SAB], stock).
Department of Orthopaedic Surgery, Duke University Medical Center, Duke University, Box 3000, Durham, NC 27710, USA
* Corresponding author.
E-mail address: matthew.crawford@duke.edu

medial compartment arthritis and/or meniscal deficiency; or increased posterior tibial slope, which can result in increased anterior tibial translation.

In the symptomatic ACL-deficient knee with varus malalignment, the degree and nature of malalignment are important to evaluate. Primary varus refers to the tibiofemoral osseous alignment, including any underlying medial meniscal damage and medial tibiofemoral articular cartilage loss. With a potential loss of proprioception and neuromuscular control after ACL injury,[1] this varus malalignment can be exacerbated dynamically. Double varus refers to elongation of the lateral soft tissue restraints, with lateral tibiofemoral compartment separation (lateral condylar liftoff). Triple varus occurs when chronic stress on the posterolateral structures leads to increased external tibial rotation and a hyperextension recurvatum deformity.[2,3] In triple-varus knees, the medial compartment tends to have a posterior medial tibial wear pattern, thought to be caused by a chronic anterior subluxation of the tibia with respect to the femur[4] (Fig. 1A). van de Pol and colleagues[5] showed a direct relationship between varus alignment and ACL tension and suggested that malalignment may lead to ACL reconstruction failure (Fig. 2).

Excess posterior tibial slope can also contribute to knee instability in the ACL-deficient knee. Dejour and Bonnin[6] and Giffin and colleagues[7] showed that an increase in tibial slope can lead to increased anterior tibial translation, resulting in symptomatic knee instability (Fig. 1B). Rodner and colleagues[8] and Agneskirchner and colleagues[9] studied cartilage and joint kinematics and showed that increasing tibial slope shifts contact pressures to the posterior plateau and a tibial flexion osteotomy can help to redistribute pressure away from the damaged posterior cartilage.

INDICATIONS/CONTRAINDICATIONS

High tibial osteotomy (HTO) is a proven procedure used to redistribute mechanical forces across the knee joint. Indications include knee instability, varus alignment of the knee with associated early medial compartment arthrosis, medial compartment overload following meniscectomy, and osteochondral defects requiring resurfacing

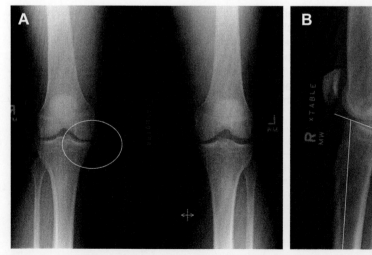

Fig. 1. Patient with symptoms of knee instability and examination findings of ACL laxity, lateral gapping, and varus thrust during gait. Anteroposterior (AP) (A) and lateral (B) radiographs show varus alignment (circle in A) with an increased posterior tibial slope (B).

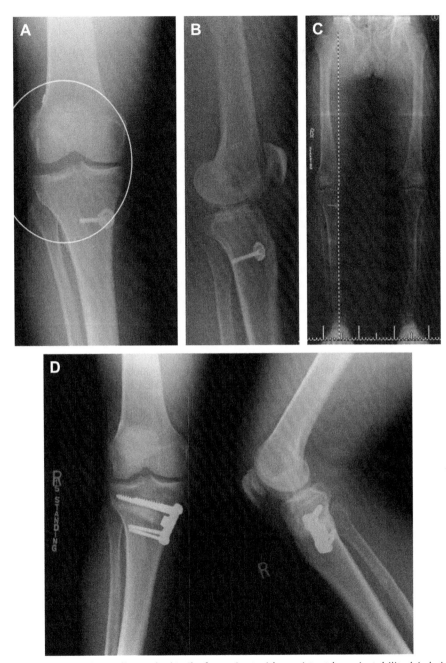

Fig. 2. Preoperative radiographs (*A–C*) of a patient with persistent knee instability (*circle in A*) 2 years after ACL reconstruction with allograft showing varus alignment. The patient underwent an opening wedge high tibial osteotomy with posteromedial placement of the plate to decrease slope and prevent anterior tibial translation. One-year postoperative film (*D*) shows maintained alignment and correction.

procedures.[10] Indications have expanded to include correcting the tibial slope in sagittal instability.[11,12]

The use of a combined ACL reconstruction and HTO in the acute setting is rarely indicated with symmetric varus alignment.

Contraindications to HTO include patellofemoral arthrosis, markedly decreased range of motion (arc of motion <120° and flexion contracture >5°),[13] severe articular damage of the medial compartment (Ahlbäck grade III or higher), tricompartmental arthritis,[14] and persons aged more than 50 years.[13,14] Relative contraindications also include obesity and smoking.[15]

During the clinical examination, it is important to evaluate lower limb alignment dynamically in all 3 planes and observe the patient's gait for any abnormalities, especially varus thrust. Knee range of motion should be assessed and any contractures noted. The patellofemoral joint should be examined for crepitus, tenderness to palpation, instability or malalignment, and signs of arthritis.

Patients commonly complain of pain on the medial aspect of the knee with tenderness along the medial joint line, the posteromedial tibial plateau, and medial femoral condyle. The use of an unloader brace can be diagnostic because it may confirm the need to unload the medial knee joint.

It is important to assess the entire clinical picture and try to differentiate the cause of a patient's complaints; for example, pain with sports activities and pivoting movements may indicate instability, versus pain with activities of daily living potentially indicating medial compartment overload. In young patients with symptoms of instability and underlying malalignment, with other meniscal or chondral disorders, ACL reconstruction should be considered in addition to an HTO. Older or less active patients are likely to respond to osteotomy alone if they have mechanical overload symptoms.[16] If the patient complains of instability after HTO, ACL reconstruction can then be considered as a secondary procedure. Conservative care should always be optimized, including bracing, physical therapy, and activity modification, before pursuing surgical treatment.

SURGICAL TECHNIQUE/PROCEDURE
Preoperative Planning

- Clinical evaluation
  - Assess physical examination findings of joint line tenderness, abnormal gait patterns (eg, varus thrust), and varus/recurvatum limb alignment in stance.
  - Perform instability tests, including Lachman, pivot shift, anterior and posterior drawer, reverse pivot shift, external rotation tests.
- Radiographs
  - Bilateral standard weight-bearing long-leg (hip to ankle) anteroposterior views.
  - Bilateral weight-bearing posteroanterior tunnel views in 30° of flexion.
  - Standard anteroposterior views in full extension, lateral views, and Merchant patellar views.
- Advanced imaging
  - MRI to confirm ACL status and evaluate for chondral, meniscal, and soft tissue injury.
- Overall factors to consider
  - Pure varus or valgus malalignment.
  - Varus thrust suggesting lateral ligament injury.
  - Excess tibial slope associated with ACL deficiency. Physiologic slope in adults has been noted to be 0° to 18°.[17] In cases of ACL deficiency or ACL

reconstruction failure, Dejour and colleagues[18] recommend correction of tibial slope if it exceeds 12°.
- ○ Triple-varus knee.
- ○ Degree of unicompartmental degeneration (ie, postmeniscectomy).
- Planning the opening wedge osteotomy in the coronal plane (as described by Dugdale and colleagues[19]) (**Fig. 3**)
  - ○ Determine the weight-bearing line (line connecting the center of the femoral head to the center of the ankle). Identify the point halfway between 50% and 75% (approximately 62.5%) of the width of the tibial plateau as measured from the tip of the medial edge of the proximal tibia. This point is slightly lateral to the tip of the lateral tibial spine and represents correction of 3° to 5° of mechanical valgus. One line is drawn from this point to the center of the femoral head and 1 line is drawn to the center of the ankle joint. The angle formed at the intersection of these lines represents the angle of correction (alpha angle).
  - ○ Draw the osteotomy line (ab). Start approximately 4 cm below the medial joint line and draw a line to the tip of the fibular head.
  - ○ Transfer this line segment to both rays of the alpha angle starting at the vertex (creating 2 line segments, a^ib^i and a^ic). Connect these segments, creating b^ic, which serves as the base of an isosceles triangle and corresponds with the opening that should be achieved medially at the osteotomy site.

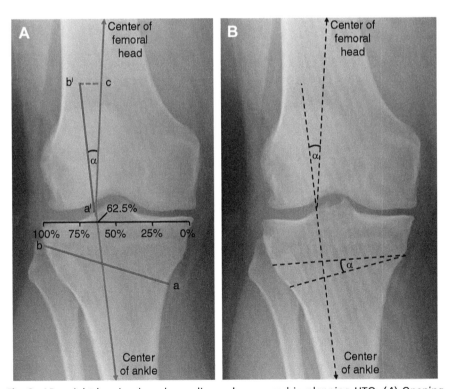

Fig. 3. AP weight-bearing long-leg radiographs are used in planning HTO. (*A*) Opening wedge. (*B*) Closing wedge. See text for planning steps. (*From* Rossi R, Bonasia DE, Amendola A. The role of high tibial osteotomy in the varus knee. J Am Acad Orthop Surg 2011;19(10):592; with permission.)

- Planning the closing wedge osteotomy
  - The alpha angle is calculated as described for the opening wedge osteotomy.
  - Draw the 2 osteotomy lines. Start approximately 2 to 2.5 cm below the medial joint line and draw the proximal osteotomy line horizontally. The distal osteotomy line should define the angle of correction (alpha angle).
- Planning the sagittal plane correction
  - Anterior tibial translation can be reduced by decreasing the tibial slope.
  - Evaluation of the slope is performed using a lateral radiograph of the knee.
  - It is important to pay careful attention to tibial slope during preoperative planning, because Marti and colleagues[20] showed that medial opening wedge osteotomy can lead to a mean increase in tibial slope. The slope can be adjusted by the type of plate (ie, rectangular or tapered) and the positioning of the plate.[21] Posteromedial placement of either a rectangular wedge plate or tapered wedge plate results in decreased slope and reduced anterior tibial translation. Care should be taken to avoid anteromedial placement of a rectangular wedge plate, which may result in increased slope and effectively increase anterior tibial translation (**Fig. 4**).
  - If the opening is greater than 1 cm anteriorly, tibial tubercle osteotomy should be considered to maintain physiologic patellar height.

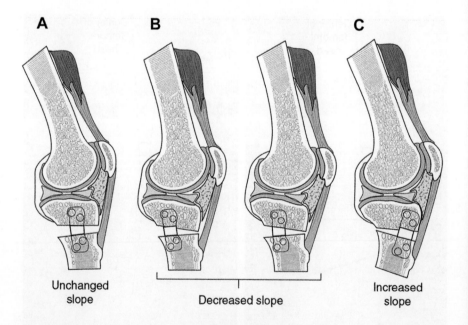

Fig. 4. Posterior tibial slope correction based on plate shape and positioning. (*A*) Medial placement of a plate with a rectangular wedge should not alter the slope. (*B*) In an ACL-deficient knee, posteromedial placement of either a rectangular wedge plate or a tapered wedge plate results in decreased slope and reduced anterior tibial translation. (*C*) In a posterior cruciate ligament–deficient knee, anteromedial placement of a rectangular wedge plate results in increased slope and reduced posterior tibial translation. (*From* Rossi R, Bonasia DE, Amendola A. The role of high tibial osteotomy in the varus knee. J Am Acad Orthop Surg 2011;19(10):596; with permission.)

The senior author prefers the medial opening wedge osteotomy to the lateral closing wedge osteotomy. It avoids osteotomy of the proximal fibula, decreasing the risk of instability through the proximal tibiofibular joint and posterolateral corner structures as well as injury to the peroneal nerve. The medial opening wedge osteotomy allows for correction in the sagittal and coronal planes, and in the setting of ACL reconstruction it can also provide access for hamstring autograft through the same incision.

Prep and Patient Positioning

- Supine on a radiolucent operating table
- C-arm is positioned for fluoroscopic guidance
- A lateral post is positioned at the level of the thigh so that the foot can be dropped out of the table and at least 120° of knee flexion can be achieved
- A tourniquet is placed around the proximal thigh
- Intravenous antibiotics are administered

Surgical Approach

- A complete diagnostic arthroscopy is performed using standard anteromedial and anterolateral portals to evaluate the condition of the articular cartilage, menisci, and cruciate ligaments. Once arthroscopy has been completed, the extremity is elevated and exsanguinated and the tourniquet remains inflated for the remainder of the osteotomy procedure.
- A 5-cm longitudinal incision is made, extending from 1 cm below the medial joint line midway between the medial border of the tibial tubercle and the posteromedial border of the tibia. If a hamstring autograft will be used during subsequent ACL reconstruction, harvesting of the graft is performed at this stage to avoid damage to the tendons during proximal tibia exposure. The sartorius fascia is exposed and the pes anserinus is retracted distally with a blunt retractor, exposing the superficial medial collateral ligament (sMCL). The distal sMCL is partially detached with a Cobb elevator and a blunt retractor is placed deep to the medial collateral ligament (MCL), between the capsule and medial gastrocnemius muscle belly, to protect the posterior neurovascular structures. The medial border of the patellar tendon is identified and retracted laterally. Subperiosteal exposure of the proximal tibia is then performed from the tibial tubercle around to its posteromedial corner, staying extra-articular.

SURGICAL PROCEDURE
Coronal Plane Osteotomy (Opening Wedge)

- Under fluoroscopic guidance, a guidewire is inserted, beginning on the anteromedial tibia at the level of the superior border of the tibial tubercle (approximately 4 cm distal to the joint line). The wire is oriented obliquely and aimed toward the tip of the fibular head (1 cm below the lateral articular surface). This trajectory keeps it proximal to the patellar tendon insertion and sufficiently inferior to the articular surface to prevent intraarticular fracture during the cut. The osteotomy takes advantage of its metaphyseal location to maximize stability and healing potential.
- The tibial osteotomy is performed immediately distal to the guidewire to avoid proximal migration of the osteotomy into the joint. The slope of the osteotomy in the sagittal plane should mimic the slope of the proximal tibia joint. A small oscillating saw is used to cut the tibial cortex from the tibial tubercle around to the posteromedial corner under direct visualization. Graduated flexible osteotomes are used to advance the osteotomy to within 1 cm of the lateral cortex

using intermittent fluoroscopy as needed. Two or three osteotomies can be stacked on top of one another. The mobility of the osteotomy is checked by gentle manipulation of the leg with a valgus force. Graduated wedges are then impacted and advanced slowly until the desired opening is achieved. Care is taken not to disrupt the lateral cortex.

- A long alignment rod, centered over the hip and ankle joints, is used to check the mechanical axis. As calculated preoperatively, the rod should lie at approximately 62.5% of the tibial width, measured from medial to lateral.
- The sagittal plane correction should also be assessed fluoroscopically and under direct visualization. Distracting the osteotomy more anteriorly or posteriorly can change the posterior tibial slope. Because the tibia has a triangular shape, if the opening at the anteromedial tibia is approximately half the size of the opening at the posteromedial tibia, the preexisting slope will be generally maintained. The wedges and plate can be moved posteriorly to decrease the slope or anteriorly to increase the slope. If the opening is more than 1 cm anterior, a tibial tubercle osteotomy is performed to advance the tubercle the same height as the osteotomy.
- Once the desired opening has been achieved, the plate is placed and the wedges are removed. There are various plating options, including conventional, locking, short or long, and with a spacer (ie, rectangular or tapered) or without a spacer.[22] The size of the spacer should match the opening created with the wedges.
- The plate is fixed proximally with 6.5-mm cancellous screws and distally with 4.5-mm cortical screws. Fluoroscopic guidance is used to assess screw positioning. Attention should be paid to positioning the proximal screws in order to have enough bone for the tibial tunnel of the ACL reconstruction (**Fig. 5**).
- Tibial slope can be further decreased when fixing the plate. One distal screw is positioned to initially fix the plate and then the knee is kept in full extension while a proximal screw is inserted. Holding the leg in extension ensures that the osteotomy gap will close anteriorly and the slope will decrease.
- An ACL reconstruction can be performed at this point in the procedure, with grafting of the osteotomy site at the conclusion of the procedure using the preferred bone graft (ie, iliac crest autograft, allograft, bone substitutes). Corticocancellous autograft or allograft is recommended for an opening measuring greater than 10 mm.[22]

Sagittal Plane Osteotomy (Anterior Closing Wedge)

- An anterior longitudinal incision is performed midline or just medial to the tibial tuberosity. The patellar tendon insertion is exposed, and then subperiosteal dissection is performed medially deep to the MCL. A sharp Hohmann is used as a retractor for the deep MCL. Laterally, dissection is performed to the tibiofibular joint
- The base of the wedge is anterior and just above the insertion of the patellar tendon. At the level of the superior edge of the wedge, 2 parallel Kirschner wires are inserted under fluoroscopic guidance on both sides of the patellar tendon until they are touching the posterior tibial cortex parallel to the articular surface. The superior cut is made with a thin microsagittal blade just below and in line with the guide pins just short of the posterior cortex. The inferior cut is made to meet the superior cut at the posterior cortex. The patellar tendon is protected from the oscillating saw using spreaders. The wedge is resected and, if remaining bone is present, small needle-nose rongeurs are used to remove it medially, laterally, and posteriorly, always trying to keep the posterior cortical hinge intact.

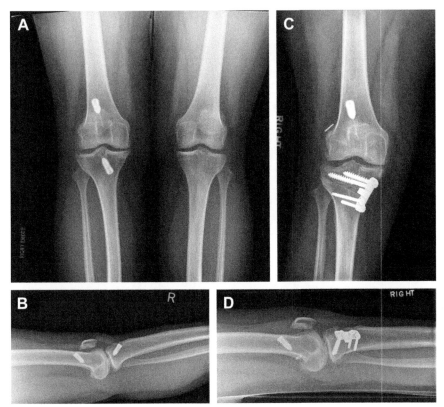

Fig. 5. Patient with persistent knee instability after ACL reconstruction. Preoperative radiographs (*A, B*) show varus deformity with increased anterior tibial translation. The patient underwent opening wedge HTO plus revision ACL reconstruction with postoperative radiographs (*C, D*) showing improved coronal and sagittal alignment.

The authors consider that 1 mm is equal to 1°. The anterior closing wedge osteotomy is compressed simply by extending the knee, thereby exerting pressure by the femoral condyles onto the anterior tibial plateau, closing the wedge. When the resected surfaces are united, fixation is achieved through 2 large staples or 2 eight plates on either side of the patellar tendon, or a small T plate (**Fig. 6**).

ANTERIOR CRUCIATE LIGAMENT RECONSTRUCTION

- The osteotomy should be performed before the ACL reconstruction. Performing the ACL reconstruction first risks damage to the graft during the tibial bone cut, loosening or tightening of the newly tensioned graft, and the possibility of creating a stress riser through the ACL tibial tunnel.
- The ACL reconstruction can be performed with the surgeon's preferred technique and graft selection, through the same anteromedial incision used for the HTO. The incision can be lengthened 3 cm proximally if the patellar tendon is harvested.
- Posterior plate positioning during the osteotomy (as previously outlined) is important to reduce tibial slope and avoid interference between the proximal screws and placement of the tibial tunnel.[23]

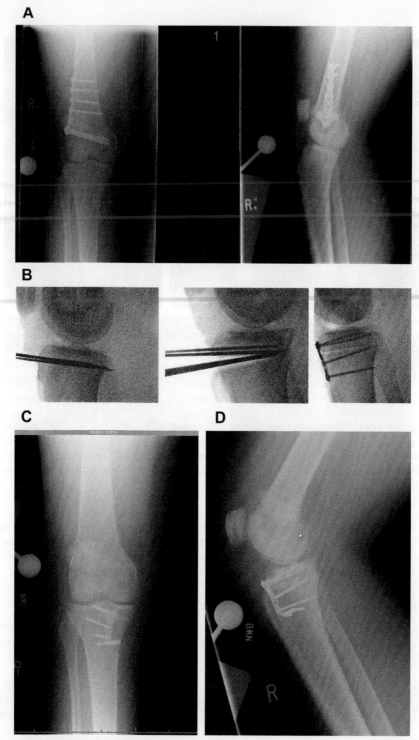

Fig. 6. Patient with knee instability and prior distal femoral osteotomy showing preoperative (*A*), intraoperative (*B*), postoperative (*C, D*) correction of excessive tibial slope with an anterior closing wedge HTO.

- Consideration is given to drilling the tibial tunnel anterior and superior to the osteotomy site. A retro drill (Arthrex) technique can be helpful to avoid the osteotomy site.
- The senior author's preference is to use extracortical button fixation on the femoral side. A tibial side interference screw is placed for primary fixation proximal to the osteotomy site. Secondary fixation can be placed distal to the osteotomy site if desired.
- At the conclusion of the procedure, the leg is placed in a hinged knee brace set at 0° to 90°.

COMPLICATIONS AND MANAGEMENT

A recent systematic review by Li and colleagues[24] reporting on simultaneous HTO with ACL reconstruction shows a 24.3% complication rate. The most common complications were deep vein thrombosis (DVT) (7.7%), stiffness (6.1%), and hematoma (2.8%). Other complications are listed here:

- Fracture: medial or lateral hinge fractures and intraarticular fractures can impair osteotomy stability and articular congruency. Matthews and colleagues[25] and Hernigou and colleagues[26] reported a fracture rate of approximately 11% in medial opening wedge HTOs and 10% to 20% in lateral closing wedge HTOs in separate studies published in the late 1980s. To avoid this complication, the senior author uses a guide pin aimed 1 cm below the joint line on the lateral side and he stays inferior to the guide pin during the osteotomy. In order to prevent lateral hinge fractures, some investigators have suggested using a temporary external fixator to hold the hinge together under compression while the osteotomy is being performed.[27] A key to avoiding tibial plateau fracture is to choose the hinge of the osteotomy at the external cortex of the proximal tibia and to carry the osteotomy to almost complete as opposed to subtotal.[27]
- Nonunion: this is more common with opening wedge techniques, especially with larger corrections and in smokers and diabetics. Risks have been reported to be from 0.7% to 4.4%.[28,29] The senior author routinely uses femoral head allograft to fill the void and decrease the risk of nonunion.
- Hardware failure: locking plate designs enhance fixation and allow earlier weight bearing in order to decrease nonunion.
- Symptomatic hardware: various plates can be utilized for the osteotomy, but in very active patients, large plates may be symptomatic on the medial side of the knee if they are prominent and from the proximity to the hamstring insertion.
- Infection: risk of infection with open reduction and internal fixation is reported to be around 4%.[30]
- Peroneal nerve palsy: this is more common in a closing wedge HTO, with incidence reported between 2% and 16%.[28]
- Compartment syndrome: the exact incidence is unknown, but concomitant arthroscopic procedures should increase concern for compartment syndrome during HTO given the risk of irrigation fluid extravasation.[31] Lower pressures should be used during arthroscopy with frequent assessments during the procedure.

POSTOPERATIVE CARE

- From 0 to 6 weeks: the patient is placed in a hinged knee brace set at 0° to 90° and kept touch-down weight bearing. Early postoperative range of motion is important to prevent stiffness.

Table 1
Publications of high tibial osteotomy plus anterior cruciate ligament reconstruction outcomes since 2000

Study	Patients Evaluated	Mean Follow-up	HTO Type	Subjective Outcome	Return to Sports	Radiographic Outcome (IKDC)	Postoperative Translation (Side-to-Side Difference)	Complications
Bonin et al,[4] 2004	30	12 y	CW 25, OW 5	78.5 postoperative IKDC	14: intense 11: moderate	2 of 30 progressed to grade D	3 mm vs contralateral	2 requiring reoperation: patella baja, stiffness Others: 7 DVTs, 3 wound hematomas, 1 delayed wound healing, 1 case of CRPS
Trojani et al,[36] 2014	29	6 y	OW	77 postoperative IKDC	23 resumed sports	2 of 29 progressed to grade D	2.65 mm vs contralateral	NP
Williams et al,[37] 2003	13	38 mo	CW	80.8 postoperative 47 preoperative Lysholm	92% resumed sports	NP	11 with grade 1 Lachmann	1 (postoperative instability on postoperative day 1)
Zaffagnini et al,[38] 2013	32	6.5 y	CW	72 postoperative 58 preoperative IKDC	NP	7 of 32 progressed to grade D	2.2 mm vs contralateral	4 (1 hardware irritation, 2 stiffness, 1 delayed union)

Abbreviations: CRPS, complex regional pain syndrome; CW, closing wedge; IKDC, International Knee Documentation Committee; NP, not provided; OW, opening wedge.

- From 6 to 10 weeks: if radiographs at 6 weeks indicate consolidation, bracing is discontinued and the patient is advanced to full weight bearing with a strengthening program.
- Ten weeks onward: if radiographs at 10 weeks show that osseous consolidation has been achieved, sport-specific rehabilitation is initiated.
- Long-leg alignment films are obtained at 6 months.

OUTCOMES

Combined HTO and ACL reconstruction for patients with ACL deficiency and early medial compartment arthrosis has been shown to restore anterior knee stability, prevent deterioration of the medial compartment, and offer improved subjective outcomes and predictable return-to-sport outcomes.[24]

Noyes and colleagues[32] published the results of 16 patients who underwent ACL reconstruction after HTO because of repeated giving-way symptoms, reporting pain reduction in 71%, elimination of giving way in 85%, and resumption of light recreational activities in 66%. Dejour and colleagues[33] reviewed 44 patients at 3.5 years after simultaneous HTO with ACL reconstruction, reporting a 91% satisfaction rate with no radiographic progression of arthritis.

More recent studies (**Table 1**) focusing on concomitant HTO and ACL reconstruction have shown an improvement in subjective outcomes, the ability to return to sport, and anterior knee translation commensurate with the contralateral knee associated with limited progression of arthritis.

Marriott and colleagues[34] studied the change in gait biomechanics after HTO and ACL reconstruction, reporting a decrease in knee adduction moment, representing a load shift toward the lateral compartment without increasing the total load. Arun and colleagues[35] reported on the importance of correcting tibial slope on patient outcomes, because patients in his 30-patient cohort who had greater than 5° of posterior slope decrease reported higher subjective functional outcomes at 2 years after concomitant ACL reconstruction and HTO.

For older patients with ACL deficiency with symptoms of arthritis as opposed to instability, Latterman and Jakob[16] report that most patients more than 40 years of age do well with HTO alone. Consideration should be given to reducing the tibial slope to decrease anterior tibial translation.

SUMMARY

Varus malalignment and an increased tibial slope can result in instability in an ACL-deficient knee. Malalignment can increase the stress on ACL reconstruction and contribute to recurrent instability. Realignment osteotomy can reduce mechanical wear in the medial compartment and decrease anterior tibial translation. High tibial osteotomies performed in conjunction with ACL reconstruction can improve alignment, restore anterior knee stability, and help prevent the advancement of arthritis.

REFERENCES

1. Clark R, Amendola A. Osteotomy and the cruciate-deficient knee. In: Scott WN, editor. Insall & Scott surgery of the knee. 5th edition. Philadelphia: Elsevier; 2012. p. 458–64.

2. Noyes FR, Barber-Westin SD, Hewett TE. High tibial osteotomy and ligament reconstruction for varus angulated anterior cruciate ligament-deficient knees. Am J Sports Med 2000;28(3):282–96.

3. Brinkman JM, Lobenhoffer P, Agneskirchner JD, et al. Osteotomies around the knee: patient selection, stability of fixation and bone healing in high tibial osteotomies. J Bone Joint Surg Br 2008;90(12):1548–57.

4. Bonin N, Ait Si Selmi T, Donell ST, et al. Anterior cruciate reconstruction combined with valgus upper tibial osteotomy: 12 years follow-up. Knee 2004;11(6):431–7.

5. van de Pol GJ, Arnold MP, Verdonschot N, et al. Varus alignment leads to increased forces in the anterior cruciate ligament. Am J Sports Med 2009;37(3):481–7.

6. Dejour H, Bonnin M. Tibial translation after anterior cruciate ligament rupture. Two radiological tests compared. J Bone Joint Surg Br 1994;76(5):745–9.

7. Giffin JR, Vogrin TM, Zantop T, et al. Effects of increasing tibial slope on the biomechanics of the knee. Am J Sports Med 2004;32(2):376–82.

8. Rodner CM, Adams DJ, Diaz-Doran V, et al. Medial opening wedge tibial osteotomy and the sagittal plane: the effect of increasing tibial slope on tibiofemoral contact pressure. Am J Sports Med 2006;34(9):1431–41.

9. Agneskirchner JD, Hurschler C, Stukenborg-Colsman C, et al. Effect of high tibial flexion osteotomy on cartilage pressure and joint kinematics: a biomechanical study in human cadaveric knees. Winner of the AGA-DonJoy Award 2004. Arch Orthop Trauma Surg 2004;124(9):575–84.

10. Rossi R, Bonasia DE, Amendola A. The role of high tibial osteotomy in the varus knee. J Am Acad Orthop Surg 2011;19(10):590–9.

11. Amendola A. The role of osteotomy in the multiple ligament injured knee. Arthroscopy 2003;19(Suppl 1):11–3.

12. Phisitkul P, Wolf BR, Amendola A. Role of high tibial and distal femoral osteotomies in the treatment of lateral-posterolateral and medial instabilities of the knee. Sports Med Arthrosc 2006;14(2):96–104.

13. Naudie D, Bourne RB, Rorabeck CH, et al. The Install Award. Survivorship of the high tibial valgus osteotomy. A 10- to -22-year followup study. Clin Orthop Relat Res 1999;(367):18–27.

14. Flecher X, Parratte S, Aubaniac JM, et al. A 12-28-year followup study of closing wedge high tibial osteotomy. Clin Orthop Relat Res 2006;452:91–6.

15. Prodromos CC, Amendola A, Jakob RP. High tibial osteotomy: indications, techniques, and postoperative management. Instr Course Lect 2015;64:555–65.

16. Lattermann C, Jakob RP. High tibial osteotomy alone or combined with ligament reconstruction in anterior cruciate ligament-deficient knees. Knee Surg Sports Traumatol Arthrosc 1996;4(1):32–8.

17. Genin P, Weill G, Julliard R. [The tibial slope. Proposal for a measurement method]. J Radiol 1993;74(1):27–33 [in French].

18. Dejour D, Saffarini M, Demey G, et al. Tibial slope correction combined with second revision ACL produces good knee stability and prevents graft rupture. Knee Surg Sports Traumatol Arthrosc 2015;23(10):2846–52.

19. Dugdale TW, Noyes FR, Styer D. Preoperative planning for high tibial osteotomy. The effect of lateral tibiofemoral separation and tibiofemoral length. Clin Orthop Relat Res 1992;(274):248–64.

20. Marti CB, Gautier E, Wachtl SW, et al. Accuracy of frontal and sagittal plane correction in open-wedge high tibial osteotomy. Arthroscopy 2004;20(4):366–72.

21. LaPrade RF, Oro FB, Ziegler CG, et al. Patellar height and tibial slope after opening-wedge proximal tibial osteotomy: a prospective study. Am J Sports Med 2010;38(1):160–70.

22. Amendola A, Bonasia DE. Results of high tibial osteotomy: review of the literature. Int Orthop 2010;34(2):155–60.
23. Imhoff AB, Linke RD, Agneskirchner J. Corrective osteotomy in primary varus, double varus and triple varus knee instability with cruciate ligament replacement. Orthopade 2004;33(2):201–7 [in German].
24. Li Y, Zhang H, Zhang J, et al. Clinical outcome of simultaneous high tibial osteotomy and anterior cruciate ligament reconstruction for medial compartment osteoarthritis in young patients with anterior cruciate ligament-deficient knees: a systematic review. Arthroscopy 2015;31(3):507–19.
25. Matthews LS, Goldstein SA, Malvitz TA, et al. Proximal tibial osteotomy. Factors that influence the duration of satisfactory function. Clin Orthop Relat Res 1988;(229):193–200.
26. Hernigou P, Medevielle D, Debeyre J, et al. Proximal tibial osteotomy for osteoarthritis with varus deformity. A ten to thirteen-year follow-up study. J Bone Joint Surg Am 1987;69(3):332–54.
27. Jacobi M, Wahl P, Jakob RP. Avoiding intraoperative complications in open-wedge high tibial valgus osteotomy: technical advancement. Knee Surg Sports Traumatol Arthrosc 2010;18(2):200–3.
28. Spahn G. Complications in high tibial (medial opening wedge) osteotomy. Arch Orthop Trauma Surg 2004;124(10):649–53.
29. Bettin D, Karbowski A, Schwering L, et al. Time-dependent clinical and roentgenographical results of Coventry high tibial valgisation osteotomy. Arch Orthop Trauma Surg 1998;117(1–2):53–7.
30. Billings A, Scott DF, Camargo MP, et al. High tibial osteotomy with a calibrated osteotomy guide, rigid internal fixation, and early motion. Long-term follow-up. J Bone Joint Surg Am 2000;82(1):70–9.
31. Marti CB, Jakob RP. Accumulation of irrigation fluid in the calf as a complication during high tibial osteotomy combined with simultaneous arthroscopic anterior cruciate ligament reconstruction. Arthroscopy 1999;15(8):864–6.
32. Noyes FR, Barber SD, Simon R. High tibial osteotomy and ligament reconstruction in varus angulated, anterior cruciate ligament-deficient knees. A two- to seven-year follow-up study. Am J Sports Med 1993;21(1):2–12.
33. Dejour H, Neyret P, Boileau P, et al. Anterior cruciate reconstruction combined with valgus tibial osteotomy. Clin Orthop Relat Res 1994;(299):220–8.
34. Marriott K, Birmingham TB, Kean CO, et al. Five-year changes in gait biomechanics after concomitant high tibial osteotomy and ACL reconstruction in patients with medial knee osteoarthritis. Am J Sports Med 2015;43(9):2277–85.
35. Arun GR, Kumaraswamy V, Rajan D, et al. Long-term follow up of single-stage anterior cruciate ligament reconstruction and high tibial osteotomy and its relation with posterior tibial slope. Arch Orthop Trauma Surg 2016;136(4):505–11.
36. Trojani C, Elhor H, Carles M, et al. Anterior cruciate ligament reconstruction combined with valgus high tibial osteotomy allows return to sports. Orthop Traumatol Surg Res 2014;100(2):209–12.
37. Williams RJ 3rd, Kelly BT, Wickiewicz TL, et al. The short-term outcome of surgical treatment for painful varus arthritis in association with chronic ACL deficiency. J Knee Surg 2003;16(1):9–16.
38. Zaffagnini S, Bonanzinga T, Grassi A, et al. Combined ACL reconstruction and closing-wedge HTO for varus angulated ACL-deficient knees. Knee Surg Sports Traumatol Arthrosc 2013;21(4):934–41.

Surgical Indications and Technique for Anterior Cruciate Ligament Reconstruction Combined with Lateral Extra-articular Tenodesis or Anterolateral Ligament Reconstruction

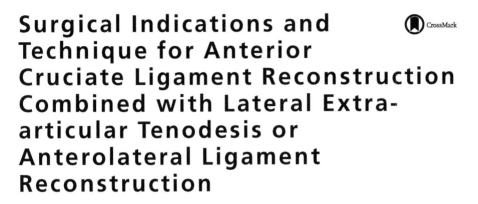 CrossMark

Bart Vundelinckx, MD, Benjamin Herman, MD, FRCSC,
Alan Getgood, MPhil, MD, FRCS (Tr&Orth), DipSEM,
Robert Litchfield, MD, FRCSC*

KEYWORDS

- Anterior cruciate ligament (ACL) • ACL reconstruction
- Lateral extra-articular tenodesis (LET) • Anterolateral ligament (ALL)

KEY POINTS

- After anterior cruciate ligament (ACL) rupture, anteroposterior and rotational instability in the knee causes clinical symptoms and possible secondary intra-articular damage.
- ACL reconstruction techniques evolved over time, trying to recreate anatomy as much as possible and address residual laxity.
- Recently, more attention has gone to combined intra-articular and extra-articular reconstruction types, in an attempt to better control rotational laxity and the pivot shift phenomenon.
- Biomechanical and clinical studies are being performed, to evaluate if the newer techniques result in superior clinical outcomes, without possible detrimental effects on the intra-articular cartilage.
- Lateral extra-articular tenodesis or anterolateral ligament reconstructions can be indicated in certain clinical settings. Clinical efficiency is not yet completely proven however.

Department of Surgery, Fowler Kennedy Sport Medicine Clinic, Western University, 3M Centre, 1151 Richmond Street, London, Ontario N6A 3K7, Canada
* Corresponding author.
E-mail address: rlitchf@uwo.ca

Clin Sports Med 36 (2017) 135–153
http://dx.doi.org/10.1016/j.csm.2016.08.009
0278-5919/17/© 2016 Elsevier Inc. All rights reserved.

INTRODUCTION

Anterior cruciate ligament (ACL) ruptures result in anterior and rotational laxity of the proximal tibia relative to the distal femur. With surgical treatment, the aim is to stabilize the knee to prevent further injury to articular cartilage and the menisci and to maximize patient function in activities of daily life and sports activity.

Historically, ACL ruptures were treated surgically by isolated extra-articular tenodesis, as described by Lemaire and Ireland, among many others.[1,2] These techniques effectively limited the rotational laxity, but provided only moderate control of the anterior translation. The overall long-term results of isolated extra-articular tenodesis are poor, with only half of the patients reporting good to excellent outcomes.[3] Moreover, increased degenerative changes of the lateral tibiofemoral compartment have been described after these procedures, possibly due to overtensioning of the graft leading to overconstraint of this compartment.[4]

The extra-articular tenodesis was largely abandoned when single-bundle, intra-articular ACL reconstruction became the gold standard. The original single-bundle reconstruction consisted of a vertical graft position resulting in poor rotational control, with some patients experiencing persistent rotatory laxity.[3,5,6]

Double-bundle ACL reconstruction was subsequently developed in the early 2000s, with the concept of the additional posterolateral bundle to the more standard anteromedial graft, better controlling rotation. Because it is technically more difficult and it did not show better clinical outcomes, the double-bundle technique has since lost popularity.[3,6]

Currently, anatomic single-bundle ACL reconstruction, with a more oblique orientation of the graft and tunnel positioning in the anatomic footprint on the femoral and tibial insertion points, is considered the gold standard. This technique results in good to excellent outcomes in most patients.[3]

However, even in the face of a well-perfumed single-bundle or double-bundle ACL reconstruction, rotational laxity has been demonstrated to persist. Two metaanalyses by Prodromos and colleagues[7] (2005) and Mohtadi[8] (2008) showed that up to 34% and 22% of patients, respectively, continue to have a positive pivot shift, the presence of which has been correlated with worsening outome.[9] This is one reason that has led to a greater interest in the anterolateral side of the knee.

Detailed anatomy of the structures at the anterolateral side of the knee have recently been described, with particular attention on the anterolateral ligament (ALL).[10–13] However, other structures have been identified as having an important role in controlling anterolateral rotational laxity, and, as such, newer techniques are being developed to reproduce original anatomy as close as possible. However, clinical advantages of these new reconstructive techniques are yet to be shown to be efficacious.

ANATOMY

The ACL is a primary restraint to anterior translation and contributes to restraint of internal tibial rotation and varus/valgus laxity. It has been described as being composed of 2 bundles, each having a different kinematic role: the anteromedial (AM) and posterolateral (PL) bundles, which are taut in flexion and extension, respectively. The AM bundle is more dominant in controlling anteroposterior stability, the PL bundle more in controlling rotational stability. The noncontact mechanism of injury involves a combination of forces, but has been described as similar to those forces involved in the pivot shift test: an axial load on the lateral compartment with a valgus force as the knee moves from flexion to extension.[14] This mechanism results in the pathognomonic bone bruising of the posterior aspect of the lateral tibial plateau and anterolateral femoral condyle that is seen on MRI or sometimes as the lateral femoral notch sign on a lateral radiograph of the knee.

This mechanism of injury often also results in additional injuries to soft tissue structures on the anterolateral side of the knee, as well as to the lateral or medial meniscus and to the articular cartilage.

Recently, interest has grown in the lateral capsuloligamentous structures. Anatomic studies have identified the ALL as a discrete lateral structure that acts as a secondary stabilizer to internal tibial rotation.[10–13] Very detailed anatomy has been described, with the origin of the ALL being shown to lie just posterior and proximal from the fibular collateral ligament (FCL) origin on the lateral femoral epicondyle. From here it runs in an oblique and distal-anterior way to its insertion point on the tibia, exactly midway between the Gerdy tubercle and the anterior border of the fibular head, approximately 6 to 11 mm distal to the articular level of the lateral tibial plateau. There seems to be a strong connection to the body of the lateral meniscus, but there are no attachments to the iliotibial band (ITB).[13]

There have been several studies in the past that have implicated various structures on the lateral side of the knee in restraining anterolateral rotational laxity.[10,12,15–18] In 1879, Segond described "a pearly, resistant, fibrous band which invariably showed extreme amounts of tension during forced internal rotation." He also described a remarkably constant avulsion fracture pattern at the anterolateral proximal tibia as a result of forced internal rotation of the knee.[19] This Segond fracture, described before the development of radiographs, was originally hypothesized to be an avulsion of the middle third of the "lateral capsular ligament" and later, after the work of Goldman and colleagues[17] and Hess and colleagues,[20] this eponymous fracture became a pathognomonic sign for ACL rupture. Hughston and colleagues[15] demonstrated that sectioning the "lateral capsular ligament" resulted in a high grade of anterolateral rotational instability and Norwood and colleagues[21] identified this ligament and/or iliotibial band injuries in 32 of 36 knees with acute anterolateral rotatory instability. It would seem that many of the structures identified in previous studies, also called the "anterior oblique band" (by Campos and colleagues[22]) or "lateral femorotibial ligament" (by Vieira and colleagues[11]) may be synonymous with the ALL and it is now with modern techniques in imaging and histology that we are able to more accurately characterize this structure. Landmark descriptions of Claes and colleagues[10] and Caterine and colleagues[13] defined the ALL as a separate existing, extra-articular ligament, with histologic properties of a real ligament and its own peripheral nervous innervation. A recent study has confirmed the ALL to be associated with the Segond fracture.[23]

It should be noted that the ALL is not the only structure that has an effect on rotational control. Posterior root tears of the lateral meniscus and meniscocapsular separations of the medial meniscus both impact the degree of rotational laxity in an ACL-deficient knee.[24–26] The iliotibial band (ITB) has also been shown to have an impact on the control of anterolateral rotation, because it attaches to the Gerdy tubercle. In particular, recent research would suggest that the capsule-osseous layer of the ITB, attaching proximally from the posterior Kaplan fibers on the distal femur, to distally on the posterior aspect of the Gerdy tubercle is a major contributor to anterolateral rotational control.[27] We can therefore surmise that anterolateral rotational control is provided by a combination of intra-articular and extra-articular structures, with the ACL, lateral meniscus, ITB, and ALL working in unison. Furthermore, ACL injury may therefore result in a combination of injuries to these structures. It is important therefore to look for peripheral injuries in addition to the ACL and address these as appropriate. The new anatomic understanding also implies that lateral extra-articular procedures may be more anatomic than previously believed.

BIOMECHANICS AND RATIONALE FOR THE LATERAL EXTRA-ARTICULAR TENODESIS
Biomechanics of Anterior Cruciate Ligament Reconstruction

The conventional intra-articular ACL reconstruction is typically successful at reducing anterior tibial translation but less so at controlling rotational stability. Recent advancements in ACL reconstruction techniques have aimed to restore normal knee kinematics, with varying degrees of success.

Double-bundle ACL reconstruction techniques have increased the complexity of the surgery and although biomechanical studies suggest the additional posterolateral bundle helps control rotational laxity, clinical studies have not shown any significant benefit over traditional single-bundle techniques.[6,28,29] The anatomic single-bundle ACL reconstruction is the most recent technique development. This places the femoral tunnel within the ACL footprint and results in a lower graft position with a more oblique angle than previous single-bundle techniques.[30] Theoretically, increased graft obliquity should provide a biomechanical advantage for controlling tibial rotation.[31] There is a growing body of literature supporting the improved rotational control and patient-reported outcomes of a more oblique graft position and furthermore, an anatomic single-bundle ACL reconstruction.[32-38]

Biomechanics of Lateral Extra-articular Tenodesis

Lateral extra-articular tenodesis (LET) techniques were developed to recreate the anterolateral capsular structures to address the laxity present in an ACL-deficient knee, before the development of intra-articular ACL reconstruction procedures.[39] Theoretically, it is thought that an extra-articular reconstruction has a biomechanical advantage over an intra-articular reconstruction with regard to anterolateral rotational control. The longer lever arm exerted by the peripherally based extra-articular reconstruction would theoretically be more able to resist torque. Ellison[40] described the ACL as "the hub of the wheel" and suggested that "it is easier to control rotation of a wheel at its rim than at its hub."

The LET has also been shown to protect the ACL graft. As previously mentioned, the obliquity of the graft is increased in the anatomic ACL reconstruction technique. This may expose the graft to higher than normal forces because it should theoretically resist more rotational torques.[36] This could lead to graft failure due to stretching or rupture. In a cadaver model, an LET has been shown to decrease the stress on an ACL graft by 43%.[41] A cadaver model has also shown a load-sharing relationship between an intra-articular ACL reconstruction and a LET during both anterior translation and internal rotation.[42] Similar benefits have been seen in an in vivo model. At the time of surgery, LET added to a single-bundle ACL reconstruction was shown to significantly reduce tibial internal rotation compared with a single-bundle ACL reconstruction alone or a double-bundle ACL reconstruction.[43] Zaffagnini and colleagues[44] also showed that patients had improved restraint to internal tibial rotation at 90° flexion in addition to improved varus-valgus laxity in full extension.

Biomechanics of the Anterolateral Ligament

The biomechanics and reconstruction of the lateral side of the knee have been more rigorously investigated in recent years. The renewed interest in the ALL resulted in the development of an anatomic ALL reconstruction with the goal of restoring rotational stability.

Kennedy and colleagues[45] examined the biomechanical properties and failure mechanisms of the ALL. They determined a mean maximum load of 175 N and stiffness of 20 N/mm. In 12 specimens, they identified 4 mechanisms of failure: ligamentous tear at the femoral attachment in 4 specimens and at the tibial insertion in 1 specimen. Mid-substance tears occurred in 4, and a bony avulsion (ie, Segond fracture) in 6, although it should be noted that the line of pull in these experiments was nonphysiologic. Regarding function, Dodds and colleagues[46] determined the ligament to be isometric from 0° to 60° of flexion, and to lengthen with internal tibial rotation, strongly suggesting a role in rotational control. Kittl and colleagues[47] studied the isometry of the native anterolateral structures, as well as potential points for the fixation of an extra-articular reconstruction. They found an ALL with an origin posterior and proximal to the FCL to be relatively isometric, whereas an ALL with a distal and anterior origin was lax approaching extension and unlikely to be effective in controlling the pivot shift. Monaco and colleagues[48] examined the effect of cutting the ACL and lateral capsular ligament using a navigation system and manually applied forces. Their description of division of the lateral capsular ligament would have involved division of the ALL. They found an increase in internal rotation in all knee flexion angles in the ACL-deficient knee following division of the lateral capsular ligament, which was significant at 30° with an increase in internal rotation of 5.5°. Spencer and colleagues[49] investigated both sectioning and reconstruction of the ALL using navigation and manually applied forces. They measured an increase in internal rotation in extension of 2° after division of the ALL in the ACL-deficient knee while performing a simulated pivot shift. Reconstruction of the ALL did not restore the kinematics of the native ALL intact state. However, when an LET was performed using a strip of the ITB and routing it under the FCL, attaching it to the distal femoral metaphysis (modified Lemaire technique), this resulted in a significant reduction in anterior translation and internal rotation in the ACL-deficient state.[49] This study showed that the LET was superior to the anatomic ALL reconstruction, which may be in part due to issues with the position of the ALL femoral attachment and tensioning of the latter structure, or to the routing of the LET under the FCL, which functions as a pulley to the internal rotation.

Parsons and colleagues,[50] using a 6° of freedom robot, found the ALL to be the primary restraint to internal rotation at knee flexion angles greater than 35°, with the ACL providing the greatest restraint closer to extension. It should be noted that the ITB was removed from all specimens in this study before testing.[50]

Biomechanics of the Iliotibial Band

In contrast to Parsons and colleagues,[50] Kittl and colleagues[27] found that the ALL played no significant role in internal rotational control. In a similar robotic experiment, they determined the superficial and deep components of the ITB to be the primary restraints to internal rotation from 30° to 90°, with the ACL having a significant contribution at 0° only. Interestingly, the ACL provided no restraint to the pivot shift.

The finding of a role for the ITB in the control of internal tibial rotation is important but not new. Fetto and Marshall[51] were able to induce a pivot shift by division of the ITB in an ACL intact knee. Jakob and colleagues[52] noted increased internal rotation but a paradoxic decrease in the pivot shift after division of Kaplan fibers, reflecting the complex and multifactorial nature of these rotational abnormalities. When they released the ITB distally by osteotomy of the Gerdy tubercle, the pivot shift became so marked in the ACL-deficient knee that the subluxation did not reduce before 60° of flexion. Gadikota and colleagues,[53] in a robotic study investigating the effect of increasing ITB load, found that internal rotation was significantly reduced between 20° and 30° of knee flexion with an ITB load of 50 N, and from 15° to 30° with a load of 100 N.

CLINICAL RESULTS OF DIFFERENT SURGICAL TECHNIQUES
Clinical Results of Isolated Anterior Cruciate Ligament Reconstruction

Current intra-articular ACL reconstruction techniques generally result in good to excellent outcomes in most patients and reliably restore the functional activities of daily life and sport.[3] According to a meta-analysis of 48 studies, 90% of participants achieved normal or nearly normal knee function.[54] However, the rate of reinjury in patients younger than 20 may be as high as 20%,[39,55–57] whereas recurrent or persistent laxity after ACL reconstruction is reported from 11% to 30%.[58–60] Many studies report a high incidence of persisting rotational laxity as measured by the pivot shift test. A positive pivot shift test correlates with decreased patient satisfaction and increased functional instability.[9,32,58] There is a growing body of literature emerging that shows that current ACL reconstruction techniques are not effective at reducing rotational laxity.[61] Furthermore, rates of return to sport to a preinjury level may be as low as 63%, whereas return to competitive sport is even lower at 44%.[54] Last, the incidence and severity of posttraumatic osteoarthritis (PTOA) seems to be higher in ACL reconstruction knees compared with the uninjured side[62] but direct causation is unclear. A positive pivot shift may be predictive of abnormal articular cartilage contact stress and the subsequent development of increased wear[63]; however, the molecular events that occur at the time of injury are most likely to be the primary factor in PTOA development.[64,65]

Although current ACL reconstruction techniques do have good patient-reported outcomes,[62] it is evident that there is a lack of consistent restoration of rotational control and clinical issues remain. Many investigators hypothesize that these clinical issues may be mitigated by addressing the rotational laxity.

Clinical Results of Isolated Lateral Extra-articular Tenodesis

Several methods for LET procedures have been developed and, initially, these procedures were done in isolation without addressing the ACL.

The original Lemaire technique was described in 1967 and used an 18 × 1-cm strip of ITB, left attached at the Gerdy tubercle. Two osseous tunnels are prepared to anchor this graft: the first in the femur, just above the lateral epicondyle and proximal to the FCL origin; the other is through the Gerdy tubercle on the proximal lateral tibia. Once the strip of ITB is harvested and the bony tunnels are prepared, the graft is passed under the FCL, through the femoral bone tunnel, and back under the FCL and finally inserted into the Gerdy tubercle via the second bone tunnel. Graft fixation is done at 30° of knee flexion, with neutral rotation.[3,66] The "modified Lemaire" technique was first described by Christel and Djian.[67] This was developed to simplify the classic technique. The length of the ITB graft was diminished, to decrease the required skin incision and soft tissue dissection. A graft of 75 mm long and 12 mm wide, again left attached distally on the Gerdy tubercle, is harvested of the ITB. On the femoral insertion site, an isometric point on the lateral femoral condyle is determined and the graft is secured in a femoral tunnel with an interference screw. To avoid possible devascularization of the FCL, the graft is not passed under the ligament. The graft is twisted 180°, to yield more homogeneous graft forces and better isometry, as shown by Draganich and colleagues.[42]

The Ellison procedure, described in 1979, harvested an ITB graft from the Gerdy tubercle with a bone plug and passed it under the proximal aspect of the FCL before stapling the bone plug anterior to the Gerdy tubercle.[68]

The MacIntosh procedure was described in 1980 and was similar to the Lemaire procedure.[69] The graft was passed on the femoral side through a subperiosteal tunnel posterior to the FCL origin and looped behind the lateral intermuscular septum before being passed distally again. A modification of the MacIntosh procedure looped the ITB graft around the lateral femoral condyle, through the notch and in a tunnel in the tibia (MacIntosh 2). Another MacIntosh iteration took a strip of the central third of quadriceps-patellar tendon dissected off the anterior patella, left it attached distally, passed the graft through the notch and secured it to the lateral aspect of the femur.[70]

Results for the various isolated LET procedures have been generally poor. Patient satisfaction in terms of good to excellent results has been reported at rates of as low as 57% to 63% for the Ellison procedure[71,72] and 52% for the Lemaire procedure.[73] Return to previous level of sport was seen in fewer than half of patients with a MacIntosh procedure despite a negative pivot shift in 84% of patients.[69] Objective testing of the pivot shift in isolated LET procedures usually found a positive result more often than not. Neyret and colleagues[71,73] reported the outcomes for an isolated Lemaire procedure in amateur skiers. Of the 33 knees operated in 31 patients, only 16 were satisfied with the result. The pivot shift was positive in 9 of 18 at 1 year, and 12 of 15 at final follow-up after 4.5 years. The outcome was noted to be dependent on the status of the medial meniscus, especially in those younger than 35 years. Ireland and Trickey[2] reported their results with the MacIntosh procedure in 50 knees at 2 years of follow-up. Anterolateral jerk was abolished in 42 of the 50 knees; however, fewer than half of their patients with excellent and satisfactory results were able to return to sports at their previous level. Amirault and colleagues[74] reported the long-term results for this procedure, examining 27 patients at more than 11 years of follow-up with 52% of patients being rated as good or excellent.

Ellison[68] reported good or excellent results in 15 of 18 knees using his procedure with up to 41 months of follow-up. Other investigators were unable to reproduce these results. Kennedy and colleagues[71] reported only 57% good or excellent results with the procedure, with 24 of 28 having a positive pivot shift at 6 months postoperatively, and all patients having a persistent anterior drawer. Fox and colleagues[72] reported 63% fair or better results in 76 knees using a modification of Ellison's technique.

In addition to the poor long-term clinical outcomes, there were other concerns that led to the abandonment of the isolated LET. The nonanatomic nature of LET procedures was thought to result in poor knee kinematics, as it did not restore the function of the ACL in preventing anterior tibial translation. Several studies have shown overconstraint in the form of abnormal resting tibial position in external rotation.[41,75–78] However, this is likely a result of tensioning the LET graft in excessive external rotation.[59] It was felt that this overconstraint would lead to either stretching of the graft over time or an increase in lateral compartment osteoarthritis.[4] Whereas graft elongation may certainly have contributed to the suboptimal clinical results, there is little evidence of increased lateral compartment degenerative change in the literature.

Clinical Results of Combined Anterior Cruciate Ligament and Lateral Extra-articular Tenodesis Reconstruction

As arthroscopic ACL reconstruction techniques improved and became the gold standard, surgeons experimented with the LET as an adjunctive procedure. Some surgeons used the MacIntosh or Lemaire procedure to compliment an intra-articular graft reconstruction.[79–83] Combined procedures are advantageous for 2 main reasons. As stated in the biomechanics section, an added lateral extra-articular procedure has a more beneficial lever arm for rotational control and it has been shown that it offloads the intra-articular graft, possibly preventing it more from failure. Even in case of failure of the intra-articular graft, it functions as a secondary restraint to rotational laxity. This combined technique is currently mostly used in the scenario of revision ACL reconstruction. There is, however, a contraindication to perform an LET: the presence of a posterolateral corner injury. In such cases, the tenodesis may tether the tibia in a posterolateral subluxated postition.[3] Results for combined intra-articular ACL reconstruction and LET procedures have been more promising.

Twelve of the 13 studies reviewed by Dodds and colleagues[84] reported good to excellent results in 80% to 90% of patients. The remaining study performed an advancement of the biceps femoris tendon as an extra-articular restraint, which is different from the extra-articular tenodesis techniques described previously. Marcacci and colleagues[85] prospectively studied 54 high-level athletes who underwent ACL reconstruction, combined with LET. They developed a technique in 1992 that used hamstring grafts, with intact tibial insertion, to reconstruct both the ACL and lateral reconstruction. After passing the ACL portion of the graft, it is then brought through the "over-the-top" position, passed deep to the ITB and over the FCL down to the Gerdy tubercle where it is secured. They reported highly satisfactory results, with 90.7% of patients classified as International Knee Documentation Committee (IKDC) A or B, 11 years postoperatively. No more knee osteoarthritis was found in this group, compared with patients who did not have an LET.[86] Bertoia and colleagues[80] reported good or excellent results in 31 of 34 knees using the MacIntosh lateral substitution over-the-top repair (MacIntosh II), with the pivot shift abolished in 91%. Zarins and Rowe[81] described a modification of the MacIntosh over-the-top procedure, with an ITB graft passing from outside-in supplemented by the addition of a distally based semitendinosus graft passing from inside-out; 88 of 100 patients reported good or excellent satisfaction with the procedure, with pivot shift reduced to grade 0 or 1+ in 91 patients.

Augmentation procedures also showed promising results. Dejour and colleagues[83] studied 251 cases operated with a patella tendon intra-articular reconstruction augmented with the Lemaire procedure; 83% had good or excellent functional results, although the pivot shift was described as equivocal in 24%. Rackemann and colleagues[82] reported the results of 714 knees treated with a medial third patella tendon reconstruction augmented with a MacIntosh procedure. At 6 years, results were satisfactory in 93%, with only one positive pivot shift.

The first comparative study of intra-articular and extra-articular reconstruction versus intra-articular reconstruction alone was published by Jensen and colleagues in 1983.[87] In this retrospective study, they found the combined procedure group showed the most marked reduction in anterolateral laxity.

Lerat and colleagues[88] published long-term results for combined procedures. They reported the results for 138 patients at a mean follow-up of 11.7 years. Patients were treated with a "MacInJones" procedure, in which an intra-articular patella tendon graft was augmented by an extra-articular reconstruction performed with a strip of quadriceps tendon in continuity with the patella tendon graft. IKDC functional results were good or excellent in 60%. The pivot shift was negative in 66%, grade 1+ in 30% and grade 2+ in 4%. There were 12 graft failures.

A recent meta-analysis by Hewison and colleagues[89] of 29 articles revealed a statistically significant reduction in the pivot shift in favor of a combination ACL reconstruction + LET compared with ACL reconstruction alone. No significant difference was seen in anterior translation as measured by KT1000/2000 arthrometry or in IKDC scores. The meta-analysis also highlights the degree of heterogeneity in the studies, as several factors were different, including type of ACL graft (bone-patellar tendon-bone [BTB] vs hamstring tendon [HT]) and method of LET. Overconstraint has not been shown in cadaver studies.[42] Clinical studies also have failed to show an increased risk of lateral compartment osteoarthritis, even with the LET graft tensioned with tibial external rotation.[86,90]

Other studies, however, challenged the superiority of combined procedures. Strum and colleagues[4] reported no benefit of combined procedures over isolated intra-articular reconstructions, stressing the importance of a well-performed intra-articular procedure. O'Brien and colleagues[91] found no difference in clinical stability for those treated with a central third patella tendon intra-articular graft with or without the addition of a lateral extra-articular sling procedure; however, 40% of the extra-articular group had chronic pain or swelling associated with the additional procedure. Anderson and colleagues[59] compared patella tendon, hamstring, and hamstring combined with lateral extra-articular procedures, and found no benefit to the addition of the extra-articular reconstruction.

Clinical Outcomes of Combined Anterior Cruciate Ligament and Anterolateral Ligament Reconstruction

With the recent, very detailed, anatomic descriptions of the ALL, surgical anatomic reconstructive techniques have been developed. However, only a few studies have been published with clinical results of these newer techniques and so far, no comparative clinical studies with differentiation between LET have been performed.

Sonnery-Cottet and colleagues[92] published a series of 92 patients with minimum 2-year follow-up. In their technique, a hamstring graft is used for the ALL reconstruction, in a triangular shape, to mimic the wider anatomy of the distal ALL. Indications for a combined ACL and ALL reconstruction are an associated Segond fracture, chronic ACL lesion, grade 3 pivot shift, high level of sporting activity, pivoting sports, and radiographic lateral femoral notch sign. Good to excellent improvement in subjective and objective scores were achieved as well as a clear decrease in pivot shift to grade 0 or grade 1 in all patients. No specific complications due to the technique were reported.[92]

Colombet[93] studied his technique of anterolateral tenodesis. This study was performed before the recent, detailed ALL descriptions. However, in retrospect, following his description and drawings of his technique, he actually performed a combined ACL and anatomic ALL reconstruction, by means of hamstring grafts. He concluded that the extra-articular addition provided no significant improvement to anterior tibial translation and improved internal tibial rotation control only at 90° of flexion. However, only time zero biomechanical testing was performed by means of computer navigation and no clinical results were reported.[93]

THE FOWLER KENNEDY APPROACH
Indications

The current practice at our institution is to perform an isolated anatomic ACL reconstruction in most primary cases with either a BTB or HT autograft. The addition of an LET procedure is considered in the setting of a revision ACL reconstruction in which no other significant pathology needs to be addressed (eg, posterolateral corner, medial collateral ligament reconstruction, meniscus transplantation), and particularly if allograft is being used. This is supported in a study by Trojani and colleagues,[94] in which a negative pivot shift was found in 80% of revision patients receiving an LET augment compared with 63% in ACL reconstruction alone. There are no clear indications for LET in the primary setting. However, consideration is given to patients who present with a combination of specific risk factors, in which case additional procedure may be recommended due to perceived increased risk of failure.

> **Risk factors to consider for addition of LET:**
>
> - Grade 2 or 3 pivot shift (high-grade rotational laxity)
> - Young age of <25 years
> - Generalized ligamentous laxity
> - Genu recurvatum >10°
> - Returning to pivoting sport (ie, soccer, basketball)

Others have proposed an individualized treatment algorithm for treating ACL ruptures based on the constellation of concomitant injuries. Musahl and colleagues[95] suggests consideration of LET in a patient with a grade 2 or 3 pivot shift test in the absence of a meniscus or collateral ligament injury. In these cases, permanent capsular strain, generalized ligamentous laxity, or underlying morphologic abnormalities may be the cause for the abnormal pivot shift. Lerat and colleagues[96] suggests that patients with differential translation of the lateral side of the knee during the Lachman test (ie, obvious internal rotation during anterior translation) may benefit from LET. Lording and colleagues[97] suggests that a significant injury to the medial meniscus may be another indication given the fact its loss increases stress within the ACL graft and negatively affects postoperative knee stability.

Surgical Technique of Lateral Extra-articular Tenodesis

Following the final tensioning of the ACL reconstruction, a modified Lemaire procedure is performed.[67,98] A 5-cm curvilinear incision is placed just posterior to the lateral femoral epicondyle. The posterior border of the ITB is identified and freed of any fascial attachments to the level of the Gerdy tubercle. An 8-cm-long × 1-cm-wide strip of ITB is harvested from the posterior half of the ITB, ensuring that the most posterior fibers of the capsulo-osseous layer remain intact. It is left attached distally at the Gerdy tubercle, freed of any deep attachments to vastus lateralis, released proximally, and a #1 Vicryl whip stitch is placed in the free end of the graft. The FCL is then identified. Small capsular incisions are made anterior and posterior to the proximal portion of the ligament and Metzenbaum scissors are placed deep to the FCL to bluntly dissect out a tract for graft passage. An attempt is made to remain extracapsular, while ensuring there is no iatrogenic damage to the popliteus tendon. The ITB graft is then passed beneath the FCL from distal to proximal. The lateral femoral supracondylar area is then cleared of the small fat pad found proximal to the lateral head of gastrocnemius using electrocautery. The attachment site should be identified just anterior and proximal to the lateral gastrocnemius tendon. The periosteum is cleared using a cob on the metaphyseal flare of the lateral femoral condyle. Care is taken not to damage the ACL graft femoral fixation as the suspensory loop button is often found close to this location. The graft is then held taught but not overtensioned, with the knee at 60° flexion and the foot in neutral rotation to avoid lateral compartment overconstraint. The graft is secured using a small Richards staple and then folded back distally and sutured to itself using the #1 Vicryl whip stitch. The wound is irrigated, hemostasis is confirmed, and closure is performed in layers. We do not close the posterior aspect of the ITB, where the graft was harvested, to avoid overtightening the lateral patellofemoral joint. Postoperative rehabilitation is the same as for any ACL reconstruction and weight bearing and range of motion are performed as tolerated as long as there is no significant meniscal repair. In **Figs. 1–5**, the stepwise technique of LET reconstruction is shown in clinical pictures.

Technical pearls

- Place the leg in **Fig. 4** position to place the FCL under tension to help identify it so as to pass the LET graft deep to it.

- Apply minimal tension to the LET graft during fixation and secure it with the knee at 60° of flexion and the foot in neutral rotation to avoid overconstraint.

- Start using the LET in the revision scenario, as this will demonstrate its ability to control anterolateral rotation. Once comfortable with the technique, it may be used in high-risk primary ACL reconstruction, such as in the young patient with generalized ligamentous laxity, genu recurvatum, and high-grade pivot shift who is wishing to return to pivoting sport.

What about anatomic anterolateral ligament reconstruction?

As mentioned in the section "Clinical Outcomes of Combined Anterior Cruciate Ligament and Anterolateral Ligament Reconstruction," so far only a very few studies reported on clinical outcomes of anatomic ALL reconstruction. Until a clear benefit of this technique over the LET is proven, it is not performed in a clinical setting at our institution. In our opinion, probably the most anatomic reconstruction is the technique described by Sonnery-Cottet and colleagues.[92]

Future Directions

The role of LET or ALL reconstruction will become more clear as studies more accurately identify those patients who are at an increased risk of failure with an isolated ACL reconstruction. Many risk factors are known with regard to graft rupture and ACL reconstruction failure. Young age, female sex, use of allograft, concomitant injuries (loss of medial meniscus), and return to high-risk sport involving pivoting or jumping have all been implicated as possible causes of failure.[99–102] It will take well-designed studies to determine who, if anyone, will benefit most from an adjunctive LET procedure.

Our center is currently leading a multicenter randomized clinical trial aimed at determining if there is a clinical benefit to performing LET in the primary setting in high-risk patients.[103] The STAbiLiTY (Standard ACL Reconstruction vs ACL + Lateral Extra-Articular Tenodesis) study has been enrolling patients at 8 centers in Canada and

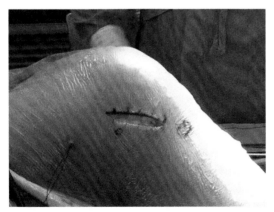

Fig. 1. Incision used for LET reconstruction. Curvilinear incision of 5 to 6 cm, centered over the lateral epicondyle.

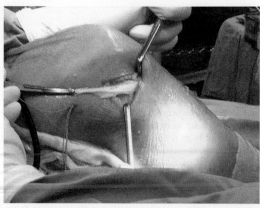

Fig. 2. Harvesting of ITB strip of 1 cm wide and 8 to 9 cm long, distally left attached to the Gerdy tubercle. Resorbable whipstitch suture at the proximal end of the ITB strip.

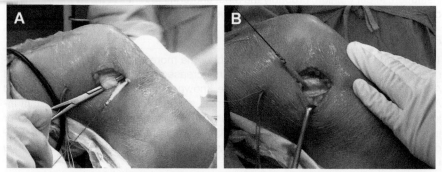

Fig. 3. (A, B) Routing of ITB strip under the fibular collateral ligament, after 2 longitudinal snap incisions just anterior and posterior to the FCL.

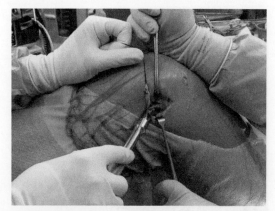

Fig. 4. Fixation of the graft onto the posterior lateral femoral condyle, with a Richards staple. The knee is held in 60° of flexion and the foot in a neutral position. Care is taken not to overtighten the graft.

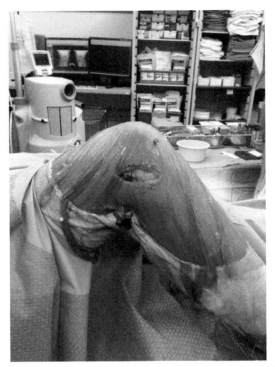

Fig. 5. The end of the graft is looped back onto itself and sutured with the end of the resorbable whipstich suture.

Europe since January 2014 and is aiming to recruit 600 participants. Patients are included if they are younger than 25 and have any 2 of the following characteristics: greater than a grade 2 pivot shift, participation in a pivoting sport, or generalized ligamentous laxity. Two-year follow-up will be performed with a primary outcome of graft failure as defined by instability requiring revision surgery or a positive pivot shift test. We are also currently setting up a cadaver laboratory study to compare LET versus anatomic ALL reconstruction in terms of anterolateral rotational stability and contact pressures in the compartments.

SUMMARY

Recent research has demonstrated the combined roles of the ACL, lateral meniscus posterior root, ALL, and ITB in controlling anterolateral rotation and the pivot shift. Although the ALL has received significant attention, it is likely that the high-grade rotational laxity that results from an ACL injury is a combination of injury to many of these structures. The literature supports the biomechanical benefits of providing an extra-articular restraint to internal tibial rotation. LET is widely accepted in the European orthopedic community and is beginning to be recognized in North America as a useful adjunct to current ACL reconstruction techniques in certain patient populations. With modern techniques, it is a low-morbidity procedure with minimal complications. However, more clinical studies are needed to determine which is the most beneficial technique, who best benefits from receiving the additional procedure, and if this will confer any benefit in the medium to long term.

REFERENCES

1. Lemaire M, Combelles F. Plastic repair with fascia lata for old tears of the anterior cruciate ligament (author's transl). Rev Chir Orthop Reparatrice Appar Mot 1980;66(8):523–5 [in French].
2. Ireland J, Trickey EL. Macintosh tenodesis for anterolateral instability of the knee. J Bone Joint Surg Br 1980;62(3):340–5.
3. Duthon V, Magnussen R, Servien E, et al. ACL reconstruction and extra-articular tenodesis. Clin Sports Med 2013;32(1):141–53.
4. Strum GM, Fox JM, Ferkel RD, et al. Intraarticular versus intraarticular and extraarticular reconstruction for chronic anterior cruciate ligament instability. Clin Orthop Relat Res 1989;245:188 08.
5. Menetrey J, Duthon VB, Laumonier T, et al. "Biological failure" of the anterior cruciate ligament graft. Knee Surg Sports Traumatol Arthrosc 2008;16:224–31.
6. Yagi M, Wong EK, Kanamori A, et al. Biomechanical analysis of an anatomic anterior cruciate ligament reconstruction. Am J Sports Med 2002;30:660–6.
7. Prodromos CC, Joyce BT, Shi K, et al. A meta-analysis of stability after anterior cruciate ligament reconstruction as a function of hamstring versus patellar tendon graft and fixation type. Arthroscopy 2005;21(10):1202.
8. Mohtadi N. Function after ACL reconstruction: a review. Clin J Sport Med 2008; 18(1):105–6.
9. Ayeni OR, Chahal M, Tran MN, et al. Pivot shift as an outcome measure for ACL reconstruction: a systematic review. Knee Surg Sports Traumatol Arthrosc 2012; 20(4):767–77.
10. Claes S, Vereecke E, Maes M, et al. Anatomy of the anterolateral ligament of the knee. J Anat 2013;223:321–8.
11. Vieira ELC, Vieira EÁ, Teixeira da Silva R, et al. An anatomic study of the iliotibial tract. Arthroscopy 2007;23(3):269–74.
12. Vincent JP, Magnussen RA, Gezmez F, et al. The anterolateral ligament of the human knee: an anatomic and histologic study. Knee Surg Sports Traumatol Arthrosc 2012;20:147–52.
13. Caterine S, Litchfield R, Johnson M, et al. A cadaveric study of the anterolateral ligament: re-introducing the lateral capsular ligament. Knee Surg Sports Traumatol Arthrosc 2015;23(11):3186–95.
14. Boden BP, Sheehan FT, Torg JS, et al. Noncontact anterior cruciate ligament injuries: mechanisms and risk factors. J Am Acad Orthop Surg 2010;18:520–7.
15. Hughston JC, Andrews JR, Cross MJ, et al. Classification of knee ligament instabilities. Part II. The lateral compartment. J Bone Joint Surg Am 1976;58:173–9.
16. Dietz GW, Wilcox DM, Montgomery JB. Segond tibial condyle fracture: lateral capsular ligament avulsion. Radiology 1986;159:467–9.
17. Goldman AB, Pavlov H, Rubenstein D. The Segond fracture of the proximal tibia: a small avulsion that reflects major ligamentous damage. Am J Roentgenol 1988;151:1163–7.
18. Johnson LL. Lateral capsular ligament complex: anatomical and surgical considerations. Am J Sports Med 1979;7:156–60.
19. Segond P. Recherches cliniques et experimentales sur les epanchements sanguins du genou par entorse. Paris: Progres Medical; 1879.
20. Hess T, Rupp S, Hopf T, et al. Lateral tibial avulsion fractures and disruptions to the anterior cruciate ligament. A clinical study of their incidence and correlation. Clin Orthop Relat Res 1994;(303):193–7.

21. Norwood LA, Andrews JR, Meisterling RC, et al. Acute anterolateral rotatory instability of the knee. J Bone Joint Surg Am 1979;61-A:704–9.
22. Campos JC, Chung CB, Lektrakul N, et al. Pathogenesis of the Segond fracture: anatomic and MR imaging evidence of an iliotibial tract or anterior oblique band avulsion. Radiology 2001;219(2):381–6.
23. Claes S, Luyckx T, Vereecke E, et al. The Segond fracture: a bony injury of the anterolateral ligament of the knee. Arthroscopy 2014;30:1475–82.
24. Bhatia S, LaPrade CM, Ellman MB, et al. Meniscal root tears: significance, diagnosis, and treatment. Am J Sports Med 2014;42:3016–30.
25. Tanaka M, Vyas D, Moloney G, et al. What does it take to have a high-grade pivot shift? Knee Surg Sports Traumatol Arthrosc 2012;20:737–42.
26. Thompson WO, Fu FH. The meniscus in the cruciate-deficient knee. Clin Sports Med 1993;12:771–96.
27. Kittl C, El Daou H, Athwayl K, et al. The role of the anterolateral structures and the ACL in controlling internal rotational knee laxity. Lyon (France): ISAKOS Bienn. Congr; 2015.
28. Zelle B, Vidal AF, Brucker PU, et al. Double-bundle reconstruction of the anterior cruciate ligament: anatomic and biomechanical rationale. J Am Acad Orthop Surg 2007;15:87–96.
29. Meredick RB, Vance KJ, Appleby D, et al. Outcome of single-bundle versus double-bundle reconstruction of the anterior cruciate ligament: a meta-analysis. Am J Sports Med 2008;36:1414–21.
30. Bedi A, Raphael B, Maderazo A, et al. Transtibial versus anteromedial portal drilling for anterior cruciate ligament reconstruction: a cadaveric study of femoral tunnel length and obliquity. Arthroscopy 2010;26:342–50.
31. Markolf KL, Jackson SR, McAllister DR. A comparison of 11 o'clock versus oblique femoral tunnels in the anterior cruciate ligament-reconstructed knee: knee kinematics during a simulated pivot test. Am J Sports Med 2010;38:912–7.
32. Lee MC, Seong SC, Lee S, et al. Vertical femoral tunnel placement results in rotational knee laxity after anterior cruciate ligament reconstruction. Arthroscopy 2007;23:771–8.
33. Loh JC, Fukuda Y, Tsuda E, et al. Knee stability and graft function following anterior cruciate ligament reconstruction: comparison between 11 o'clock and 10 o'clock femoral tunnel placement. Arthroscopy 2003;19:297–304.
34. Scopp JM, Jasper LE, Belkoff SM, et al. The effect of oblique femoral tunnel placement on rotational constraint of the knee reconstructed using patellar tendon autografts. Arthroscopy 2004;20:294–9.
35. Jepsen CF, Lundberg-Jensen AK, Faunoe P. Does the position of the femoral tunnel affect the laxity or clinical outcome of the anterior cruciate ligament-reconstructed knee? A clinical, prospective, randomized, double-blind study. Arthroscopy 2007;23:1326–33.
36. Kato Y, Ingham SJM, Kramer S, et al. Effect of tunnel position for anatomic single-bundle ACL reconstruction on knee biomechanics in a porcine model. Knee Surg Sports Traumatol Arthrosc 2009;18:2–10.
37. Kato Y, Maeyama A, Lertwanich P, et al. Biomechanical comparison of different graft positions for single-bundle anterior cruciate ligament reconstruction. Knee Surg Sports Traumatol Arthrosc 2012;21:816–23.
38. Kondo E, Merican AM, Yasuda K, et al. Biomechanical comparison of anatomic double-bundle, anatomic single-bundle, and nonanatomic single-bundle anterior cruciate ligament reconstructions. Am J Sports Med 2011;39:279–88.

39. Schindler OS. Surgery for anterior cruciate ligament deficiency: a historical perspective. Knee Surg Sports Traumatol Arthrosc 2012;20:5–47.

40. Ellison A. Anterolateral rotatory instability. In: Funk F Jr, editor. Symp. Athlete's knee, surg. Repair reconstr. St Louis/Toronto/London: Mosby; 1978. p. 178–93.

41. Engebretsen L, Lew WD, Lewis JL, et al. The effect of an iliotibial tenodesis on intraarticular graft forces and knee joint motion. Am J Sports Med 1990;18: 169–76.

42. Draganich LF, Reider B, Ling M, et al. An in vitro study an intraarticular and extraarticular reconstruction in the anterior cruciate ligament deficient knee. Am J Sports Med 1990;18:262–6.

43. Monaco E, Labianca L, Conteduca F, et al. Double bundle or single bundle plus extraarticular tenodesis in ACL reconstruction? A CAOS study. Knee Surg Sports Traumatol Arthrosc 2007;15:1168–74.

44. Zaffagnini S, Signorelli C, Lopomo N, et al. Anatomic double-bundle and over-the-top single-bundle with additional extra-articular tenodesis: an in vivo quantitative assessment of knee laxity in two different ACL reconstructions. Knee Surg Sports Traumatol Arthrosc 2012;20:153–9.

45. Kennedy MI, Claes S, Fuso FAF, et al. The anterolateral ligament: an anatomic, radiographic, and biomechanical analysis. Am J Sports Med 2015;43(7): 1606–15.

46. Dodds AL, Halewood C, Gupte CM, et al. The anterolateral ligament: anatomy, length changes and association with the Segond fracture. Bone Joint J 2014; 96-B(3):325–31.

47. Kittl C, Halewood C, Stephen JM, et al. Length change patterns in the lateral extra-articular structures of the knee and related reconstructions. Am J Sports Med 2015;43(2):354–62.

48. Monaco E, Ferretti A, Labianca L, et al. Navigated knee kinematics after cutting of the ACL and its secondary restraint. Knee Surg Sports Traumatol Arthrosc 2011;20(5):870–7.

49. Spencer L, Burkhart TA, Tran MN, et al. Biomechanical analysis of simulated clinical testing and reconstruction of the anterolateral ligament of the knee. Am J Sports Med 2015;43(9):2189–97.

50. Parsons EM, Gee AO, Spiekerman C, et al. The biomechanical function of the anterolateral ligament of the knee. Am J Sports Med 2015;43(3):669–74.

51. Fetto JF, Marshall JL. Injury to the anterior cruciate ligament producing the pivot-shift sign. J Bone Joint Surg Am 1979;61(5):710–4.

52. Jakob RP, Hassler H, Staeubli HU. Observations on rotatory instability of the lateral compartment of the knee. Experimental studies on the functional anatomy and the pathomechanism of the true and the reversed pivot shift sign. Acta Orthop Scand Suppl 1981;191:1–32.

53. Gadikota HR, Kikuta S, Qi W, et al. Effect of increased iliotibial band load on tibiofemoral kinematics and force distributions: a direct measurement in cadaveric knees. J Orthop Sports Phys Ther 2013;43(7):478–85.

54. Ardern CL, Webster KE, Taylor NF, et al. Return to sport following anterior cruciate ligament reconstruction surgery: a systematic review and meta-analysis of the state of play. Br J Sports Med 2011;45:596–606.

55. Strickler FP. A satisfactory method of repairing crucial ligaments. Ann Surg 1937;105(6):912–6.

56. Lemaire M. Ruptures anciennes du ligament croise anterieur du genou. J Chir 1967;93:311–20.

57. Lemaire M. Instabilité chronique du genou. Techniques et résultats des plasties ligamentaires en traumatologie sportive. J Chir (Paris) 1975;110(4):281–94.
58. Kocher MS, Steadman JR, Briggs K, et al. Determinants of patient satisfaction with outcome after anterior cruciate ligament reconstruction. J Bone Joint Surg Am 2002;84-A:1560–72.
59. Anderson AF, Snyder RB, Lipscomb AB. Anterior cruciate ligament reconstruction. A prospective randomized study of three surgical methods. Am J Sports Med 2001;29:272–9.
60. Eriksson E. How good are the results of ACL reconstruction? Knee Surg Sports Traumatol Arthrosc 1997;5:137.
61. Mohtadi NG, Chan DS, Dainty KN, et al. Patellar tendon versus hamstring tendon autograft for anterior cruciate ligament rupture in adults. Cochrane Database Syst Rev 2011;(9):CD005960.
62. Leiter JRS, Gourlay R, McRae S, et al. Long-term follow-up of ACL reconstruction with hamstring autograft. Knee Surg Sports Traumatol Arthrosc 2014;22:1061–9.
63. Jonsson H, Riklund-Ahlström K, Lind J. Positive pivot shift after ACL reconstruction predicts later osteoarthrosis: 63 patients followed 5-9 years after surgery. Acta Orthop Scand 2004;75:594–9.
64. Catterall JB, Stabler TV, Flannery CR, et al. Changes in serum and synovial fluid biomarkers after acute injury. Arthritis Res Ther 2010;12:R229.
65. Natoli RM, Scott CC, Athanasiou KA. Temporal effects of impact on articular cartilage cell death, gene expression, matrix biochemistry, and biomechanics. Ann Biomed Eng 2008;36:780–92.
66. Losee RE, Johnson TR, Southwick WO. Anterior subluxation of the lateral tibial plateau. A diagnostic test and operative repair. J Bone Joint Surg Am 1978;60:1015–30.
67. Christel P, Djian P. Anterio-lateral extra-articular tenodesis of the knee using a short strip of fascia lata. Rev Chir Orthop Reparatrice Appar Mot 2002;88:508–13 [in French].
68. Ellison AE. Distal iliotibial-band transfer for anterolateral rotatory instability of the knee. J Bone Joint Surg Am 1979;61-A:330–7.
69. Ireland J, Trickey E. MacIntosh tenodesis for anterolateral instability of the knee. J Bone Jt Surg Br 1980;62-B:340–5.
70. McCulloch PC, Lattermann C, Boland AL, et al. An illustrated history of anterior cruciate ligament surgery. J Knee Surg 2007;20:95–104.
71. Kennedy JC, Stewart R, Walker DM. Anterolateral rotatory instability of the knee joint. J Bone Joint Surg Am 1978;60-A:1031–9.
72. Fox JM, Blazina ME, Del Pizzo W, et al. Extra-articular stabilization of the knee joint for anterior instability. Clin Orthop Relat Res 1980;(147):56–61.
73. Neyret P, Palomo JR, Donell ST, et al. Extra-articular tenodesis for anterior cruciate ligament rupture in amateur skiers. Br J Sports Med 1994;28:31–4.
74. Amirault JD, Cameron JC, MacIntosh DL, et al. Chronic anterior cruciate ligament deficiency. Long-term results of MacIntosh's lateral substitution reconstruction. J Bone Joint Surg Br 1988;70(4):622–4.
75. Sydney S, Haynes D, Hungerford D, et al. The altered kinematic effect of an ilitotibial band tenodesis on the anterior cruciate deficient knee. Trans Orthopd Res Soc Annu Meet 1987;340.
76. Draganich LF, Reider B, Miller PR. An in vitro study of the Muller anterolateral femorotibial ligament tenodesis in the anterior cruciate ligament deficient knee. Am J Sports Med 1989;17:357–62.

77. Amis AA, Scammell BE. Biomechanics of intra-articular and extra-articular reconstruction of the anterior cruciate ligament. J Bone Joint Surg Br 1993;75: 812–7.

78. Tavlo M, Eljaja S, Jensen JT, et al. The role of the anterolateral ligament in ACL insufficient and reconstructed knees on rotatory stability: a biomechanical study on human cadavers. Scand J Med Sci Sports 2015;26(8):960–6.

79. Dandy DJ. Some clinical aspects of reconstruction for chronic anterior cruciate ligament deficiency. Ann R Coll Surg Engl 1995;77:290–8.

80. Bertoia JT, Urovitz EP, Richards RR, et al. Anterior cruciate reconstruction using the MacIntosh lateral-substitution over-the-top repair. J Bone Joint Surg Am 1985;67–S:1183–8.

81. Zarins B, Rowe CR. Combined anterior cruciate-ligament reconstruction using semitendinosus tendon and iliotibial tract. J Bone Joint Surg Am 1986;68-A: 160–77.

82. Rackemann S, Robinson A, Dandy DJ. Reconstruction of the anterior cruciate ligament with an intra-articular patellar tendon graft and an extra-articular tenodesis: results after six years. J Bone Joint Surg Br 1991;73-B:368–73.

83. Dejour H, Walsh G, Neyret P, et al. Resultats des laxites chroniques anterieures operees. Rev Chir Orthop Reparatrice Appar Mot 1988;74:622–36.

84. Dodds AL, Gupte CM, Neyret P, et al. Extra-articular techniques in anterior cruciate ligament reconstruction: a literature review. J Bone Joint Surg Br 2011; 93(11):1440–8.

85. Marcacci M, Zaffagnini S, Iacono F, et al. Arthroscopic intra- and extra-articular anterior cruciate ligament reconstruction with gracilis and semitendinosus tendons. Knee Surg Sports Traumatol Arthrosc 1998;6:68–75.

86. Marcacci M, Zaffagnini S, Giordano G, et al. Anterior cruciate ligament reconstruction associated with extra-articular tenodesis: a prospective clinical and radiographic evaluation with 10- to 13-year follow-up. Am J Sports Med 2009; 37:707–14.

87. Jensen JE, Slocum DB, Larson RL, et al. Reconstruction procedures for anterior cruciate ligament insufficiency: a computer analysis of clinical results. Am J Sports Med 1983;11(4):240–8.

88. Lerat J-L, Chotel F, Besse JL, et al. The results after 10-16 years of the treatment of chronic anterior laxity of the knee using reconstruction of the anterior cruciate ligament with a patellar tendon graft combined with an external extra-articular reconstruction. Rev Chir Orthop Reparatrice Appar Mot 1998;84(8):712–27 [in French].

89. Hewison CE, Tran MN, Kaniki N, et al. Lateral extra-articular tenodesis reduces rotational laxity when combined with anterior cruciate ligament reconstruction: a systematic review of the literature. Arthroscopy 2015;31(10):2022–34.

90. Zaffagnini S, Marcacci M, Lo Presti M, et al. Prospective and randomized evaluation of ACL reconstruction with three techniques: a clinical and radiographic evaluation at 5 years follow-up. Knee Surg Sports Traumatol Arthrosc 2006;14: 1060–9.

91. O'Brien SJ, Warren RF, Wickiewicz TL, et al. The iliotibial band lateral sling procedure and its effect on the results of anterior cruciate ligament reconstruction. Am J Sports Med 1991;19(1):21–4 [discussion: 24–5].

92. Sonnery-Cottet B, Thaunat M, Freychet B, et al. Outcome of a combined anterior cruciate ligament and anterolateral ligament reconstruction technique with a minimum 2-year follow-up. Am J Sports Med 2015;43(7):1598–605.

93. Colombet P. Knee laxity control in revision anterior cruciate ligament reconstruction versus anterior cruciate ligament reconstruction and lateral tenodesis: clinical assessment using computer-assisted navigation. Am J Sports Med 2011; 39(6):1248–54.
94. Trojani C, Beaufils P, Burdin G, et al. Revision ACL reconstruction: influence of a lateral tenodesis. Knee Surg Sports Traumatol Arthrosc 2012;20(8):1565–70.
95. Musahl V, Kopf S, Rabuck S, et al. Rotatory knee laxity tests and the pivot shift as tools for ACL treatment algorithm. Knee Surg Sports Traumatol Arthrosc 2012;20:793–800.
96. Lerat JL, Moyen BL, Cladière F, et al. Knee instability after injury to the anterior cruciate ligament. Quantification of the Lachman test. J Bone Joint Surg Br 2000;82:42–7.
97. Lording TD, Lustig S, Servien E, et al. Lateral reinforcement in anterior cruciate ligament reconstruction. Sports Med Arthrosc Rehabil Ther Technol 2014;1: 3–10.
98. Getgood A. Lateral extra-articular tenodesis (LET) - indications and technique [Internet]. VuMedi. 2014. Available at: https://www.vumedi.com/video/lateral-extra-articular-tenodesis-let-indications-and-technique/. Accessed March, 2014.
99. Shelbourne K, Gray T, Haro M. Incidence of subsequent injury to either knee within 5 years after anterior cruciate ligament reconstruction with patellar tendon autograft. Am J Sports Med 2009;37:246–51.
100. Salmon L, Russell V, Musgrove T, et al. Incidence and risk factors for graft rupture and contralateral rupture after anterior cruciate ligament reconstruction. Arthroscopy 2005;21:948–57.
101. Wright RW, Dunn WR, Amendola A, et al. Risk of tearing the intact anterior cruciate ligament in the contralateral knee and rupturing the anterior cruciate ligament graft during the first 2 years after anterior cruciate ligament reconstruction: a prospective MOON cohort study. Am J Sports Med 2007;35:1131–4.
102. Brophy R, Schmitz L, Wright RW. Return to play and future ACL injury risk after ACL reconstruction in soccer athletes from the Multicenter Orthopaedic Outcomes Network (MOON) group. Am J Sports Med 2012;40:2517–22.
103. Getgood A. Standard ACL Reconstruction vs ACL + Lateral Extra-Articular Tenodesis Study (STAbiLiTY). ClinicalTrials.gov. 2013. Available at: https://clinicaltrials.gov/ct2/show/NCT02018354. Accessed December 10, 2014.

Etiologic Factors That Lead to Failure After Primary Anterior Cruciate Ligament Surgery

James D. Wylie, MD, MHS[a], Lucas S. Marchand, MD[b],
Robert T. Burks, MD[b],*

KEYWORDS

- Anterior cruciate ligament • Reconstruction • Failure • Revision • Etiologic factors

KEY POINTS

- Primary anterior cruciate ligament (ACL) surgery failure can be grouped into stiffness, infection, instability, and poor patient-reported outcomes without objective failure, such as pain.
- Proper diagnosis and treatment of associated injuries and bony malalignment, as well as proper timing of surgery, can limit failures and contribute to optimizing patient outcomes.
- Improper graft choices and technical errors during surgery that are avoidable can lead to stiffness and/or graft failure.
- Biological failure of ligamentization of grafts can lead to graft failure even in the absence of other identifiable errors.

INTRODUCTION

The anterior cruciate ligament (ACL) is the most commonly injured ligament in the knee and among the most commonly treated sporting injuries. The reported incidence is between 37 and 69 per 100,000 persons each year, with the highest incidence in patients between the ages of 14 and 25 years of age.[1–3] In the United States alone, there are 200,000 ACL ruptures per year.[1–4] This number has been increasing annually over the last 2 decades.[1] With the increasing incidence of this injury, there also is an inevitable increase in the number of failures and revision surgeries. Recent prospective studies

Disclosure Statement: J.D. Wylie and L.S. Marchand have nothing to disclose. R.T. Burks is an unpaid consultant and receives royalties from Arthrex, receives research support from DePuy, and is a paid consultant for VirtaMed and Mitek.
Funding: There was no outside funding for this article.
[a] Department of Orthopedic Surgery, University of Connecticut, Farmington, CT, USA;
[b] Department of Orthopedic Surgery, University of Utah, 590 Wakara Way, Salt Lake City, UT 84108, USA
* Corresponding author.
E-mail address: Robert.Burks@hsc.utah.edu

Clin Sports Med 36 (2017) 155–172
http://dx.doi.org/10.1016/j.csm.2016.08.007
0278-5919/17/© 2016 Elsevier Inc. All rights reserved.

sportsmed.theclinics.com

from the Multicenter Orthopedic Outcomes Network (MOON) group reported a failure rate of 4.4% at minimum 2-year follow-up and 7.7% at 6-year follow-up.[5,6] The classic teaching is that the mechanism of failure is technical failure of the operation in most cases.[7] However, the Multicenter ACL Revision Study (MARS) has recently published that the cause of ACL failure is most commonly repeat trauma, followed by technical errors, lack of biological healing or fixation, or some combination of these causes.[8] Causes for failure are outlined in **Box 1**. When faced with a failure and revision is required, revision ACL reconstruction compared with primary ACL reconstruction have significantly poorer outcomes.[9] This includes a graft failure rate that can approach 4 times that of primary ACL reconstruction, depending on the study.[9] In addition to graft failure causing recurrent instability, significant pain or stiffness, patient reported poor knee function, and/or inability to return to sport all should be considered failure of primary ACL reconstruction. Given the inferior outcomes reported in revision ACL reconstruction, this article reviews the common etiologic factors leading to the failure of primary ACL reconstruction in hopes of preventing future failures and poor patient outcomes.

FAILURE OF PRIMARY ANTERIOR CRUCIATE LIGAMENT RECONSTRUCTION
Stiffness or Arthrofibrosis

A common postoperative complication seen after ACL reconstruction is stiffness.[10] This outcome ranges from a small decrease in terminal flexion or extension to a marked overall decrease in range of motion, the end result of which can be disabling.[11,12] Arthrofibrosis is a significant loss of flexion and extension with fibrosis of the medial and lateral gutters, prepatellar fat pad, and suprapatellar pouch. Paulos

---

Box 1
Common causes of failure of anterior cruciate ligament reconstruction

Arthrofibrosis and stiffness
  Early surgery
  Prolonged immobilization
  Graft impingement and errors in tunnel placement

Infection

Instability
  Concomitant ligamentous Injury
  Meniscal injury
  Bony malalignment
  Graft impingement and errors in tunnel placement
  Traumatic graft failure
  Failure of fixation
  Graft tension and isometry
  Failure of graft incorporation

Pain
  Anterior knee pain
  Meniscal injury
  Chondral injury
  Joint degeneration

Subjective and patient-reported failure
  Patient-reported outcome scores
  Patient satisfaction
  Failure to return to sport

---

and colleagues[13] described it as infrapatellar contraction causing significant reduction of both flexion and extension, with an associated decrease in patellar mobility characterized as patellar entrapment and patellar infera. This is caused by exaggerated pathologic fibrous hyperplasia of the anterior soft tissues. Loss of extension is usually more symptomatic compared with loss of flexion, and it is associated with patellofemoral pain, quadriceps weakness, and overall poor knee function.[13,14] Treatment of arthrofibrosis should be directed at improving range of motion and limb function. Conservative management can be successful but arthroscopic debridement, releases, and manipulation are often needed.[15] However, prevention should be the primary goal in dealing with arthrofibrosis or even mild motion loss.[16] Several surgical factors have been implicated as contributors to arthrofibrosis or stiffness following ACL reconstruction, including reconstruction performed in an acute setting before regaining normal range of motion, prolonged postoperative immobilization, infection, development of a cyclops lesion, and graft impingement.

Early surgery

An initial report from Shelbourne and colleagues[17] noted that patients undergoing reconstruction within the first week of injury had a significant increase in arthrofibrosis compared with those who had surgery greater than 21 days from injury. Passler and colleagues[18] assessed the timing of surgical intervention and noted a much higher rate of arthrofibrosis (18%) in patients undergoing ACL reconstruction within 7 days of injury compared with patients who waited at least 4 weeks (6%). Furthermore, the irritability of the knee (eg, swelling, effusion, hyperthermia), and preoperative deficits in knee extension and flexion range of motion have a strong association with arthrofibrosis.[19]

Contradicting studies demonstrated no difference in final knee range of motion when evaluating early versus delayed reconstruction. These studies included surgeries that were only bone-patella tendon-bone and military recruit subjects and, therefore, may have limited generalizability.[20,21] A recent meta-analysis evaluated pooled data from 8 studies and revealed no significant increase in risk of adverse outcomes, including arthrofibrosis with early surgery using a variety of time-point cutoffs.[22] These investigators concluded that with modern surgical technique and an accelerated rehabilitation protocol, early ACL reconstruction does not increase the risk of complication. Therefore, the optimal timing of ACL reconstruction has been the subject of much interest and debate. In the investigators' opinion, a knee that is not inflamed or painful, with full ability to easily have full extension and flexion, is desirable when considering ACL reconstruction and that the potential risks associated with early surgery is not warranted.[19,23]

Prolonged immobilization

Prolonged immobilization following ACL reconstruction is a well-established risk factor for developing stiffness. Immobilization for 2 weeks following surgery results in significant motion loss in nearly half of patients.[24] Immobilization in extension is preferable if needed for a short period of time because regaining lost extension is more difficult than lost flexion. Additional early range-of-motion protocols provide favorable outcomes in this regard.[24] Early joint movement inhibits the expression of proinflammatory genes that may play a role in the development of scar tissue.[24,25] Furthermore, early range of motion following an injury reduces the formation of adhesions and provides nutrition for joint surfaces.[26–28]

Impingement

Another purely intra-articular cause of lost range of motion following ACL reconstruction is cyclops syndrome.[29] This manifests itself not as global arthrofibrosis but rather as an isolated extension loss after ACL reconstruction caused by a mechanical block from hypertrophic fibrous tissue attached to the tibial insertion point of the ACL graft.[30] This most likely results from anterior graft placement in the tibia causing repetitive trauma of the graft against bone from impingement on the top of the notch and graft hypertrophy with fibrous tissue proliferation.[24] See later discussion of other consequences of nonanatomic tunnel placement and instability.

Other sources

There are other factors leading to stiffness in the postoperative period following ACL reconstruction, including persistent synovitis, complex regional pain syndrome, and genetic risk factors.[10,24,31] Although, unrelated to surgical technique, these complications lead to the same end result and functional limitations for patients.

Infection

Infections are uncommon after ACL reconstruction, occurring in less than 1% of cases.[32] The outcomes of deep infection following ACL reconstruction are mixed. Overall outcomes are much worse for patients with postoperative infection and stiffness.[33–37] Infection needs to be evaluated emergently and addressed with prompt irrigation and debridement and antibiotic management to prevent devastating long-term consequences. Grafts can be preserved with rapid diagnosis and treatment but failure to respond to treatment should warrant consideration of graft and fixation removal. Even with prompt treatment, stiffness following infection may be the most devastating of complications and thus the need for careful management in this arena is emphasized.

Instability

Misdiagnosed or undiagnosed secondary injuries

Although ACL tears commonly occur in isolation, one has to be vigilant in the diagnosis of concomitant injuries to the knee or mechanical factors that may have contributed to the primary ACL failure. These injuries include other ligamentous injuries that further destabilize the knee, meniscal injuries that can lead to altered secondary stabilization of the knee, and bony malalignment that may lead to increased stress on the ACL reconstruction.

Concomitant ligamentous injuries are not uncommon in the setting of an ACL rupture. Potential injuries include medial collateral ligament tears, posterolateral corner injuries, and posterior cruciate ligament tears. More recently, there has been increased interest in the importance of anterolateral capsular thickening in knee stability that some now refer to as the anterolateral ligament (ALL) of the knee. The anterolateral capsule has long been recognized as an important structure in ACL tears in which a Segond fragment on radiographs was diagnostic for an ACL injury.[38] In ACL graft failures, 15% were found to have some type of untreated ligamentous laxity that contributed to the failure of the primary reconstruction.[39] In addition, the MARS group attributed 7% of the technical errors seen in their revision cohort to untreated concomitant ligamentous laxity or bony malalignment.[8]

Medial collateral ligament injuries occur in approximately 20% of ACL tears.[40] These commonly heal with nonoperative measures; however, if there is continued valgus laxity, this will lead to increased loads on the ACL graft that could predispose it to failure. In this setting, medial collateral ligament reconstruction is recommended to restore stability to the medial side of the knee. Posterolateral laxity is common in the chronic ACL deficient knee, being present in up to 15% of cases.[41] LaPrade and colleagues[42] demonstrated that ACL graft forces increase with sequential sectioning of the structures in the posterolateral corner. In addition, reconstruction of the ACL with either a single-bundle or double-bundle technique cannot recreate normal knee kinematics in the absence of the lateral collateral ligament.[43] Therefore, physical examination and detailed imaging evaluation of the posterolateral corner should be undertaken in any patient with an ACL tear. If posterolateral laxity is noted, then either primary repair or reconstruction of the posterolateral structures should be performed to restore normal knee kinematics and protect the ACL reconstruction. Recent biomechanical studies have suggested that in the setting of combined ACL and ALL tears, reconstruction of both ligaments may help to restore normal knee kinematics.[44,45] Future clinical studies of ACL failures and combined ACL-ALL reconstructions will be important to further delineate the importance of the ALL in the ACL injured knee.

The medial meniscus is an important secondary stabilizer of anterior translation of the tibia.[46] In turn, meniscal deficiency can affect stresses on the ACL graft after reconstruction.[46] Missed medial posterior horn or posterior meniscal root injury that is not repaired at the time of index surgery or meniscectomy could lead to abnormal forces in the ACL graft, making it susceptible to failure.[47] This missed injury can also lead to continued knee pain, abnormal loading of the articular cartilage, and potentially early degenerative changes in the joint.

Bony malalignment

Bony malalignment is another concomitant pathologic condition that can easily be missed in the setting of an ACL tear. More specifically, either varus malalignment and/or an increase in tibial slope both may contribute to failure of ACL reconstruction. Varus malalignment increases the stress in the ACL.[48] This is most severe in the setting of varus malalignment with a dynamic varus thrust on ambulation. In this setting, a valgus producing high tibial osteotomy may be indicated to protect the ACL graft from chronic repeated stress and elongation.[49] Increased tibial slope also causes alterations in the resting position of the tibiofemoral joint.[50,51] Studies have found that increasing tibial slope leads to more anterior translation of the tibia. Recent clinical studies have identified increasing lateral tibial plateau slope as a risk factor for early graft failure after ACL reconstruction.[52] In addition, patients with increased tibial slope and history of ACL revision had improved knee stability and graft survival with re-revision of their ACL and deflexion osteotomy of the tibial plateau.[53,54] More research is needed to fully understand the influence of tibial slope on the failure of ACL reconstruction.

Errors in tunnel placement

As a result of inaccurate surgical technique with tunnel placement, excessive graft forces and strain may result in inadequate incorporation and failure.[10] Errors in tunnel placement may lead to postoperative loss of motion secondary to impingement or persistent instability with graft failure given the lack of anatomic reconstruction. As a result of inaccurate surgical technique, excessive graft forces and strain may lead to inadequate incorporation and/or result in early instability.[55] Recent studies have suggested that technical error, most commonly poor tunnel placement, is thought to contribute to failure in 22% to 79% of cases.[10] Failure to replicate the native ACL anatomic footprints can lead to increased graft stress and, eventually, excessive laxity, loss of motion, or injury to other structures (**Table 1**).[10,55–57] Technical error in this arena is thought to be the most likely culprit of early ACL graft laxity and failure.[10] Anatomic tunnel placement is the most important technical step in ACL reconstruction. The authors' preferred technique is creation of the tibial and femoral tunnel at the midpoint of the ACL remnant on each.

Table 1
Errors in tunnel placement and resultant problems

Tunnel	Error in Placement	Result
Femoral	Anterior	Excessive graft tension in flexion
		Loss of flexion or stretching and laxity of graft
	Posterior	Excessive graft tension in extension
		Graft laxity in flexion
	Vertical	Less rotational stability
		Can predispose to anterior impingement of the graft
Tibial	Anterior	Impingement against the intercondylar notch
		Loss of extension
	Posterior	Impingement against the posterior cruciate ligament
		Loss of flexion or stretching and laxity of graft
		Less control of anterior translation
	Medial or lateral	Impingement of the graft on the intercondylar notch
		Injury to the tibial plateau articular cartilage
		Injury to the meniscal roots

Traumatic graft failure

Several investigations have been completed to evaluate the short-term and long-term risks of failure per graft type used. Initial studies associated the use of hamstring grafts,[58] single-bundle reconstruction,[59,60] younger age,[58,61,62] higher activity level, female patients,[58,63–66] smaller hamstring autograft size (<8 mm),[64] and contact mechanisms of the initial injury with graft rupture.[65] However, the difficulties with drawing conclusions from these studies include the inconsistent definition of graft failure, smaller cohort sizes, and lack of control for confounding variables. Furthermore, there is concern that these studies lacked adequate reporting of failure events given their largely retrospective nature. In an effort to address the pitfalls in prior studies, Mohtadi and colleagues[67] performed a prospective randomized clinical trial comparing 3 graft types (patellar tendon, quadruple-stranded hamstring tendon, and double-bundle hamstring tendon autografts) for ACL reconstruction. With a minimum of 2-year follow-up and 300 subjects included in the study, the investigators identified that more traumatic reinjuries occurred with hamstrings tendon autograft, double-bundle grafts, and subjects with higher Tegner activity levels. Younger age was an independent predictor of complete traumatic rerupture and traumatic reinjury, irrespective of graft type.[67]

More recently, both the Swedish and Norwegian ACL reconstruction registries reported multivariable analyses controlling for factors such as sex, age, and surgical characteristics, including autograft type used for reconstruction. In the Swedish study, Andernord and colleagues[68] demonstrated that graft selection, graft width, a single-bundle or a double-bundle technique, femoral graft fixation, the injury-to-surgery interval, and meniscus injury were not predictors of early revision surgery in a cohort of 13,102 subjects. The Norwegian study by Persson and colleagues[69] included 12,643 subjects and noted that subjects with hamstring tendon grafts had twice the risk of revision compared with subjects with patellar tendon grafts. Younger age was noted to be the most important risk factor for revision and no effect was seen for sex.

Data from the MOON group was used to further investigate subsequent ACL injury after primary ACL reconstruction in the United States.[6] In this prospective longitudinal cohort study of 2683 subjects, younger age, higher activity level, and allograft type were predictors of increased odds of ipsilateral graft failure. The odds of ACL graft failure were 5.2 times greater for an allograft compared with autograft. There was no difference noted between patellar tendon and hamstring tendon autografts. Furthermore, higher activity level and younger age were risk factors for contralateral ACL tears. Many similarities exist between the MOON study and Scandinavia registries, including prospective collection of data, overlapping time periods of enrollment, near-equivalent sex distribution, and use of multivariable analysis to control for confounding factors. Evaluation of all 3 studies yields 2 consistent results: younger age is a primary risk factor for revision ACL reconstruction and sex is not a risk factor. Additional data, such as the risk of reinjury in hamstring versus patellar tendon autograft, remain discordant between studies. Possible explanations for this finding include differences in size of graft used but further investigation in this arena is warranted.

Failure of fixation

Many options for graft fixation exist and the strength afforded by the various methods differs significantly between fixation types.[70] In clinical practice, these variations may manifest as differences in postoperative laxity; however, most clinical trials comparing different fixation devices have not found major differences.[69,71–79] In vitro biomechanical studies have demonstrated that most graft fixation devices investigated have sufficient fixation strength to withstand the estimated forces calculated for the ACL during various normal day activities.[80–86] Complicating in vitro biomechanical studies, however, is that in vivo incorporation is a complex biological event. It has been suggested that the weakest link in the early postoperative phase is the graft fixation technique; however, few comparative studies about the role of different fixation techniques and graft incorporation have been done.[87]

In a nonrandomized study comparing interference screw versus transcondylar cross-pins, no difference in radiographic or objective laxity outcome was noted.[88] However, Ibrahim and colleagues[89] conducted a randomized clinical trial comparing femoral intratunnel cross-pin fixation with bio absorbable Rigidfix pins (Mitek, Raynham, MA) versus extra-tunnel fixation with an Endobutton (Smith & Nephew, Andover, MA). They noted no failure in the intra-tunnel fixation cohort (n = 34) but 4 failures in the extra-tunnel fixation cohort (n = 32). A separate randomized trial compared aperture fixation (bone-patellar tendon-bone with intra-articular screw fixation) to suspensory fixation (cortical button for quadrupled hamstring grafts) and noted that aperture fixation increases overall construct stiffness in the early postoperative period but demonstrates no long-term superiority in regard to patient outcome or rate of revision.[90,91]

Some surgeons favor the use of aperture fixation methods to avoid problems related to the windshield wiper effect from micromotion as seen with suspensory fixation.[92] The use of suspensory fixation has been coupled with tunnel widening[93–95] but several studies have reported no clinical effect of this phenomenon.[93,96,97]

In a large registry study, fixation methods, including femoral extra-tunnel fixation constructs had hazards ratio for revision at 2 years, were significantly greater than that of femoral intra-tunnel fixation constructs.[98] However, a separate registry study also evaluated the effect of femoral-sided graft fixation and noted no significant difference between constructs used.[68] Recent data from the Norwegian registry showed the highest revision rates in hamstring tendons with suspensory fixation in the femur along with bioabsorbable interference screws in the tibia.[98]

The tibial graft fixation site is known to have a lower fixation strength than the femoral sided fixation site.[99–101] Bioabsorable screws are often used but they may not be degraded several years after surgery.[102] Given the association between tunnel widening on the femoral side with bioabsorbable screws, some investigators suggest other alternatives for fixation on the tibial side be considered.

Graft tensioning and isometry

Applying the appropriate tension to a reconstructed ACL graft is often performed by surgeons based on experience and their perception of applied tension.[103] Initial tensioning of graft is typically done without objective measuring devices and with a presumably variable force applied by the surgeon.[104] However, there are inherent problems with manual application of tension to the ACL reconstruction, such as under-tightening or over-tightening the reconstruction.[103] The concern with under-tightening is that this may lead to persistent instability, whereas over-tightening may have deleterious effects on cartilage by increasing joint contact forces.[105,106] Furthermore, with manual surgeon tensioning concerns about inconsistent tension application between patients persists and, hence, the development of commercially designed tensioning devices.[103] Commercial devices are available to aid in the application of a fixed tension force in a reproducible manner but data are scarce regarding the clinical benefit of these instruments. Data regarding the use of a tensioning device must be interpreted within the context that little consensus on the amount of tension required to produce an optimal outcome exists.[107,108]

Failure of graft incorporation

A subset of patients that have failures of their ACL reconstruction despite appropriate diagnosis, tunnel placement, graft choice, and graft fixation. These patients have failure of graft incorporation or ligamentization. This failure occurs due to multiple reasons. True failure of graft incorporation is a diagnosis of exclusion because the mechanisms of failure explained previously must be ruled out before a diagnosis of failure of graft incorporation or ligamentization can be made.[109]

Graft incorporation starts early after implantation. The first phase is necrosis, in which the avascular graft undergoes necrosis due to lack of blood supply. This stimulates revascularization of the graft by 2 months postoperatively.[110] Revascularization happens primarily from the bone tunnels, as well as from the fat-pad distally and the posterior synovial tissues proximally. Therefore, care must be taken to not excessively debride these tissues during reconstruction.[111] Revascularization can be inhibited by smoking, cocaine use, and diabetes.[109] Autograft has more rapid and complete vascularization compared with allograft tissue.[112] Allografts can also generate an immune reaction to the graft that leads to a longer and less complete incorporation of the graft.[113] This may explain higher failure rates with allograft but an increased rate of biological failure has not been shown definitively with allograft compared with autograft if no secondarily sterilized grafts are considered. Sterilization of allografts is also an important factor in failure. Graft irradiation greater than 1.8 mrad and BioCleanse graft (RTI Surgical, Alachua, FL) processing is associated with graft failure.[114] After the graft has revascularized, it undergoes cellular repopulation and proliferation, which is generally complete by 3 months after surgery and correlates with growth factor production by cells populating the graft.[115] The graft then undergoes collagen remodeling and ligamentization. A proper mechanical environment is important for the ligamentization process and, therefore, the technical errors outlined previously can lead to abnormal or incomplete biological healing of the graft.

Pain

Anterior knee pain

Pain is not uncommon after ACL reconstruction. Anterior knee pain can occur in up to half of patients after surgery.[116] This may be more common in patients in the setting of patella tendon grafts. Stiffness and arthrofibrosis are common causes of anterior knee pain and are previously described in detail. Shelbourne and colleagues[117] think that anterior knee pain is due to patients not regaining the natural hyperextension of the knee joint postoperatively and reported that, if subjects with patellar tendon grafts regain this motion, then they have no increased incidence of anterior knee pain compared with a control population. Proper rehabilitation and return of full quadriceps function is important in preventing and treating anterior knee pain. In the setting of recalcitrant anterior knee pain and failure of conservative measures, an interval release may help alleviate pain and loss of function.[118]

Meniscal tears

Meniscal tears are common in ACL-injured knees. Meniscal preservation or repair is preferred over meniscectomy because loss of meniscal tissue can lead to joint degeneration. Prior partial meniscectomy is a risk factor for a higher rate of chondral changes at the time of revision ACL reconstruction.[119] In addition, a history of meniscal repair is associated with less chondral changes at revision compared with a partial menisectomy.[119] A recent report from the MOON cohort reported that small peripheral tears left untreated at the time of ACL surgery were unlikely to undergo further surgery at 6 years follow-up.[120] This supports meniscal preservation by avoiding partial meniscectomy in small peripheral tears.

Chondral injuries

Femoral chondral defects diagnosed at the time of ACL reconstruction are also predictive of poor outcomes. Data from the MOON cohort report worse patient-reported outcomes at 6 years in patients with chondral injuries at the time of ACL reconstruction.[121] In 24-year follow-up of a cohort of patients, Pernin and colleagues[122] found that femoral chondral defects and medial meniscus status was predictive of the onset of radiographic osteoarthritis postoperatively. Similarly, Filardo and colleagues[123] systematically reviewed the literature and found that the presence, depth, and location of cartilage lesions influence subjective, objective, and radiographic outcomes of ACL reconstruction. Interestingly, only 9% of cartilage lesions were treated in the studies they reviewed.[123] In the setting of revision ACL reconstruction, there is an increased incidence of chondral lesions compared with primary and this further increases with prior menisectomy.[124] Although chondral defects are associated with earlier onset arthritis and poorer outcomes after ACL reconstruction, there is no definitive evidence that treating these with chondral restoring procedures improves that natural history of these injuries.

Joint degeneration

Concomitant chondral and meniscal injuries at initial ACL injury lead to osteoarthritic change over time. Most patients with ACL injuries have bony edema at the time of injury, which likely represents an impact injury to the chondral surface, even in the absence of a focal chondral defects.[125] Traditionally, reconstruction of the ACL was thought to protect the joint from degenerative change by restoring stability. However, the joint preserving function of ACL reconstruction is controversial. A recent longitudinal cohort study suggests a decrease in secondary meniscal injuries, diagnoses of osteoarthritis, and subsequent joint arthroplasty in patients undergoing acute reconstruction compared with delayed reconstruction or nonoperative treatment.[1] Osteoarthritic progression at a young age can lead to a painful and stiff joint, requiring knee arthroplasty for pain relief and return of function.

Patient-Reported Outcomes, Patient Satisfaction, and Return to Sport

Outcomes reporting in orthopedic surgery transitioned over the last 30 years from clinician-centered measures to patient-reported outcomes scores. With this, there are at times disparity between what the surgeon determines to be a good outcome and the patient-reported outcome. In the setting of ACL reconstruction, an example of this would be the patient with a stable ACL with return of full lower extremity strength who reports a poor outcome on patient-reported measures and/or cannot return to sport. Some patient-reported measures, such as the Knee injury and Osteoarthritis Outcome Score (KOOS) that measures multiple dimensions (ie, pain, function, activities of daily living) of patient-reported outcome, can be useful to decipher why the patient reports a poor outcome from an ACL reconstruction that when measured by objective measures seems like a success. Poor patient-reported outcomes could also be influenced by unrealistic expectations of the patient preoperatively, causing an inability for the intervention to meet the patient's goals.[39] In addition, patient-reported outcomes measures could be influenced by patient comorbid factors, such as psychosocial factors and patient mental health, which could influence the patient's perceived outcome.[126] The inability to return to sport also is confounded because high school or college seniors who suffer ACL tears may not be able to return to the same level of play due to there not being an opportunity to return to that same level. Rather, if they want to return to play, then they have to be able to propel themselves to a higher level of play; that is, the high school senior must be able to play in college, or the college senior must be able to play professionally. These factors may create an outcome that the patient or physician perceives to be worse due to the measurement tool used to judge the outcome.

SUMMARY

ACL reconstruction can fail in multiple ways that can be grouped into 3 main categories: stiffness, pain, and instability. Although graft failure is the most common form of failure associated with failure of ACL reconstruction, other modes of failure can also lead to poor patient outcomes. Proper prehabilitation, intraoperative tunnel placement, graft choice, graft fixation, graft tensioning, identification and treatment of concomitant meniscal, chondral and ligamentous injuries, and proper rehabilitation can optimize the outcomes of primary ACL reconstruction and, it is hoped, avoid the inferior patient outcomes associated with revision ACL reconstruction.

REFERENCES

1. Sanders TL, Maradit Kremers H, Bryan AJ, et al. Incidence of anterior cruciate ligament tears and reconstruction: a 21-year population-based study. Am J Sports Med 2016;44(6):1502–7.
2. Gianotti SM, Marshall SW, Hume PA, et al. Incidence of anterior cruciate ligament injury and other knee ligament injuries: a national population-based study. J Sci Med Sport 2009;12(6):622–7.
3. Parkkari J, Pasanen K, Mattila VM, et al. The risk for a cruciate ligament injury of the knee in adolescents and young adults: a population-based cohort study of 46 500 people with a 9 year follow-up. Br J Sports Med 2008;42(6):422–6.
4. Griffin LY, Albohm MJ, Arendt EA, et al. Understanding and preventing noncontact anterior cruciate ligament injuries: a review of the Hunt Valley II meeting, January 2005. Am J Sports Med 2006;34(9):1512–32.
5. Hettrich CM, Dunn WR, Reinke EK, et al. The rate of subsequent surgery and predictors after anterior cruciate ligament reconstruction: two- and 6-year follow-up results from a multicenter cohort. Am J Sports Med 2013;41(7):1534–40.
6. Kaeding CC, Pedroza AD, Reinke EK, et al, MOON Consortium. Risk factors and predictors of subsequent ACL injury in either knee after ACL

reconstruction: prospective analysis of 2488 primary ACL reconstructions from the MOON cohort. Am J Sports Med 2015;43(7):1583–90.

7. George MS, Dunn WR, Spindler KP. Current concepts review: revision anterior cruciate ligament reconstruction. Am J Sports Med 2006;34(12):2026–37.

8. The MARS Group, Wright RW, Huston LJ, Spindler KP, et al. Descriptive epidemiology of the multicenter ACL revision study (MARS) cohort. Am J Sports Med 2010;38(10):1979–86.

9. Wright RW, Gill CS, Chen L, et al. Outcome of revision anterior cruciate ligament reconstruction: a systematic review. J Bone Joint Surg Am 2012;94(6):531–6.

10. Kamath GV, Redfern JC, Greis PE, et al. Revision anterior cruciate ligament reconstruction. Am J Sports Med 2011;39(1):199–217.

11. Shelbourne KD, Patel DV, Martini DJ. Classification and management of arthrofibrosis of the knee after anterior cruciate ligament reconstruction. Am J Sports Med 1996;24(6):857–62.

12. Laubenthal KN, Smidt GL, Kettelkamp DB. A quantitative analysis of knee motion during activities of daily living. Phys Ther 1972;52(1):34–43.

13. Paulos LE, Rosenberg TD, Drawbert J, et al. Infrapatellar contracture syndrome. An unrecognized cause of knee stiffness with patella entrapment and patella infera. Am J Sports Med 1987;15(4):331–41.

14. Aglietti P, Buzzi R, D'Andria S, et al. Patellofemoral problems after intraarticular anterior cruciate ligament reconstruction. Clin Orthop Relat Res 1993;288: 195–204.

15. Paulos LE, Wnorowski DC, Greenwald AE. Infrapatellar contracture syndrome. Diagnosis, treatment, and long-term followup. Am J Sports Med 1994;22(4): 440–9.

16. Shelbourne KD, Patel DV. Treatment of limited motion after anterior cruciate ligament reconstruction. Knee Surg Sports Traumatol Arthrosc 1999;7(2):85–92.

17. Shelbourne KD, Wilckens JH, Mollabashy A, et al. Arthrofibrosis in acute anterior cruciate ligament reconstruction. The effect of timing of reconstruction and rehabilitation. Am J Sports Med 1991;19(4):332–6.

18. Passler JM, Schippinger G, Schweighofer F, et al. [Complications in 283 cruciate ligament replacement operations with free patellar tendon transplantation. Modification by surgical technique and surgery timing]. Unfallchirurgie 1995; 21(5):240–6.

19. Mayr HO, Weig TG, Plitz W. Arthrofibrosis following ACL reconstruction–reasons and outcome. Arch Orthop Trauma Surg 2004;124(8):518–22.

20. Bottoni CR, Liddell TR, Trainor TJ, et al. Postoperative range of motion following anterior cruciate ligament reconstruction using autograft hamstrings: a prospective, randomized clinical trial of early versus delayed reconstructions. Am J Sports Med 2008;36(4):656–62.

21. Almekinders LC, Moore T, Freedman D, et al. Post-operative problems following anterior cruciate ligament reconstruction. Knee Surg Sports Traumatol Arthrosc 1995;3(2):78–82.

22. Kwok CS, Harrison T, Servant C. The optimal timing for anterior cruciate ligament reconstruction with respect to the risk of postoperative stiffness. Arthroscopy 2013;29(3):556–65.

23. Evans S, Shaginaw J, Bartolozzi A. Acl reconstruction - it's all about timing. Int J Sports Phys Ther 2014;9(2):268–73.

24. Magit D, Wolff A, Sutton K, et al. Arthrofibrosis of the knee. J Am Acad Orthop Surg 2007;15(11):682–94.

25. Dossumbekova A, Anghelina M, Madhavan S, et al. Biomechanical signals inhibit IKK activity to attenuate NF-kappaB transcription activity in inflamed chondrocytes. Arthritis Rheum 2007;56(10):3284–96.

26. Madhavan S, Anghelina M, Rath-Deschner B, et al. Biomechanical signals exert sustained attenuation of proinflammatory gene induction in articular chondrocytes. Osteoarthritis Cartilage 2006;14(10):1023–32.

27. Nam J, Perera P, Liu J, et al. Transcriptome-wide gene regulation by gentle treadmill walking during the progression of monoiodoacetate-induced arthritis. Arthritis Rheum 2011;63(6):1613–25.

28. O'Driscoll SW, Keeley FW, Salter RB. Durability of regenerated articular cartilage produced by free autogenous periosteal grafts in major full-thickness defects in joint surfaces under the influence of continuous passive motion. A follow-up report at one year. J Bone Joint Surg Am 1988;70(4):595–606.

29. Jackson DW, Schaefer RK. Cyclops syndrome: loss of extension following intra-articular anterior cruciate ligament reconstruction. Arthroscopy 1990;6(3):171–8.

30. Fullerton LR, Andrews JR. Mechanical block to extension following augmentation of the anterior cruciate ligament. A case report. Am J Sports Med 1984;12(2):166–8.

31. Skutek M, Elsner H-A, Slateva K, et al. Screening for arthrofibrosis after anterior cruciate ligament reconstruction: analysis of association with human leukocyte antigen. Arthroscopy 2004;20(5):469–73.

32. Gobbi A, Karnatzikos G, Chaurasia S, et al. Postoperative infection after anterior cruciate ligament reconstruction. Sports Health 2016;8(2):187–9.

33. Williams RJ, Laurencin CT, Warren RF, et al. Septic arthritis after arthroscopic anterior cruciate ligament reconstruction. Diagnosis and management. Am J Sports Med 1997;25(2):261–7.

34. McAllister DR, Parker RD, Cooper AE, et al. Outcomes of postoperative septic arthritis after anterior cruciate ligament reconstruction. Am J Sports Med 1999;27(5):562–70.

35. Viola R, Marzano N, Vianello R. An unusual epidemic of Staphylococcus-negative infections involving anterior cruciate ligament reconstruction with salvage of the graft and function. Arthroscopy 2000;16(2):173–7.

36. Keays SL, Newcombe PA, Bullock-Saxton JE, et al. Factors involved in the development of osteoarthritis after anterior cruciate ligament surgery. Am J Sports Med 2010;38(3):455–63.

37. Judd D, Bottoni C, Kim D, et al. Infections following arthroscopic anterior cruciate ligament reconstruction. Arthroscopy 2006;22(4):375–84.

38. Goldman AB, Pavlov H, Rubenstein D. The Segond fracture of the proximal tibia: a small avulsion that reflects major ligamentous damage. AJR Am J Roentgenol 1988;151(6):1163–7.

39. Getelman MH, Friedman MJ. Revision anterior cruciate ligament reconstruction surgery. J Am Acad Orthop Surg 1999;7(3):189–98.

40. Yoon KH, Yoo JH, Kim K-I. Bone contusion and associated meniscal and medial collateral ligament injury in patients with anterior cruciate ligament rupture. J Bone Joint Surg Am 2011;93(16):1510–8.

41. Gersoff WK, Clancy WG. Diagnosis of acute and chronic anterior cruciate ligament tears. Clin Sports Med 1988;7(4):727–38.

42. LaPrade RF, Resig S, Wentorf F, et al. The effects of grade III posterolateral knee complex injuries on anterior cruciate ligament graft force. A biomechanical analysis. Am J Sports Med 1999;27(4):469–75.

43. Zantop T, Schumacher T, Schanz S, et al. Double-bundle reconstruction cannot restore intact knee kinematics in the ACL/LCL-deficient knee. Arch Orthop Trauma Surg 2010;130(8):1019–26.
44. Nitri M, Rasmussen MT, Williams BT, et al. An in vitro robotic assessment of the anterolateral ligament, Part 2: anterolateral ligament reconstruction combined with anterior cruciate ligament reconstruction. Am J Sports Med 2016;44(3):593–601.
45. Rasmussen MT, Nitri M, Williams BT, et al. An in vitro robotic assessment of the anterolateral ligament, Part 1: secondary role of the anterolateral ligament in the setting of an anterior cruciate ligament injury. Am J Sports Med 2016;44(3):585–92.
46. Papageorgiou CD, Gil JE, Kanamori A, et al. The biomechanical interdependence between the anterior cruciate ligament replacement graft and the medial meniscus. Am J Sports Med 2001;29(2):226–31.
47. Trojani C, Sbihi A, Djian P, et al. Causes for failure of ACL reconstruction and influence of meniscectomies after revision. Knee Surg Sports Traumatol Arthrosc 2011;19(2):196–201.
48. van de Pol GJ, Arnold MP, Verdonschot N, et al. Varus alignment leads to increased forces in the anterior cruciate ligament. Am J Sports Med 2009;37(3):481–7.
49. Noyes FR, Barber-Westin SD, Hewett TE. High tibial osteotomy and ligament reconstruction for varus angulated anterior cruciate ligament-deficient knees. Am J Sports Med 2000;28(3):282–96.
50. Giffin JR, Vogrin TM, Zantop T, et al. Effects of increasing tibial slope on the biomechanics of the knee. Am J Sports Med 2004;32(2):376–82.
51. Fening SD, Kovacic J, Kambic H, et al. The effects of modified posterior tibial slope on anterior cruciate ligament strain and knee kinematics: a human cadaveric study. J Knee Surg 2008;21(3):205–11.
52. Christensen JJ, Krych AJ, Engasser WM, et al. Lateral tibial posterior slope is increased in patients with early graft failure after anterior cruciate ligament reconstruction. Am J Sports Med 2015;43(10):2510–4.
53. Dejour D, Saffarini M, Demey G, et al. Tibial slope correction combined with second revision ACL produces good knee stability and prevents graft rupture. Knee Surg Sports Traumatol Arthrosc 2015;23(10):2846–52.
54. Sonnery-Cottet B, Mogos S, Thaunat M, et al. Proximal tibial anterior closing wedge osteotomy in repeat revision of anterior cruciate ligament reconstruction. Am J Sports Med 2014;42(8):1873–80.
55. Carson EW, Anisko EM, Restrepo C, et al. Revision anterior cruciate ligament reconstruction: etiology of failures and clinical results. J Knee Surg 2004;17(3):127–32.
56. Woo SLY, Kanamori A, Zeminski J, et al. The effectiveness of reconstruction of the anterior cruciate ligament with hamstrings and patellar tendon. A cadaveric study comparing anterior tibial and rotational loads. J Bone Joint Surg Am 2002;84-A(6):907–14.
57. Muneta T, Yamamoto H, Ishibashi T, et al. The effects of tibial tunnel placement and roofplasty on reconstructed anterior cruciate ligament knees. Arthroscopy 1995;11(1):57–62.
58. Barrett AM, Craft JA, Replogle WH, et al. Anterior cruciate ligament graft failure: a comparison of graft type based on age and Tegner activity level. Am J Sports Med 2011;39(10):2194–8.
59. Aglietti P, Giron F, Losco M, et al. Comparison between single-and double-bundle anterior cruciate ligament reconstruction: a prospective, randomized, single-blinded clinical trial. Am J Sports Med 2010;38(1):25–34.

60. Suomalainen P, Järvelä T, Paakkala A, et al. Double-bundle versus single-bundle anterior cruciate ligament reconstruction: a prospective randomized study with 5-year results. Am J Sports Med 2012;40(7):1511–8.
61. Magnussen RA, Lawrence JTR, West RL, et al. Graft size and patient age are predictors of early revision after anterior cruciate ligament reconstruction with hamstring autograft. Arthroscopy 2012;28(4):526–31.
62. Kamien PM, Hydrick JM, Replogle WH, et al. Age, graft size, and Tegner activity level as predictors of failure in anterior cruciate ligament reconstruction with hamstring autograft. Am J Sports Med 2013;41(8):1808–12.
63. Barrett G, Stokes D, White M. Anterior cruciate ligament reconstruction in patients older than 40 years: allograft versus autograft patellar tendon. Am J Sports Med 2005;33(10):1505–12.
64. Magnussen RA, Spindler KP. Anterior cruciate ligament reconstruction: two-incision technique. Oper Tech Sports Med 2013;21(1):34–9.
65. Salmon L, Russell V, Musgrove T, et al. Incidence and risk factors for graft rupture and contralateral rupture after anterior cruciate ligament reconstruction. Arthroscopy 2005;21(8):948–57.
66. Salmon LJ, Refshauge KM, Russell VJ, et al. Gender differences in outcome after anterior cruciate ligament reconstruction with hamstring tendon autograft. Am J Sports Med 2006;34(4):621–9.
67. Mohtadi N, Chan D, Barber R, et al. Reruptures, Reinjuries, and Revisions at a Minimum 2-year follow-up: a randomized clinical trial comparing 3 graft types for ACL reconstruction. Clin J Sport Med 2016;26(2):96–107.
68. Andernord D, Björnsson H, Petzold M, et al. Surgical predictors of early revision surgery after anterior cruciate ligament reconstruction: results from the Swedish National Knee Ligament Register on 13,102 patients. Am J Sports Med 2014; 42(7):1574–82.
69. Persson A, Fjeldsgaard K, Gjertsen J-E, et al. Increased risk of revision with hamstring tendon grafts compared with patellar tendon grafts after anterior cruciate ligament reconstruction: a study of 12,643 patients from the Norwegian Cruciate Ligament Registry, 2004-2012. Am J Sports Med 2014;42(2):285–91.
70. Sherman SL, Chalmers PN, Yanke AB, et al. Graft tensioning during knee ligament reconstruction: principles and practice. J Am Acad Orthop Surg 2012; 20(10):633–45.
71. Drogset JO, Straume LG, Bjørkmo I, et al. A prospective randomized study of ACL-reconstructions using bone-patellar tendon-bone grafts fixed with bioabsorbable or metal interference screws. Knee Surg Sports Traumatol Arthrosc 2011;19(5):753–9.
72. Drogset JO, Strand T, Uppheim G, et al. Autologous patellar tendon and quadrupled hamstring grafts in anterior cruciate ligament reconstruction: a prospective randomized multicenter review of different fixation methods. Knee Surg Sports Traumatol Arthrosc 2010;18(8):1085–93.
73. Frosch S, Rittstieg A, Balcarek P, et al. Bioabsorbable interference screw versus bioabsorbable cross pins: influence of femoral graft fixation on the clinical outcome after ACL reconstruction. Knee Surg Sports Traumatol Arthrosc 2012;20(11):2251–6.
74. Harilainen A, Sandelin J. A prospective comparison of 3 hamstring ACL fixation devices–Rigidfix, BioScrew, and Intrafix–randomized into 4 groups with 2 years of follow-up. Am J Sports Med 2009;37(4):699–706.
75. Laxdal G, Kartus J, Eriksson BI, et al. Biodegradable and metallic interference screws in anterior cruciate ligament reconstruction surgery using hamstring

tendon grafts: prospective randomized study of radiographic results and clinical outcome. Am J Sports Med 2006;34(10):1574–80.

76. Moisala A-S, Järvelä T, Paakkala A, et al. Comparison of the bioabsorbable and metal screw fixation after ACL reconstruction with a hamstring autograft in MRI and clinical outcome: a prospective randomized study. Knee Surg Sports Traumatol Arthrosc 2008;16(12):1080–6.

77. Nebelung W, Becker R, Merkel M, et al. Bone tunnel enlargement after anterior cruciate ligament reconstruction with semitendinosus tendon using Endobutton fixation on the femoral side. Arthroscopy 1998;14(8):810–5.

78. Rahr-Wagner L, Thillemann TM, Pedersen AB, et al. Comparison of hamstring tendon and patellar tendon grafts in anterior cruciate ligament reconstruction in a nationwide population-based cohort study: results from the danish registry of knee ligament reconstruction. Am J Sports Med 2014;42(2):278–84.

79. Rose T, Hepp P, Venus J, et al. Prospective randomized clinical comparison of femoral transfixation versus bioscrew fixation in hamstring tendon ACL reconstruction–a preliminary report. Knee Surg Sports Traumatol Arthrosc 2006; 14(8):730–8.

80. Aga C, Rasmussen MT, Smith SD, et al. Biomechanical comparison of interference screws and combination screw and sheath devices for soft tissue anterior cruciate ligament reconstruction on the tibial side. Am J Sports Med 2013;41(4):841–8.

81. Brown CH, Wilson DR, Hecker AT, et al. Graft-bone motion and tensile properties of hamstring and patellar tendon anterior cruciate ligament femoral graft fixation under cyclic loading. Arthroscopy 2004;20(9):922–35.

82. Kousa P, Järvinen TLN, Vihavainen M, et al. The fixation strength of six hamstring tendon graft fixation devices in anterior cruciate ligament reconstruction. Part I: femoral site. Am J Sports Med 2003;31(2):174–81.

83. Kousa P, Järvinen TLN, Vihavainen M, et al. The fixation strength of six hamstring tendon graft fixation devices in anterior cruciate ligament reconstruction. Part II: tibial site. Am J Sports Med 2003;31(2):182–8.

84. Holden JP, Grood ES, Korvick DL, et al. In vivo forces in the anterior cruciate ligament: direct measurements during walking and trotting in a quadruped. J Biomech 1994;27(5):517–26.

85. Brand J, Weiler A, Caborn DN, et al. Graft fixation in cruciate ligament reconstruction. Am J Sports Med 2000;28(5):761–74.

86. Harvey A, Thomas NP, Amis AA. Fixation of the graft in reconstruction of the anterior cruciate ligament. J Bone Joint Surg Br 2005;87(5):593–603.

87. Ekdahl M, Wang JH-C, Ronga M, et al. Graft healing in anterior cruciate ligament reconstruction. Knee Surg Sports Traumatol Arthrosc 2008;16(10):935–47.

88. Kawano CT, de Moraes Barros Fucs PM, Severino NR. Pretensioning of quadruple flexor tendon grafts in two types of femoral fixation: quasi-randomised controlled pilot study. Int Orthop 2011;35(4):521–7.

89. Ibrahim SAR, Abdul Ghafar S, Marwan Y, et al. Intratunnel versus extratunnel autologous hamstring double-bundle graft for anterior cruciate ligament reconstruction: a comparison of 2 femoral fixation procedures. Am J Sports Med 2015;43(1):161–8.

90. Feller JA, Webster KE. A randomized comparison of patellar tendon and hamstring tendon anterior cruciate ligament reconstruction. Am J Sports Med 2003;31(4):564–73.

91. Webster KE, Feller JA, Hartnett N, et al. Comparison of patellar tendon and hamstring tendon anterior cruciate ligament reconstruction: A 15-year follow-up of a randomized controlled trial. Am J Sports Med 2016;44(1):83–90.

92. Brucker PU, Lorenz S, Imhoff AB. Aperture fixation in arthroscopic anterior cruciate ligament double-bundle reconstruction. Arthroscopy 2006;22(11):1250.e1-6.
93. Baumfeld JA, Diduch DR, Rubino LJ, et al. Tunnel widening following anterior cruciate ligament reconstruction using hamstring autograft: a comparison between double cross-pin and suspensory graft fixation. Knee Surg Sports Traumatol Arthrosc 2008;16(12):1108–13.
94. Fauno P, Kaalund S. Tunnel widening after hamstring anterior cruciate ligament reconstruction is influenced by the type of graft fixation used: a prospective randomized study. Arthroscopy 2005;21(11):1337–41.
95. Kamelger FS, Onder U, Schmoelz W, et al. Suspensory fixation of grafts in anterior cruciate ligament reconstruction: a biomechanical comparison of 3 implants. Arthroscopy 2009;25(7):767–76.
96. Buelow J-U, Siebold R, Ellermann A. A prospective evaluation of tunnel enlargement in anterior cruciate ligament reconstruction with hamstrings: extracortical versus anatomical fixation. Knee Surg Sports Traumatol Arthrosc 2002;10(2):80–5.
97. Clatworthy MG, Annear P, Bulow JU, et al. Tunnel widening in anterior cruciate ligament reconstruction: a prospective evaluation of hamstring and patella tendon grafts. Knee Surg Sports Traumatol Arthrosc 1999;7(3):138–45.
98. Persson A, Kjellsen AB, Fjeldsgaard K, et al. Registry data highlight increased revision rates for endobutton/biosure HA in ACL reconstruction with hamstring tendon autograft: a nationwide cohort study from the Norwegian Knee Ligament Registry, 2004-2013. Am J Sports Med 2015;43(9):2182–8.
99. Scheffler SU, Südkamp NP, Göckenjan A, et al. Biomechanical comparison of hamstring and patellar tendon graft anterior cruciate ligament reconstruction techniques: The impact of fixation level and fixation method under cyclic loading. Arthroscopy 2002;18(3):304–15.
100. Steiner ME, Hecker AT, Brown CH, et al. Anterior cruciate ligament graft fixation. Comparison of hamstring and patellar tendon grafts. Am J Sports Med 1994;22(2):240–6 [discussion: 246–7].
101. Ma CB, Francis K, Towers J, et al. Hamstring anterior cruciate ligament reconstruction: a comparison of bioabsorbable interference screw and endobutton-post fixation. Arthroscopy 2004;20(2):122–8.
102. Watson JN, McQueen P, Kim W, et al. Bioabsorbable interference screw failure in anterior cruciate ligament reconstruction: a case series and review of the literature. Knee 2015;22(3):256–61.
103. Grunau PD, Arneja S, Leith JM. A randomized clinical trial to assess the clinical effectiveness of a measured objective tensioning device in hamstring anterior cruciate ligament reconstruction. Am J Sports Med 2016;44(6):1482–6.
104. O'Neill BJ, Byrne FJ, Hirpara KM, et al. Anterior cruciate ligament graft tensioning. Is the maximal sustained one-handed pull technique reproducible? BMC Res Notes 2011;4:244.
105. Mae T, Shino K, Nakata K, et al. Optimization of graft fixation at the time of anterior cruciate ligament reconstruction. Part I: effect of initial tension. Am J Sports Med 2008;36(6):1087–93.
106. Mae T, Shino K, Nakata K, et al. Optimization of graft fixation at the time of anterior cruciate ligament reconstruction. Part II: effect of knee flexion angle. Am J Sports Med 2008;36(6):1094–100.
107. Arneja S, McConkey MO, Mulpuri K, et al. Graft tensioning in anterior cruciate ligament reconstruction: a systematic review of randomized controlled trials. Arthroscopy 2009;25(2):200–7.

108. Fleming BC, Fadale PD, Hulstyn MJ, et al. The effect of initial graft tension after anterior cruciate ligament reconstruction: a randomized clinical trial with 36-month follow-up. Am J Sports Med 2013;41(1):25–34.

109. Ménétrey J, Duthon VB, Laumonier T, et al. "Biological failure" of the anterior cruciate ligament graft. Knee Surg Sports Traumatol Arthrosc 2008;16(3):224–31.

110. Amiel D, Kleiner JB, Roux RD, et al. The phenomenon of "ligamentization": anterior cruciate ligament reconstruction with autogenous patellar tendon. J Orthop Res 1986;4(2):162–72.

111. Arnoczky SP, Warren RF, Ashlock MA. Replacement of the anterior cruciate ligament using a patellar tendon allograft. An experimental study. J Bone Joint Surg Am 1986;68(3):376–85.

112. Hunt P, Scheffler SU, Unterhauser FN, et al. A model of soft-tissue graft anterior cruciate ligament reconstruction in sheep. Arch Orthop Trauma Surg 2005; 125(4):238–48.

113. Jackson DW, Grood ES, Goldstein JD, et al. A comparison of patellar tendon autograft and allograft used for anterior cruciate ligament reconstruction in the goat model. Am J Sports Med 1993;21(2):176–85.

114. Tejwani SG, Chen J, Funahashi TT, et al. Revision risk after allograft anterior cruciate ligament reconstruction: association with graft processing techniques, patient characteristics, and graft type. Am J Sports Med 2015;43(11): 2696–705.

115. Kuroda R, Kurosaka M, Yoshiya S, et al. Localization of growth factors in the reconstructed anterior cruciate ligament: immunohistological study in dogs. Knee Surg Sports Traumatol Arthrosc 2000;8(2):120–6.

116. Samitier G, Marcano AI, Alentorn-Geli E, et al. Failure of anterior cruciate ligament reconstruction. Arch Bone Jt Surg 2015;3(4):220–40.

117. Shelbourne KD, Trumper RV. Preventing anterior knee pain after anterior cruciate ligament reconstruction. Am J Sports Med 1997;25(1):41–7.

118. Steadman JR, Dragoo JL, Hines SL, et al. Arthroscopic release for symptomatic scarring of the anterior interval of the knee. Am J Sports Med 2008;36(9): 1763–9.

119. Brophy RH, Wright RW, David TS, et al. Association between previous meniscal surgery and the incidence of chondral lesions at revision anterior cruciate ligament reconstruction. Am J Sports Med 2012;40(4):808–14.

120. Duchman KR, Westermann RW, Spindler KP, et al. The fate of meniscus tears left in situ at the time of anterior cruciate ligament reconstruction: A 6-year follow-up study from the MOON cohort. Am J Sports Med 2015;43(11):2688–95.

121. Cox CL, Huston LJ, Dunn WR, et al. Are articular cartilage lesions and meniscus tears predictive of IKDC, KOOS, and Marx activity level outcomes after anterior cruciate ligament reconstruction? A 6-year multicenter cohort study. Am J Sports Med 2014;42(5):1058–67.

122. Pernin J, Verdonk P, Si Selmi TA, et al. Long-term follow-up of 24.5 years after intra-articular anterior cruciate ligament reconstruction with lateral extra-articular augmentation. Am J Sports Med 2010;38(6):1094–102.

123. Filardo G, de Caro F, Andriolo L, et al. Do cartilage lesions affect the clinical outcome of anterior cruciate ligament reconstruction? A systematic review. Knee Surg Sports Traumatol Arthrosc 2016. [Epub ahead of print].

124. Borchers JR, Kaeding CC, Pedroza AD, et al. Intra-articular findings in primary and revision anterior cruciate ligament reconstruction surgery: a comparison of the MOON and MARS study groups. Am J Sports Med 2011; 39(9):1889–93.

125. Speer KP, Spritzer CE, Bassett FH, et al. Osseous injury associated with acute tears of the anterior cruciate ligament. Am J Sports Med 1992;20(4):382–9.

126. Dunn WR, Lincoln AE, Hinton RY, et al. Occupational disability after hospitalization for the treatment of an injury of the anterior cruciate ligament. J Bone Joint Surg Am 2003;85-A(9):1656–66.

Surgical Pearls in Revision Anterior Cruciate Ligament Surgery: When Must I Stage?

Dustin L. Richter, MD*, Brian C. Werner, MD, Mark D. Miller, MD

KEYWORDS

- Revision ACL • Tunnel osteolysis • Two-stage ACL • ACL failure

KEY POINTS

- The cause of anterior cruciate ligament failure must be critically evaluated to allow for a successful outcome after a revision reconstruction.
- In a revision setting, although collagen fibers may be present on MRI, this does not mean that the tissue is functional. History and physical examination are critically important.
- With significant tunnel osteolysis (>14 mm) or if the proposed revision tunnel(s) are within the borders of the current tunnel(s), a 2-stage revision may be best. The sports surgeon must have several tricks and tools readily available to address the tunnel osteolysis.

INTRODUCTION

Anterior cruciate ligament (ACL) reconstruction is among the most commonly performed and studied surgeries in orthopedic sports medicine. The incidence of primary ACL reconstruction (ACLR) rose from an estimated 87,000 cases in 1994 to nearly 130,000 in 2006.[1] The increased number of reconstructions was most prominent in those younger than 20 or older than 40, and in the female population. The incidence of recurrent instability or failure rate after primary ACLR varies from 3% to 10%.[2–6] In the patient with a failed ACLR, a systematic approach must be used starting with identification of the cause for graft failure or recurrent instability, obtaining the appropriate imaging if needed to evaluate for malalignment or tunnel osteolysis, and deciding whether the patient may be treated with a single-stage revision or if a 2-stage revision is more appropriate. The surgeon must have several tricks and tools readily available for this potentially technically demanding revision reconstruction.

No outside research support or funding is pertinent to this review. No conflicts of interest to disclose.

Department of Orthopaedic Surgery, University of Virginia, 400 Ray C. Hunt Drive, Suite 300, Charlottesville, VA 22903, USA

* Corresponding author. 400 Ray C. Hunt Drive, Suite 330, Charlottesville, VA 22903.

E-mail address: dustin.richter1818@gmail.com

ETIOLOGY OF ANTERIOR CRUCIATE LIGAMENT FAILURES

Without addressing the likely cause of primary ACLR failure, the risk for recurrent failure and instability is high. Harner and colleagues[7] divided the causes of failure of ACLRs into 3 groups: new trauma, technical errors or failure to recognize concomitant injuries, and failure of graft incorporation (**Fig. 1**). Early failure is often associated with incomplete graft incorporation and failure at one of the fixation points, whereas late failure (the most common source for rerupture) typically occurs from noncontact trauma and may be the result of a suboptimal reconstruction.[8]

Errors in surgical technique account for most primary ACLR failures.[9] The most common technical error is placement of the tibial or femoral tunnels outside of the native ACL footprint. In the past, this was most evident with the "vertical" tunnel placement associated with transtibial ACLR.[10] Vertical femoral tunnel placement may normalize the anterior-posterior stability (ie, Lachman maneuver); however, a significant degree of rotational instability may still be present (ie, positive pivot shift). To remedy this problem, independent drilling of the tibial and femoral tunnels has been used, either through an accessory anteromedial portal or less commonly via a 2-incision (outside-in) technique. Flexible reamer systems allow an additional way of uncoupling the tibial and femoral tunnels to clearly visualize and establish an anatomic starting point within the femoral footprint of the native ACL while avoiding the complications associated with knee hyperflexion and straight reamers with the far anteromedial portal.[11] Although the literature is replete with ACL failures due to tunnel malposition, the reader should recognize that these data are becoming more obsolete with updated surgical techniques that allow anatomic tunnel placement. New information regarding ACLR failures in the setting of proper tunnel positions using accessory medial or double bundle reconstructions will need to be further investigated.

Other sources of failure include failure to recognize a concomitant injury, such as a posterolateral corner injury. Lower extremity malalignment, particularly varus, or

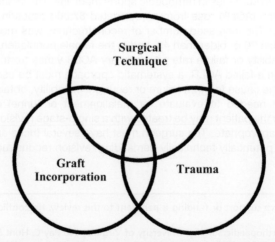

Fig. 1. Illustration showing that the causes of graft failure include surgical error, failure of graft incorporation, and trauma, either alone or in conjunction with one another. (*Reproduced from* Maday MG, Harner CD, Fu FH. Revision ACL surgery: evaluation and treatment. In: Feagin JA Jr, editor. The crucial ligaments: diagnosis and treatment of ligamentous injuries about the knee. 2nd edition. New York: Churchill Livingstone; 1994. p. 712; with permission.)

excessive posterior tibial slope can place additional stress on the graft and may warrant a simultaneous or staged osteotomy to reduce the risk of graft rerupture.[12] Fixation device failure, increased screw-tunnel divergence angle, and graft selection are all sources of potential graft compromise.

HISTORY AND PHYSICAL EXAMINATION

It is rare that the evaluation of a failed ACLR is easy. A comprehensive history and physical examination are critical in planning for a revision reconstruction. Advanced imaging such as an MRI may demonstrate the presence of collagen in the location of the ACL graft; however, imaging studies are not able to discern whether this tissue is functional, which further emphasizes the importance of a thorough examination.

The history should include not only the mechanism of injury, but whether the patient's knee ever felt stable after the index ACLR. Asking the patient if he or she "trusts the knee" can be valuable because it is often difficult for patients to verbalize instability symptoms. Did the patient develop any signs of infection after surgery? What was the rehabilitation protocol? Was there a discrete, new injury? Also, obtaining the operative report can be extremely beneficial to identify the graft used, other concomitant injuries that were treated and status of the menisci, as well as the fixation devices for both the femoral and tibial side.

The physical examination should document range of motion, prior skin incisions, presence of an effusion, and ACL ligamentous laxity (Lachman). Performing a pivot shift maneuver is especially important in a patient with a seemingly intact graft and negative Lachman, but symptoms of rotatory instability, as may be seen with vertical graft placement. Evaluating the other ligamentous structures compared with the contralateral extremity is critical to rule out a concomitant injury, such as a posterolateral corner injury that can be elucidated with the prone dial test. In the revision setting, the patient's overall lower extremity alignment and gait pattern (ie, varus thrust) should be documented. Any significant malalignment or other missed ligamentous injury should be addressed in the operative plan for the revision ACLR.

Finally, the possibility of an infection must always be entertained. If there is any concern, systemic inflammatory laboratories, including a white blood cell count, C-reactive protein, and erythrocyte sedimentation rate, should be obtained. If any of these laboratories are concerning, the patient's knee also should be aspirated and the fluid sent for cell count and culture.

IMAGING

There is typically a reason why the graft failed and a very careful assessment must be performed, including long leg alignment radiographs, possible varus or valgus stress radiographs, an MRI scan to look at the position of the previous ACLR graft tunnels as well as the status of the meniscus and articular cartilage of the joint, and a computed tomography (CT) scan when assessing for the extent of tunnel osteolysis.

Plain radiographs allow for an initial evaluation as to gross tunnel placement and type of fixation present (**Fig. 2**). Weight-bearing radiographs document degenerative changes that are not uncommon in a revision setting. Long leg alignment films specifically evaluate for any underlying varus or valgus malalignment that may benefit from an osteotomy. Varus and valgus stress radiographs are particularly useful when the physical examination is concerning for a concomitant collateral or corner injury.[13,14]

As noted previously, an MRI may demonstrate the presence of collagen in the location of the ACL graft; however, it is not able to discern whether this tissue is functional (**Fig. 3**). MRI is useful for identifying other meniscal, cartilage, or ligamentous

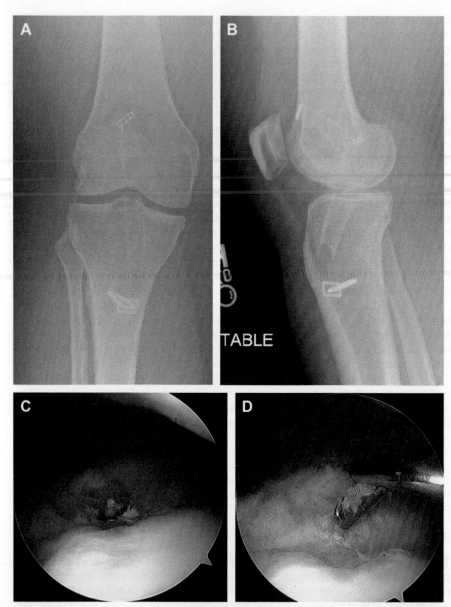

Fig. 2. (*A, B*) Anteroposterior (AP) and lateral radiographs demonstrating an ACLR using a transtibial technique and resultant vertical placement of the femoral tunnel. (*C, D*) Arthroscopic correlation of the vertical femoral tunnel with the button visible in the suprapatellar pouch just proximal to the trochlea.

injury; however, its effectiveness may be reduced in the presence of metal hardware due to artifact.

Widening of the tibial and/or femoral tunnels can present a substantial obstacle during revision ACLR because of the associated bone loss and potential for poor graft fixation. Delayed incorporation of soft tissue grafts into bone and decreased graft stability

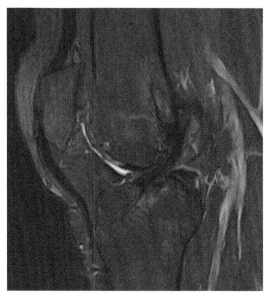

Fig. 3. Sagittal MRI demonstrating an apparently intact ACL graft in a patient with gross instability and a positive pivot shift examination finding.

are of particular concern.[15] Several methods to measure tunnel widening using plain radiographs have been proposed.[16,17] Klein and colleagues[18] described 4 primary tunnel shapes: linear, cavitary, mushroom, and conical. However, in our experience, when there is concern about tunnel osteolysis, CT evaluation has proven effective in planning for a revision ACLR, as it allows for multiplanar evaluation of the femoral and tibial tunnel bony architecture (with or without 3D reconstruction) with accurate determination of both the amount of tunnel osteolysis and tunnel position (**Fig. 4**).

SINGLE VERSUS 2-STAGE REVISION: TECHNICAL CONSIDERATIONS

A staged approach with autograft reconstruction is recommended when a single-stage approach may result in suboptimal graft selection, tunnel position, graft fixation, or biological milieu for tendon-bone healing.[19] Most ACLR failures in the past have been attributed to technical error, namely tunnel malposition. In these cases, a single-stage revision is often feasible as an accessory anteromedial portal can be used for anatomic bone tunnel placement without concern about encroaching on the prior tunnel placement. As more surgeons are now striving for anatomic ACLR, we must look more critically at other factors, such as graft selection, options for addressing tunnel osteolysis, and when to stage a revision reconstruction, and the role of backup fixation.

Graft Selection

Prior studies of ACLR show higher failure rates when allograft tissue is selected for grafts in the young, high-activity patient population.[20] Similarly, the Multicenter ACL Revision Study (MARS) group demonstrated that in the revision ACLR setting, patients reconstructed with autograft compared with allograft demonstrated improved sports function and patient-reported outcome measures.[21] Furthermore, they showed that the use of an autograft for revision reconstruction resulted in patients 2.78 times

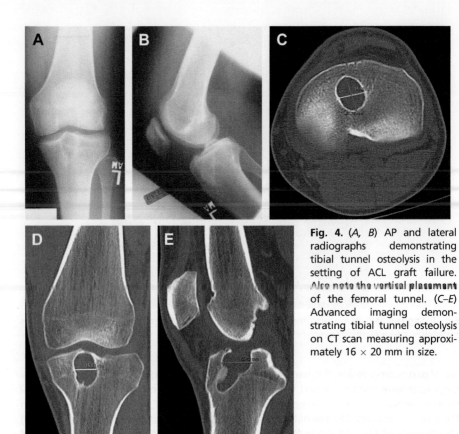

Fig. 4. (*A, B*) AP and lateral radiographs demonstrating tibial tunnel osteolysis in the setting of ACL graft failure. Also note the vertical placement of the femoral tunnel. (*C–E*) Advanced imaging demonstrating tibial tunnel osteolysis on CT scan measuring approximately 16 × 20 mm in size.

less likely to sustain a graft rerupture within 2 years than if allograft is used. Although graft diameter for hamstring tendon grafts has been shown to impact ACLR success rates, supplementation of autograft tissue with allograft to increase graft size (hybrid graft) may lead to increased graft failure as well when compared with autograft-only ACLR.[22,23] We prefer to use all autograft tissue for reconstruction. This may require draping out both legs to either supplement a hamstring autograft with hamstrings from the contralateral extremity, using a contralateral bone-patella tendon-bone (BPTB) autograft if the initial reconstruction used an ipsilateral BPTB, or tripling the semitendinosus graft to make a 5-strand graft if the tissue length allows. Occasionally, we will also use a quadriceps tendon autograft depending on what grafts have previously been used.

Management of Tunnel Osteolysis

The presence of tunnel osteolysis greater than 14 to 15 mm in the setting of anatomic or nonanatomic tunnels is our primary indication for staging a revision ACLR. Tunnel expansion makes the placement of a new ligament and rigid fixation difficult. For these cases, we recommend the liberal use of intraoperative fluoroscopy and good bone grafting technique. To ensure incorporation and consolidation of the bone graft, all residual tissue and foreign material (eg, prior screws) must be completely removed from the tibial and femoral tunnels with exposed bone cylindrically (**Fig. 5**). For significant osteolysis, the standard ACL reamers are usually not large enough in diameter to remove the remnant tissue; thus, we will typically use intramedullary reamers (from intramedullary rod fixation set) or total joint arthroplasty reamers (**Fig. 6**). A variety of graft choices are available, including autogenous bone (ie, iliac crest bone graft), allograft bone (ie, bone dowels or croutons), or other commercially available bone substitutes. We prefer to use allograft cylindrical bone dowels, which come prepackaged and provide an excellent fit and bony contact with the tunnel walls (**Fig. 7**). These allograft bone plugs are available in diameters from 10 to 18 mm with variable lengths and can be inserted using arthroscopically assisted techniques.[24] To obtain a good press fit, some investigators have advocated that the tunnel should be 1 mm smaller in diameter than the bone plug. However, we have discovered that the allograft dowels can be brittle and thus reaming the tunnel line-to-line is often necessary to avoid damage during impaction and seating of the bone dowel while still providing excellent fixation. The second stage reconstruction should be delayed for 4 to 6 months until radiographic evidence of bony consolidation is present.

Anterior Cruciate Ligament Tunnel Overlap

Whenever tunnel overlap is encountered (expectedly or unexpectedly), staging the revision ACLR is always an option. However, if there is not significant tunnel osteolysis present, then other revision options exist.[2,14] It is often beneficial to use a different technique than the index procedure to allow for tunnel divergence. The divergent tunnel (funnel) technique is used for a widened but anatomically placed tunnel in a patient with good bone quality, in which the aperture of the new tunnel is unchanged but the angle and direction of the tunnel are new. This can also be accomplished by using a 2-incision outside-in technique. For some single-stage revisions, it is possible to retain prior interference screws (ie, no removal) and drill a new tunnel immediately adjacent to the screw because the stainless steel drill bit is stronger than the titanium interference screws.[25]

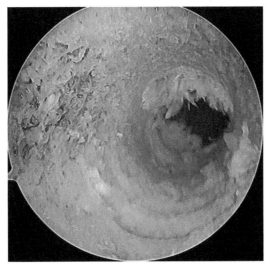

Fig. 5. Arthroscopic view looking up the tibial tunnel demonstrating complete removal of previous graft and soft tissue with good surrounding bone.

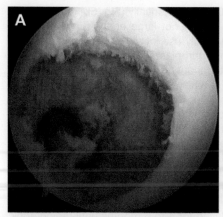

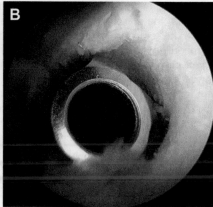

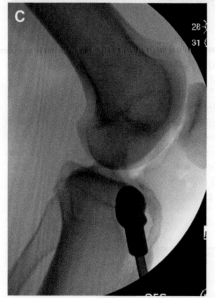

Fig. 6. (*A*) Arthroscopic view of tibial tunnel osteolysis using a 70° arthroscope to view down the old tibial tunnel from proximal to distal. Notice the significant widening proximally and then tapering to a more typical tibial tunnel distally. (*B*) Arthroscopic view demonstrating utilization of a femoral reamer (size 18) to prepare the defect for allograft bone dowel. (*C*) Lateral radiograph correlating to the arthroscopic view in **Fig. 6**B.

For patients with poor bone quality or concern regarding graft fixation, the use of stacking interference screws to provide fixation can be used. This option is useful in the setting of prior aperture fixation and requires initial removal of the old screw, drilling of a new tunnel, then reinsertion of the old screw and a new screw for improved aperture fixation and filling of the defect. Another option is the matchstick grafting technique in which small cortical allograft pieces are stacked into the tunnel before graft placement and fixation. We routinely use cannulated osteochondral allograft bone dowels for concurrent reconstruction and bone grafting of the widened tunnel. After inserting the bone graft, the guidewire is repositioned for drilling of the new tunnel; hence, the bone graft may provide stability for one of the walls of the new drilled tunnel.[26]

A recent biomechanical study evaluated the impact of 4 different tibial fixation techniques on single-stage ACL revision with confluent tibial tunnels. This study found that filling an incomplete and incorrect tibial tunnel with a press-fit bone plug or a

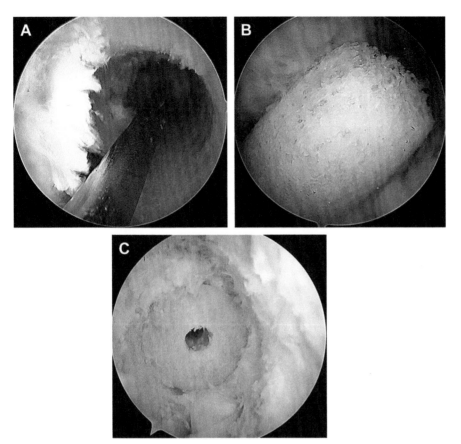

Fig. 7. (*A–C*) Demonstration of the use of a cannulated allograft bone dowel to fill a previously drilled femoral bone tunnel after an ACL graft failure.

biodegradable interference screw in a standardized laboratory situation provided initial biomechanical properties and knee stability comparable with those of primary ACLR. In contrast, the dilatation technique or leaving the malpositioned tunnel open did not restore knee kinematics adequately in this model. Furthermore, the investigators noted that backup extracortical fixation should be considered because the load to failure depends on the extracortical fixation when an undersized interference screw is used for aperture fixation.[27] (**Fig. 8**).

Graft Fixation

Secure graft fixation is critical in ensuring a successful revision ACLR. In the patient with good bone quality and when new tunnels are able to be made without difficulty or bone loss, standard graft fixation methods can be used. When the surgeon is concerned about posterior wall blow out or soft bone quality on the femoral side, an extended button may be used or the construct may be backed up by tying sutures over a screw-and-washer construct. On the tibial side, an expanded tunnel or soft bone quality may jeopardize the tibial screw purchase. In this instance, it is easy to use backup fixation with a metal staple or a cortical button. The surgeon should

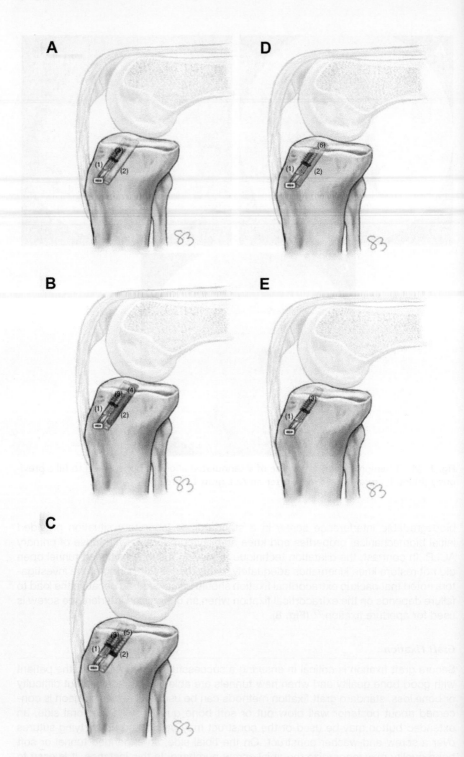

Fig. 8. Different strategies of tibial tunnel management, shown in a right knee from the medial side. (*A*) Open tunnel. The anterior tibial tunnel (1) is in an anatomic position

consider double fixation in all revisions and have a low threshold for using it if there is any question about graft fixation strength or security.

OTHER CONSIDERATIONS

ACLR alone may not be sufficient to control rotational instability in all cases. Despite a technically well-done ACLR, some patients may continue to feel instability postoperatively. In a revision setting, consideration should be given to the addition of an extra-articular procedure in a patient who either has persistent rotatory instability, or in the patient with a grade 3 pivot shift. The anterolateral ligament (ALL) is theorized to provide anterolateral stability to the knee, preventing the proximal-lateral tibia from subluxation anteriorly relative to the femur. This function may play an important role in preventing the pivot-shift phenomenon.[28] Although promising results of combined ACL and ALL reconstructions have been published, the indications and specific role for ALL reconstruction in the revision ACL setting still needs to be studied in greater detail.[29] A multicenter study by Getgood and colleagues[30] (STAbiLiTY [Standard ACL Reconstruction vs ACL + Lateral Extra-Articular Tenodesis Study]) comparing ACLR with and without lateral extra-articular tenodesis in individuals who are deemed to be at high risk of reinjuring their ACL may help address this question.

Almekinders and colleagues[31–33] have published extensively on the topic of ACL graft failure and tibia subluxation. Their studies showed that anteriorization of the tibia is evident in knees with failed ACLRs. When compared with a control group, the ACLR group was unable to achieve a reduced position secondary to a fixed anterior subluxation. However, untreated ACL ruptures did not show this phenomenon. Thus, the investigators concluded that surgical intervention may play a role in the development of the fixed tibia displacement and proposed that violation of the posterior cruciate ligament synovial sheath with subsequent fibrosis and contracture may account for this phenomenon. Tanaka and colleagues[34] used MRI measurements to further quantify the anterior-posterior and rotational motion in ACL-deficient knees. They concluded that patients who require revision ACLR have an abnormal tibiofemoral relationship noted on MRI that is most pronounced in the lateral compartment and should be taken into account during revision surgery. They go on to note that 12.5% of their cases had anterior displacement greater than 15 mm and noted this may not only help explain suboptimal clinical results after revision ACLR, but that patients with extreme tibia subluxation may be poor candidates for attempted revision ACLR. At a minimum, a modification of technique should be considered in the revision setting such as an

---

with the ACL graft (3), and the posterior, incompletely malplaced tibial tunnel (2) is left open. (B) Bone plug technique. The anterior tibial tunnel (1) is in an anatomic position with the ACL graft (3), and the posterior, incompletely malplaced tibial tunnel (2) is filled with a 10 × 30 mm femoral bone plug (4). (C) Biodegradable interference screw. The anterior tibial tunnel (1) is in an anatomic position with the ACL graft (3), and the posterior, incompletely malplaced tibial tunnel (2) is filled with a biodegradable interference screw (10 × 28 mm) (5). (D) Dilatation technique. The anterior tibial tunnel (1) is in an anatomic position created using dilators of increasing size, resulting in a thin bone bridge (6) between the 2 tunnels and collapse of the posterior, incompletely malplaced tibial (2). (E) Primary ACLR. The anterior tibial tunnel (1) is in an anatomic position (3, ACL graft). (*Reproduced from* Schliemann B, Treder M, Schulze M, et al. Influence of different tibial fixation techniques on initial stability in single-stage anterior cruciate ligament revision with confluent tibial tunnels: a biomechanical laboratory study. Arthroscopy 2016;32(1):80; with permission.)

expanded notchplasty, extra-articular tenodesis, or the role of meniscal transplant to provide the restoration of a secondary stabilizer.

CLINICAL OUTCOMES

It is important to counsel a patient regarding expected outcomes after a revision ACLR. Given the complexity of such surgery, a return to the same level of play as before ever sustaining an ACL injury is not the expected outcome.[35] Battaglia and colleagues[36] reported that only 59% of patients returned to the same degree of activity as their preinjury state. Only one study in the literature has reported a greater than 90% return to play after revision ACL reconstruction.[37] Revision ACL reconstructions also have a 3 to 4 times higher failure rate when compared with primary ACLR. A systematic review of 21 studies with a minimum of 2-year follow-up by Wright and colleagues[38] demonstrated a 13.7% failure rate in revision ACLR. Data from the MARS group regarding repeat (ie, second or third) revisions is especially dismal. Their analysis of additional predictors for graft rerupture demonstrated that the number of previous revisions significantly predicted risk for future graft rupture. Specifically, patients undergoing revision number 3 or higher were 25.8 times more likely to sustain a subsequent graft rerupture by 2 years after their enrollment surgery.[71]

As discussed earlier, a 2-stage revision may be needed when tunnel expansion or osteolysis makes a single-stage revision difficult, if not impossible. However, 2-stage revisions are not benign either. Two-stage revision groups have been shown to have higher rates of chondral and meniscal lesions, as well as inferior outcomes.[39] Furthermore, increased time to revision correlates with development of radiographic arthritis and increased meniscal and chondral lesions.[40]

SUMMARY

Failed ACLR is a challenging clinical entity and revision ACLR is a technically challenging procedure. Although MRI may demonstrate an intact ACL, this does not mean that the tissue is functional; thus, history and physical examination are of utmost importance. The cause of ACL failure must be critically evaluated to allow for a successful outcome in a revision reconstruction. The goals of knee stability and prevention of further articular cartilage or meniscal damage must be candidly discussed with the patient, as opposed to a goal of returning to a high level of athletic competition.

A single-stage revision is possible in most cases. However, a staged approach is recommended when a single-stage revision may result in suboptimal graft selection, tunnel position, graft fixation, or tendon-bone healing. Our primary indication for a 2-stage revision is when tunnel osteolysis exceeding 14 to 15 mm is present. The sports surgeon must have several tools and tricks readily available in a revision setting to address any pathology or difficulties that may be encountered.

REFERENCES

1. Mall NA, Chalmers PN, Moric M, et al. Incidence and trends of anterior cruciate ligament reconstruction in the United States. Am J Sports Med 2014;42(10): 2363-70.
2. Bach BR Jr. Revision anterior cruciate ligament surgery. Arthroscopy 2003; 19(Suppl 1):14-29.
3. Baer GS, Harner CD. Clinical outcomes of allograft versus autograft in anterior cruciate ligament reconstruction. Clin Sports Med 2007;26:661-81.

4. Liden M, Ejerhed L, Sernert N, et al. Patellar tendon or semitendinosus tendon autografts for anterior cruciate ligament reconstruction: a prospective, randomized study with a 7-Year follow-up. Am J Sports Med 2007;35(5):740–8.
5. Biau DJ, Tournoux C, Katsahian S, et al. Bone-patellar tendon-bone autografts versus hamstring autografts for reconstruction of anterior cruciate ligament: meta-analysis. BMJ 2006;332:995–1001.
6. Spindler KP, Kuhn JE, Freedman KB, et al. Anterior cruciate ligament reconstruction autograft choice: bone-tendon-bone versus hamstring: does it really matter? A systematic review. Am J Sports Med 2004;32:1986–95.
7. Harner CD, Giffin JR, Dunteman RC, et al. Evaluation and treatment of recurrent instability after anterior cruciate ligament reconstruction. Instr Course Lect 2001; 50:463–74.
8. Chen JL, Allen CR, Stephens TE, et al. Differences in mechanisms of failure, intraoperative findings, and surgical characteristics between single- and multiple-revision ACL reconstructions: a MARS cohort study. Am J Sports Med 2013;41: 1571–8.
9. Wolf RS, Lemak LJ. Revision anterior cruciate ligament reconstruction surgery. J South Orthop Assoc 2002;11:25–32.
10. Howell SM, Gittins ME, Gottlieb JE, et al. The relationship between the angle of the tibial tunnel in the coronal plane and loss of flexion and anterior laxity after anterior cruciate ligament reconstruction. Am J Sports Med 2001;29:567–74.
11. Fitzgerald J, Saluan P, Richter DL, et al. Anterior cruciate ligament reconstruction using a flexible reamer system: technique and pitfalls. Orthop J Sports Med 2015; 3(7):1–6.
12. Christensen JJ, Krych AJ, Engasser WM, et al. Lateral tibial posterior slope is increased in patients with early graft failure after anterior cruciate ligament reconstruction. Am J Sports Med 2015;43(10):2510–4.
13. Gwathmey FW Jr, Tompkins MA, Gaskin CM, et al. Can stress radiography of the knee help characterize posterolateral corner injury? Clin Orthop Relat Res 2012; 470(3):768–73.
14. Sawant M, Narasimha Murty A, Ireland J. Valgus knee injuries: evaluation and documentation using a simple technique of stress radiography. Knee 2004; 11(1):25–8.
15. Maak TG, Voos JE, Wickiewicz TL, et al. Tunnel widening in revision anterior cruciate ligament reconstruction. J Am Acad Orthop Surg 2010;18(11):695–706.
16. Clatworthy MG, Annear P, Bulow JU, et al. Tunnel widening in anterior cruciate ligament reconstruction: A prospective evaluation of hamstring and patella tendon grafts. Knee Surg Sports Traumatol Arthrosc 1999;7(3):138–45.
17. Laxdal G, Kartus J, Eriksson BI, et al. Biodegradable and metallic interference screws in anterior cruciate ligament reconstruction surgery using hamstring tendon grafts: prospective randomized study of radiographic results and clinical outcome. Am J Sports Med 2006;34(10):1574–80.
18. Klein JP, Lintner DM, Downs D, et al. The incidence and significance of femoral tunnel widening after quadrupled hamstring anterior cruciate ligament reconstruction using femoral cross pin fixation. Arthroscopy 2003;19(5):470–6.
19. Wilde J, Bedi A, Altchek DW. Revision anterior cruciate ligament reconstruction. Sports Health 2014;6(6):504–18.
20. Kaeding CC, Aros B, Pedroza A, et al. Allograft versus autograft anterior cruciate ligament reconstruction: predictors of failure from a MOON prospective longitudinal cohort. Sports Health 2011;3(1):73–81.

21. MARS Group The, Wright RW, Huston LJ, et al. Effect of graft choice on the outcome of revision anterior cruciate ligament reconstruction in the Multicenter ACL Revision Study (MARS) cohort. Am J Sports Med 2014;42(10): 2301–10.

22. Conte EJ, Hyatt AE, Gatt CJ Jr, et al. Hamstring autograft size can be predicted and is a potential risk factor for anterior cruciate ligament reconstruction failure. Arthroscopy 2014;30(7):882–90.

23. Burrus MT, Werner BC, Crow AJ, et al. Increased failure rates after anterior cruciate ligament reconstruction with soft-tissue autograft-allograft hybrid grafts. Arthroscopy 2015;31:2342–51.

24. Battaglia TC, Miller MD. Management of bony deficiency in revision anterior cruciate ligament reconstruction using allograft bone dowels: surgical technique. Arthroscopy 2005;21(6):767.

25. Miller MD. Revision cruciate ligament surgery with retention of femoral interference screws. Arthroscopy 1998;14(1):111–4.

26. Werner BC, Gilmore CJ, Hamann JC, et al. Revision ACL reconstruction: results of a single-stage approach using allograft dowel bone grafting for femoral defects. J Am Acad Orthop Surg 2016;24:581–7.

27. Schliemann B, Treder M, Schulze M, et al. Influence of different tibial fixation techniques on initial stability in single-stage anterior cruciate ligament revision with confluent tibial tunnels: a biomechanical laboratory study. Arthroscopy 2016; 32(1):78–89.

28. Musahl V, Hoshino Y, Ahlden M, et al. The pivot shift: a global user guide. Knee Surg Sports Traumatol Arthrosc 2012;20:724–31.

29. Sonnery-Cottet B, Thaunat M, Freychet B, et al. Outcome of a combined anterior cruciate ligament and anterolateral ligament reconstruction technique with a minimum 2-year follow-up. Am J Sports Med 2015;43(7):1598–605.

30. Getgood A. Standard ACL reconstruction vs ACL + lateral extra-articular tenodesis study (STAbiLiTY). Available at: https://clinicaltrials.gov/ct2/show/NCT02018354? term=stability+AND+getgood&rank=1. Accessed February 1, 2016.

31. Almekinders LC, Chiavetta JB, Clarke JP. Radiographic evaluation of anterior cruciate ligament graft failure with special reference to tibial tunnel placement. Arthroscopy 1998;14(2):206–11.

32. Almekinders LC, de Castro D. Fixed tibial subluxation after successful anterior cruciate ligament reconstruction. Am J Sports Med 2001;29(3):280–3.

33. Almekinders LC, Pandarinath R, Rahusen FT. Knee stability following anterior cruciate ligament rupture and surgery: the contribution of irreducible tibial subluxation. J Bone Joint Surg Am 2004;86-A(5):983–7.

34. Tanaka MJ, Jones KJ, Gargiulo AM, et al. Passive anterior tibial subluxation in anterior cruciate ligament-deficient knees. Am J Sports Med 2013;41(10):2347–52.

35. Cheatham SA, Johnson DL. Anticipating problems unique to revision ACL surgery. Sports Med Arthrosc Rev 2013;21(2):129–34.

36. Battaglia MJ 2nd, Cordasco FA, Hannafin JA, et al. Results of revision anterior cruciate ligament surgery. Am J Sports Med 2007;35:2057–66.

37. Garofalo R, Djahangiri A, Siegrist O. Revision anterior cruciate ligament reconstruction with quadriceps tendon-patellar bone autograft. Arthroscopy 2006;22: 205–14.

38. Wright RW, Gill CS, Chen L, et al. Outcome of revision anterior cruciate ligament reconstruction: a systematic review. J Bone Joint Surg Am 2012;94:531–6.

39. Thomas NP, Kankate R, Wandless F, et al. Revision anterior cruciate ligament reconstruction using a 2-stage technique with bone grafting of the tibial tunnel. Am J Sports Med 2005;33(11):1701–9.
40. Ohly NE, Murray IR, Keating JF. Revision anterior cruciate ligament reconstruction: timing of surgery and the incidence of meniscal tears and degenerative change. J Bone Joint Surg Br 2007;89(8):1051–4.

Rehabilitation Principles of the Anterior Cruciate Ligament Reconstructed Knee

Twelve Steps for Successful Progression and Return to Play

Kevin E. Wilk, PT, DPT[a,b,*], Christopher A. Arrigo, MS, PT, ATC[c]

KEYWORDS

• Proprioception • Neuromuscular training • Return to play • Functional rehabilitation

KEY POINTS

• Rehabilitation after anterior cruciate ligament reconstruction is a gradual and progressive progress.
• When available and appropriate use objective criteria to advance from one phase to another.
• Emphasize restoration of full knee extension and flexion after surgery.
• Stabilization for the knee joint occurs from above (hip/core) and from below (foot/ankle).
• Use objective criteria to progress a patient to return to sports activities.

INTRODUCTION

Anterior cruciate ligament (ACL) injuries often require surgical intervention followed by an extensive course of rehabilitation because without treatment they frequently result in functional and athletic limitations. Approximately 200,000 ACL injuries occur annually in the United States, making the nearly 150,000 ACL reconstruction surgeries one of the most common orthopedic procedures performed.[1–9] An evidence-based and well-designed rehabilitation program plays a critical role in any successful outcome after ACL reconstruction. Excellent outcomes after ACL surgery, including a return to unrestricted activities and preinjury levels, are generally expected.[10–12]

[a] Champion Sports Medicine, 805 Saint Vincent's Drive, Suite G100, Birmingham, AL 35205, USA; [b] American Sports Medicine Institute, Birmingham, AL, USA; [c] Advanced Rehabilitation, Tampa, FL, USA
* Corresponding author. 805 Saint Vincent's Drive, Suite G100, Birmingham, AL 35205
E-mail address: kwilkpt@hotmail.com

Clin Sports Med 36 (2017) 189–232
http://dx.doi.org/10.1016/j.csm.2016.08.012   sportsmed.theclinics.com
0278-5919/17/© 2016 Elsevier Inc. All rights reserved.

However, in reality, ACL injuries and surgery are so common and frequent that the seriousness of the pathology is often forgotten. The severity is evident in studies demonstrating that between 40% to 90% of patients exhibit radiographic osteoarthritis (OA) 7 to 12 years after ACL surgery,[13,14] and that there is a 10 times greater rate of OA in the ACL injured knee.[15] The disabling impact that ACL injuries can have on athletes is evident by reported statistics showing that only 78% of NBA players return to competition after ACL surgery and of those 44% exhibited a decrease in standard statistical performance categories and player efficiency ratings.[16] Similarly adverse return to play statistics have been reported in professional football players showing careers altered and even shortened by approximately 2 years with an overall decrease in performance of 20%.[1,17,18] Additionally, a systematic review of 48 studies reporting return to sport parameters demonstrated that 82% of patients undergoing ACL reconstruction returned to some form of sports, whereas only 63% returned to preinjury levels of participation and a mere 44% to competitive athletics.[11] Although generally present more often in low-level athletes, Kinesiophobia, the fear of movement or reinjury, is the most common reason cited for not being able to return to a preinjury level of participation.[11,19]

The frequency with which ACL injuries occur during strenuous work and athletic activity coupled with the severity of these knee injuries and the difficulty exhibited returning athletes to unrestricted, high-level activity demonstrates the need for a sequential, progressive, and structured approach to the rehabilitation program after ACL surgery. Current programs emphasize full passive knee extension,[20–24] immediate motion,[20,23–29] immediate partial weight bearing (WB),[23,24,30,31] and functional exercises.[23,32,33]

The current trend in ACL rehabilitation began in 1990 when Shelbourne and Nitz[21] reported improved clinical outcomes in patients who followed an accelerated rehabilitative approach rather than a conservative one. These patients exhibited better strength and range of motion (ROM) with fewer postoperative complications. Furthermore, the accelerated group had fewer patellofemoral pain complaints and an earlier return to sport. Numerous authors, including the two of us, have used components of an accelerated approach to ACL rehabilitation with excellent results since 1994.[24,34–39] Howe and colleagues[40] has also demonstrated improved outcomes—greater motion, improved muscular strength, and enhanced earlier function—with formal, supervised rehabilitation when compared with patients receiving no supervised rehabilitation.

Herein we provide a scientific basis for the rationale behind our ACL rehabilitation program and outline the 12 critical steps essential to the process of the successful rehabilitation and return to play after an ACL reconstruction (**Box 1**). The ultimate goal of any sound rehabilitation program is not only a successful outcome today, but also an asymptomatic knee 5 to 10 years later.

ANTERIOR CRUCIATE LIGAMENT REHABILITATION: TWELVE CRITICAL STEPS FOR SUCCESS

Using a criteria-based, evidence-based constructed approach to rehabilitation after ACL surgery is essential to systematically and successfully progress a patient through the rehabilitation process and maximize their odds of an uncomplicated and complete recovery. This type of approach strives to combine a stable knee that is functionally asymptomatic. The rehabilitation program phases, goals, and criteria for progression from phase to phase after an ACL reconstruction are outlined in **Box 2**.

Box 1
Twelve steps critical to successful anterior cruciate ligament rehabilitation
1. Preparation of both the patient and their knee for surgery
2. Restore full passive knee extension
3. Reduce postoperative inflammation
4. Gradual restoration of full knee flexion
5. Restore complete patellar mobility
6. Individualize and adjust the rehabilitation program based on the status of the knee
7. Reestablish quadriceps activation
8. Restoration of dynamic functional stability of the knee complex
9. Knee stability and dynamic control must be provided from both above and below
10. Protect the knee both now and later
11. Objective return to running
12. Objective progressing beyond running and back to sport

We use 4 different rehabilitation programs for patients with an isolated ACL reconstruction: (1) an accelerated program for patellar tendon reconstructions, (2) a regular program for patellar tendon reconstructions, (3) a separate protocol for hamstring reconstructions, and (4) ACL reconstruction with concomitant surgeries (such as meniscus repair, or articular cartilage procedures). The accelerated approach is used in the younger and/or athletic population. The main differences between each of the programs is the rate of progression through the various phases of rehabilitation and the recovery time necessary before the initiation of running and a return to full athletic activities.

Each of these programs is a criteria-based and formulated in a 6 phase approach that includes: (1) preoperative phase, (2) immediate postoperative phase (days 1–7), (3) early rehabilitation phase (weeks 2–4), (4) progressive strengthening/neuromuscular control phase (weeks 4–10), (5) advanced activity phase (weeks 10–16), and a return to activity phase (weeks >16) Our accelerated rehabilitation program after ACL reconstruction with an ipsilateral patellar tendon autograft is provided in **Box 3**. We begin rehabilitation before surgery when possible. It is imperative to reduce swelling, inflammation, and pain, restore normal ROM, normalize gait, and prevent muscle atrophy before surgery. In addition, we want to prevent the patient from further injury to their knee (ie, meniscus, articular cartilage). The goal is to return the knee to its preinjury, normalized state and to obtain tissue homeostasis. Full motion is restored before surgery to reduce the risk of postoperative arthrofibrosis.[22] Patient education, a critical aspect of preoperative rehabilitation, informs and prepares the patient for the surgical procedure and postoperative rehabilitation.

The preoperative phase, which we believe is critical to a successful outcome, may require up to several weeks, but generally 21 days is adequate.[22,41] We have found that patients undergoing a preoperative rehabilitation program progress more readily through the postoperative rehabilitation program, particularly the earlier phases, and regain their ROM with diminished symptoms.

Postoperative rehabilitation begins with passive ROM (PROM) and WB activities immediately after surgery. Full passive knee extension is emphasized while gradually

Box 2
Rehabilitation phases, program goals and criteria for progression after anterior cruciate ligament reconstruction

1. Preoperative phase
   a. Goals: Diminish inflammation, swelling and pain
      i. Restore normal ROM (especially knee extension)
      ii. Restore voluntary muscle activation
      iii. Provide patient education to prepare for surgery

2. Immediate postoperative phase (days 1–7)
   a. Goals: Restore full passive knee extension
      i. Diminish joint swelling and pain
      ii. Restore patellar mobility
      iii. Gradually improve knee flexion
      iv. Reestablish quadriceps control
      v. Restore independent ambulation
   b. Criteria to progress to early rehabilitation phase
      i. Quadriceps control (ability to perform good quadriceps set and straight leg raises)
      ii. Full passive knee extension
      iii. PROM: 0° to 90°
      iv. Good patellar mobility
      v. Minimal joint effusion
      vi. Independent ambulation

3. Early rehabilitation phase (weeks 2–4)
   a. Goals: maintain full passive knee extension ($\geq$0 to 5–7 hyperextension)
      i. Gradually increase knee flexion
      ii. Diminish remaining swelling and pain
      iii. Improve muscle control and activation
      iv. Restore proprioception/neuromuscular control
      v. Normalize patellar mobility
   b. Criteria to progress to strengthening/neuromuscular control phase
      i. Active ROM 0$\geq$ to 115°
      ii. Quadriceps strength 60% greater than the contralateral side (isometric test at 60° of knee flexion)
      iii. Unchanged KT test bilateral values ($\leq$1)
      iv. Minimal to no knee joint effusion
      v. No joint line or patellofemoral pain

4. Progressive strengthening/neuromuscular control phase (Weeks 4–10)
   a. Goals: restore full knee ROM (0°–125°)
      i. Improve lower extremity strength
      ii. Enhance proprioception, balance and neuromuscular control
      iii. Improve muscular endurance
      iv. Restore limb confidence and function
   b. Criteria to progress to advanced activity phase
      i. AROM 0° to 125° or greater
      ii. Quadriceps strength 75% of contralateral side
      iii. Knee extension flexor: extensor ratio 70% to 75%
      iv. No change in KT values (comparable with contralateral side, within 2 mm)
      v. No pain or effusion
      vi. Satisfactory clinical examination
      vii. Satisfactory isokinetic test (values at 180°/s)
         1. Quadriceps bilateral comparison 75%
         2. Hamstring strength equal bilaterally
         3. Quadriceps peak torque/body weight ratios
            a. 65% males
            b. 55% females
         4. Single leg hop test 80% of contralateral leg
         5. Subjective knee scoring (modified Noyes system) 80 points or better

5. Advanced activity phase (weeks 10–16)
    a. Goals: normalize lower extremity strength
    b. Enhance muscular poser and endurance
    c. Improve neuromuscular control
    d. Perform selected sport-specific drills
    e. Criteria to enter return to activity phase
        i. Full ROM
        ii. Unchanged KT test (within 2.5 mm of opposite side)
        iii. Isokinetic test that fulfills criteria
            1. Quadriceps bilateral comparison 80% or greater
            2. Hamstring bilateral comparison 110% or greater
            3. Quadriceps torque/body weight ratio 55% or greater
            4. Hamstring/quadriceps ratio 70% or greater
        iv. Proprioceptive test 100% of contralateral leg
        v. Functional test 85% or greater of contralateral side
        vi. Satisfactory clinical examination
        vii. Subjective knee scoring (modified Noyes system) 90 points or better

6. Return to activity phase (Weeks 16–22)
    a. Goals: gradual return to full unrestricted sports
    b. Achieve maximal strength and endurance
    c. Normalize neuromuscular control
        i. Progress skill training

Abbreviations: AROM, active range of motion; KT, knee arthrometer; PROM, passive range of motion; ROM, range of motion.

restoring knee flexion. Immediately after surgery, WB as tolerated in a locked knee brace in full extension is allowed, and the patient is progressed to full WB without crutches 10 to 14 days after surgery. Despite conflicts in the literature, we recommend a drop-lock knee brace during ambulation to emphasize full knee extension and assist the patient during the gait cycle while the quadriceps are inhibited.[6,42,43] The locked brace is used while ambulating and sleeping during the first 2 weeks after surgery. Studies have also shown that patients achieve improved functional knee scores and proprioception when using a brace after surgery.[44,45]

WB and non-WB activities, proprioceptive training, and strengthening exercises are also initiated during the first 2 weeks and progressed as tolerated. Neuromuscular control drills are gradually advanced to include dynamic stabilization and controlled perturbation training 2 or 3 weeks after surgery. Once satisfactory strength and neuromuscular control can be demonstrated, functional activities such as running and cutting may begin. Timeframes for initiating running activities range from 10 to 18 weeks after surgery, depending on the surgical procedure performed and overall patient presentation. A gradual return to athletic competition for running and cutting sports, such as baseball, football, tennis, and soccer, occurs approximately 6 months after surgery, once the patient is capable of demonstrating at least 85% of contralateral quadriceps and hamstring strength.[46] Return to jumping sports such as basketball and volleyball, however, may be delayed until 6 to 9 months after surgery.

Our postoperative programs have been designed with several key principles of ACL rehabilitation to ensure satisfactory outcomes and to return the athlete to sport as quickly and safely as possible. These principles are used to control and direct the rehabilitation program after ACL reconstruction and can be viewed as 12 critical steps crucial to successful ACL rehabilitation. These 12 steps are presented one by one and are all important factors in the rehabilitation program that need to be carefully considered, appropriately assessed, and then ensure that they happen during rehabilitation.

Box 3
Accelerated rehabilitation after anterior cruciate ligament-PTG reconstruction

Immediate Postoperative Phase (Days 1–7)

Goals
  Restore full passive knee extension
  Diminish joint swelling and pain
  Restore patellar mobility
  Gradually improve knee flexion
  Reestablish quadriceps control
  Restore independent ambulation

Postoperative day 1
  Brace
    Brace/immobilizer applied to knee, locked in full extension during ambulation and sleeping
    Unlock brace while sitting, and so on
  Weight bearing
    Two crutches, weight bearing as tolerated
  Exercises
  • Ankle pumps
  • Overpressure into full, passive knee extension
  • Active and passive knee flexion (90° by day 5)
  • Straight leg raises (flexion, abduction, adduction)
  • Quadriceps isometric setting
  • Hamstring stretches
  • Closed kinetic chain exercises: mini squats, weight shifts
  Muscle stimulation
    Use muscle stimulation during active muscle exercises (4–6 h/d)
  Continuous passive motion
    As needed, 0° to 45°/50° (as tolerated and as directed by physician)
  Ice and evaluation
    Ice 20 minutes out of every hour and elevate with knee in full extension

Postoperative Days 2 to 3
  Brace
    Brace/immobilizer, locked at 0° extension for ambulation and unlocked for sitting, and so on
  Weight bearing
    Two crutches, weight bearing as tolerated
  ROM
    Remove brace perform ROM exercises 4 to 6 times a day
  Exercises
  • Multiangle isometrics at 90° and 60° (knee extension)
  • Knee extension 90° to 40°
  • Overpressure into extension (knee extension should be ≥0° to slight hyperextension)
  • Patellar mobilization
  • Ankle pumps
  • Straight leg raises (3 directions)
  • Mini squats and weight shifts
  • Quadriceps isometric setting
  Muscle stimulation
    Electrical muscle stimulation to quads (6 h/d)
  Continuous passive motion
    0° to 90°, as needed
  Ice and evaluation
    Ice 20 minutes out of every hour and elevate leg with knee in full extension

Postoperative days 4 to 7
  Brace
    Brace/immobilizer, locked at 0° extension for ambulation and unlocked for sitting, and so on

Weight bearing
   Two crutches weight bearing as tolerated
ROM
   Remove brace to perform ROM exercises 4 to 6 times per day, knee flexion 90° by day 5,
   approximately 100° by day 7
Exercises
- Multiangle isometrics at 90° and 60° (knee extension)
- Knee extension 90° to 40°
- Overpressure into extension (full extension 0° to 5°–7° hyperextension)
- Patellar mobilization (5–8 times daily)
- Ankle pumps
- Straight leg raises (3 directions)
- Mini squats and weight shifts
- Standing hamstring curls
- Quadriceps isometric setting
- Proprioception and balance activities
Neuromuscular training/proprioception
   Open kinetic chain passive/active joint repositioning at 90°, 60°
   Closed kinetic chain squats/weight shifts with repositioning
Muscle stimulation
   Electrical muscle stimulation (continue 6 h/d)
Continue passive motion
   0° to 90°, as needed
Ice and elevation
   Ice 20 minutes of every hour and elevate leg with knee full extension

Early rehabilitation phase (weeks 2–4)

Criteria to progress to phase II
1) Quadriceps control (ability to perform good quadriceps set and straight leg raises)
2) Full passive knee extension
3) PROM 0°–90°
4) Good patellar mobility
5) Minimal joint effusion
6) Independent ambulation

Goals
   Maintain full passive knee extension (at least 0° to 5°–7° hyperextension)
   Gradually increase knee flexion
   Diminish swelling and pain
   Muscle control and activation
   Restore proprioception/neuromuscular control
   Normalize patellar mobility

Week 2
   Brace
      Continue locked brace for ambulation and sleeping
   Weight bearing
      As tolerated (goal is to discontinue crutches 10–14 days postoperatively)
   PROM
      Self-ROM stretching (4–5 times daily), emphasis on maintaining full PROM
      - Restore patient's symmetric extension
   KT 2000 test (15 lb; anterior-posterior test only)
   Exercises
   - Muscle stimulation to quadriceps exercises
   - Isometric quadriceps sets
   - Straight leg raises (4 planes)
   - Leg press (0°–60°)
   - Knee extension 90° to 40°
   - Half squats (0°–40°)
   - Weight shifts
   - Front and side lunges

- Hamstring curls standing (active ROM)
- Bicycle (if ROM allows)
- Proprioception training
- Overpressure into extension
- PROM from 0° to 100°
- Patellar mobilization
- Well leg exercises
- Progressive resistance extension program; start with 1 lb, progress 1 lb/wk

Proprioception/neuromuscular training
- Open kinetic chain passive/active joint repositioning 90°, 60°, and 30°
- Closed kinetic chain joint repositioning during squats/lunges
- Initiate squats on tilt board

Swelling control
  Ice, compression, elevation

Week 3
  Brace
    Discontinue locked brace (some patients use ROM brace for ambulation)
    If patient continues to use brace, unlock brace for ambulation
  PROM
    Continue ROM stretching and overpressure into extension (ROM should be 0°–100°/105°)
    ● Restore patient's symmetric extension
  Exercises
- Continue all exercises as in week 2
- PROM 0° to 105°
- Bicycle for ROM stimulus and endurance
- Pool walking program (if incision is closed)
- Eccentric quadriceps program 40° to 100° (isotonic only)
- Lateral lunges (straight plane)
- Front step downs
- Lateral step-overs (cones)
- Stair-stepper machine
- Progress proprioception drills, neuromuscular control drills
- Continue passive/active reposition drills (closed kinetic chain, open kinetic chain)

Progressive strengthening/neuromuscular control phase (weeks 4–10)

Criteria to enter phase III
1. Active ROM 0°–115°
2. Quadriceps strength 60% greater than contralateral side (isometric test at 60° knee flexion)
3. Unchanged KT test bilateral values (+1 or less)
4. Minimal to no full joint effusion
5. No joint line or patellofemoral pain

Goals
  Restore full knee ROM (5°–0° to 125°) symmetric motion
  Improve lower extremity strength
  Enhance proprioception, balance, and neuromuscular control
  Improve muscular endurance
  Restore limb confidence and function

Brace
  No immobilizer or brace, may use knee sleeve to control swelling/support

ROM
  Self-ROM (4–5 times daily using the other leg to provide ROM), emphasis on maintaining
  0° passive extension
- PROM 0° to 125° at 4 weeks

KT 2000 Test (Week 4, 20 lb anterior and posterior test)

Week 4
  Exercises
- Progress isometric strengthening program
- Leg press (0°–100°)

- Knee extension 90° to 40°
- Hamstring curls (isotonics)
- Hip abduction and adduction
- Hip flexion and extension
- Lateral step-overs
- Lateral lunges (straight plane and multiplane drills)
- Lateral step ups
- Front step downs
- Wall squats
- Vertical squats
- Standing toe calf raises
- Seated toe calf raises
- Biodex stability system (balance, squats, etc)
- Proprioception drills
- Bicycle
- Stair stepper machine
- Pool program (backward running, hip and leg exercises)
- Unloading treadmill walking

Proprioception/neuromuscular drills

- Tilt board squats (perturbation)
- Passive/active reposition Open kinetic chain
- Closed kinetic chain repositioning on tilt board

Week 6

KT 2000 Test

20 and 30 lb anterior and posterior tests

Exercises

- Continue all exercises
- Pool running (forward) and agility drills
- Balance on tilt boards
- Progress to balance and ball throws
- Wall slides/squats

Week 8

KT 2000 Test

20 and 30 lb anterior and posterior test

Exercises

- Continue all exercises listed in weeks 4 to 6
- Leg press sets (single leg) 0° to 100° and 40° to 100°
- Plyometric leg press
- Perturbation training
- Isokinetic exercises (90°–40°) (120°–240°/s)
- Walking program
- Bicycle for endurance
- Stair stepper machine for endurance
- Biodex stability system
- Training on tilt board

Week 10

KT 2000 test

20 and 30 lb and manual maximum test

Isokinetic Test

Concentric knee extension/flexion at 180° and 300°/s

Exercises

- Continue all exercises listed in weeks 6, 8, and 10
- Continue stretching drills
- Progress strengthening exercises and neuromuscular training

Advanced activity phase (weeks 10–16)

Criteria to enter phase IV

1. AROM 0°–125° or greater
2. Quadriceps strength 75% of contralateral side, knee extension flexor: extensor ratio of 70% to 75%

3. No change in KT values (comparable with contralateral side, within 2 mm)
4. No pain or effusion
5. Satisfactory clinical examination
6. Satisfactory isokinetic test (values at 180°)
   - Quadriceps bilateral comparison 75%
   - Hamstrings equal bilateral
   - Quadriceps peak torque/body weight 65% at 180°/s (males) 55% at 180°/s (females)
   - Hamstrings/quadriceps ratio 66% to 75%
7. Hop test (80% of contralateral leg)
8. Subjective knee scoring (modified Noyes system) 80 points or better

Goals
   Normalize lower extremity strength
   Enhance muscular power and endurance
   Improve neuromuscular control
   Perform selected sport-specific drills

Exercises
- May initiate running program (weeks 10–12) (physician decision)
- May initiate light sport program (golf) (physician decision)
- Continue all strengthening drills
  - Leg press
  - Wall squats
  - Hip abduction/adduction
  - Hip flexion/extension
  - Knee extension 90° to 40°
  - Hamstring curls
  - Standing toe calf
  - Seated toe calf
  - Step down
  - Lateral step ups
  - Lateral lunges
  - Plyometric leg press
- Neuromuscular training
  - Lateral step overs (cones)
  - Lateral lunges
  - Tilt board drills

Weeks 14 to 16
- Progress program
- Continue all drills above
- May initiate lateral agility drills
- Backward running

Return to activity phase (months 16–22)

Criteria to enter phase V
1. Full ROM
2. Unchanged KT 2000 test (within 2.5 mm of opposite side)
3. Isokinetic test that fulfills criteria
4. Quadriceps bilateral comparison ($\geq$80%)
5. Hamstring bilateral comparison ($\geq$110%)
6. Quadriceps torque/body weight ratio ($\geq$55%)
7. Hamstrings/quadriceps ratio ($\geq$70%)
8. Proprioceptive test (100% of contralateral leg)
9. Functional test ($\geq$85% of contralateral side)
10. Satisfactory clinical examination
11. Subjective knee scoring (modified Noyes system; $\geq$90 points)

Goals
   Gradual return to full-unrestricted sports
   Achieve maximal strength and endurance
   Normalize neuromuscular control
   Progress skill training

Tests
  KT 2000, isokinetic, and functional tests before return

Exercises
- Continue strengthening exercises
- Continue neuromuscular control drills
- Continue plyometrics drills
- Progress running and agility program
- Progress sport specific training
  - Running/cutting/agility drills
  - Gradual return to sport drills

6-month follow-up

Isokinetic test

KT 2000 test

Functional test

12-month follow-up

Isokinetic test

KT 2000 test

Functional test

Abbreviations: AROM, active range of motion; KT, knee arthrometer; PROM, passive range of motion; PTG, patellar tendon graft; ROM, range of motion.

Step 1: Preparation of Both the Patient and Their Knee for Surgery

The preoperative component of rehabilitation after an acute ACL injury is critical to the overall success of the upcoming ACL reconstruction procedure. The preoperative phase serves 5 key purposes: (1) physical preparation of the patient for surgery, (2) psychological preparation of the patient for surgery, (3) reduction of the risk of postoperative complications, (4) improved likelihood of a successful return to high-level activity and sport after surgery, and (5) minimization of the risk of a second ACL injury.

After the acute diagnosis of an ACL tear, the initial critical choice of proper timing for the surgery must be determined. This timing choice falls into 1 of 2 categories, either acute or delayed surgery. With the acute surgery choice, an ACL reconstruction is performed as soon as possible after the diagnosis when the knee is often swollen, with decreased ROM, hemarthrosis, and painful quadriceps inhibition. If delayed surgical reconstruction is chosen, the patient waits to undergo surgery until the knee is in a "normal" state.

Shelbourne and colleagues[22] reported on the rate of developing arthrofibrosis in a retrospective analysis of 169 ACL reconstructions divided into 3 groups based on their time from injury to surgery. There was a 17% rate of arthrofibrosis in patients undergoing surgery between 0 and 7 days after injury and an 11% rate in patients who were operated on 8 to 21 days after ACL injury, and 0% when surgery was performed greater than 21 days after injury. Hunter and colleagues[47] showed that timing of surgery after injury had no significant difference in postoperative ROM in a study of 185 acute knee injuries. Additionally, Guerra and colleagues[48] investigating the link between surgical timing and the incidence of arthrofibrosis showed an approximately 4% rate of arthrofibrosis in patients regardless of the timing of surgery, noting instead that the timing of the surgical reconstruction should be individualized to the patient and not based solely on any single period of time after ACL injury.

Short-term progressive rehabilitation has been shown to be well-tolerated after acute ACL injury and assists in improving knee function before reconstruction or the first step in nonoperative management.[49] Our clinical opinion is that rehabilitation before surgery should be undertaken when possible and necessary to reduce swelling, inflammation, and pain; restore normal ROM; normalize gait; and prevent muscle atrophy before surgery. The goal is to return the knee to its preinjury, normalized state and to obtain tissue homeostasis before further insult to the knee complex. Satisfactory motion is restored before surgery to reduce the risk of postoperative arthrofibrosis.[22] We believe the necessary PROM to achieve before surgery is approximately 0° to 120°/125°. Patient education, a critical aspect of preoperative rehabilitation, informs and prepares the patient for the surgical procedure and postoperative rehabilitation. The preoperative phase, which we believe is critical to a successful outcome, may require several weeks; however, approximately 21 days are typically adequate to achieve these goals.[22,41] The complete preoperative program is outlined in detail in **Box 4**.

Step 2: Restore Full Passive Knee Extension

The most common complication that produces poor functional outcomes after ACL reconstruction is motion loss, particularly a loss of full knee extension.[22,50–53] The inability to fully extend the knee results in abnormal joint arthrokinematics,[54–57] scar tissue formation in the anterior aspect of the knee, and subsequent increases in patellofemoral/tibiofemoral joint contact pressure.[58] Therefore, 2 of our goals are to achieve some degree of hyperextension during the first few days after surgery and eventually to work to restore symmetric motion.

Specific exercises include PROM exercises performed by the rehabilitation specialist, supine hamstring stretches with a wedge under the heel, and gastrocnemius stretches with a towel. Passive overpressure of 5 to 10 lb (2.25–4.5 kg) just proximal to the patella may be used for a low-load, long-duration stretch as needed (**Fig. 1**A). The patient is instructed to lie supine while the low-load, long-duration stretch is applied for 12 to 15 minutes 4 times per day, with the total low-load, long-duration stretch time per day equaling at least 60 minutes.[59] We use this technique immediately after surgery to maintain and improve knee extension and prevent a flexion contracture.

The amount of hyperextension we attempt to restore depends on the uninjured knee. During the first week after surgery, for patients who exhibit 10° or more of hyperextension on the uninjured knee, we will restore approximately 7° of hyperextension on the surgical side. We gradually restore the remaining hyperextension once joint inflammation is reduced and muscular control is restored over the following several weeks. We often use extension devices to create overpressure into extension, as seen in **Fig. 1**B. These authors feel that restoring hyperextension is imperative to a successful outcome and an asymptomatic knee.[6]

Step 3: Reduce Postoperative Inflammation

It is imperative to control postoperative pain, inflammation, and swelling during the first week of rehabilitation. Calming the knee down initially, starting slow, will allow the rehabilitation to accelerate faster in the long run. There is no way that a reactive—swollen, painful—knee can be accelerated under any circumstances. Reduce the swelling and pain, restore full knee extension, activate the quadriceps musculature, and then progress.

Box 4
Preoperative phase of anterior cruciate ligament injury rehabilitation

Preoperative phase

Goals
  Diminish inflammation, swelling, and pain
  Restore normal ROM (especially knee extension)
  Restore voluntary muscle activation
  Protect the knee from further injury, especially menisci
  Provide patient education to prepare patient for surgery

Brace
  Elastic wrap or knee sleeve to reduce swelling and drop locked brace in extension for
  ambulation

Weight bearing
  As tolerated with or without crutches

Exercises
• Ankle pumps
• Passive knee extension to 0°
• Passive knee flexion to tolerance
• Straight leg raises (3-way, flexion, abduction, adduction)
• Quadriceps setting
• Closed kinetic chain exercises: mini squats, lunges, step ups
  Hip external rotation/internal rotation with resistance band

Muscle stimulation
  Electrical muscle stimulation to quadriceps during voluntary quadriceps exercises (4–6 h/d)

Neuromuscular/proprioception training
  ○ Eliminate quadriceps avoidance gait
  ○ Retro stepping drills
  ○ Balance training drills
       Single leg stance (perform exercise bilaterally)

Cryotherapy/elevation
  Apply ice 20 minutes of every hour, elevate leg with knee in full extension (knee must be
  above heart)

Patient education
  Review postoperative rehabilitation program
  Review instructional video (optional)
  Select appropriate surgical date

Abbreviation: ROM, range of motion.

Pain may play a role in the inhibition of muscle activity commonly observed after ACL reconstruction. Young and colleagues[60] examined quadriceps activity in the acutely swollen and painful knee by using local anesthesia provided during medial meniscectomy. Patients in the control group had significant postoperative pain and quadriceps inhibition (30%-76%). In contrast, patients with local anesthesia reported minimal pain and only mild quadriceps inhibition (5%-31%).

DeAndrade et al[61] reported a progressive decrease in quadriceps activity as knee joint distention was increased progressively with the injection of saline solution. Spencer and colleagues[62] found a similar decrease in quadriceps activation with joint effusion. They reported the threshold for inhibition of the vastus medialis to be approximately 20 to 30 mL of joint effusion, and 50 to 60 mL for inhibition of the rectus femoris and vastus lateralis. Others have reported similar results.[63–67]

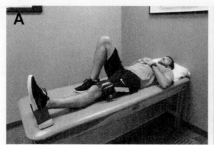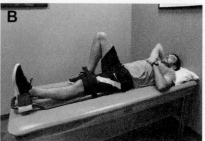

Fig. 1. (*A*) A low-load, long-duration stretch to restore the patient's full passive knee extension. A 4.5-kg weight is used for 10 to 15 minutes, with a bolster placed under the ankle to create a stretch. (*B*) Commercial device to improve extension range of motion and prevent compensatory hip external rotation. ([*B*] Extensionater; ERMI, Inc, Atlanta, GA.)

Pain after surgery can be reduced through the use of cryotherapy, analgesic medication, electrical stimulation,[68,69] and PROM.[70,71] We also use various therapeutic lasers to aid in the healing response.[72–74]

Treatment options for swelling include cryotherapy,[75–79] high-voltage stimulation,[80] and joint compression through the use of a knee sleeve or compression wrap.[81] A commercial cold device (**Fig. 2**) providing continuous cold therapy and compression may also be beneficial.

Pain and swelling may also be affected by the quick progression of a patient's WB status and ROM. In general, our patients are allowed to bear weight, as tolerated, with 2 crutches and a brace locked into extension immediately after surgery. The brace is worn until voluntary quadriceps control is demonstrated. Typically, the patient should be able to perform a straight leg raise without a lag, have no increases in pain or

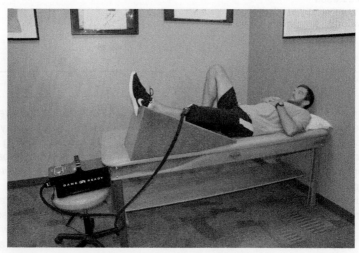

Fig. 2. A commercial cold wrap applied to the knee immediately after surgery to control pain and swelling. (Game Ready, Concord, CA.)

swelling, and demonstrate adequate quadriceps control while present in the physical therapy clinic to advance their WB status.

A critical goal of the second week is to train the patient to assume full WB. Two crutches are used for the first 7 to 10 days after surgery, progressing to 1 crutch and finally to full WB without crutches after 10 to 14 days. This WB progression is altered as needed to ensure that increased pain and swelling do not develop secondary to excessive WB forces. Also, the WB progression is altered if concomitant surgeries are performed (meniscus repair, articular cartilage procedures, etc) or if a bone bruise is present. In such cases, WB is either delayed or slowed to allow adequate healing before allowing full WB.

Step 4: Gradual Restoration of Full Knee Flexion

Unlike extension, knee flexion is gradually restored during the rehabilitation process. If flexion is pushed to aggressively, swelling will result but the goal must be a restoration of full knee flexion eventually pushing the heel to the glutes passively. Flexion ROM should be gradually progressed during the first week with the patient exhibiting 0° to 90° of knee ROM 5 to 7 days after surgery and 0° to 100° of knee ROM 7 to 10 days after surgery. However, the rate of progression must be based on the patient's unique response to surgery. If a substantial effusion exists, ROM is advanced at a slower pace. We prefer to move the knee slower the first 5 to 7 days after surgery to work on reducing swelling and pain rather than aggressively pushing knee flexion at the expense of an increase in symptoms.

It should be noted that Cosgarea and colleagues[82] compared the effects of postoperative bracing and ROM exercises on the incidence of arthrofibrosis after ACL reconstruction between 2 groups of patients. The group that was braced at 45° of knee flexion and waited 1 week before beginning ROM exercises had a 23% incidence of motion complications, compared with a rate of 3% in the group that was braced at 0° of knee extension and initiated ROM exercises immediately after surgery. Similarly, several other authors have all reported that immediate motion is essential to avoid ROM complications.[22,82–85]

Although the initial primary focus is on obtaining full knee extension, the recovery of knee flexion is a much more gradual process, starting with 90° in the first week and progressing by approximately 10° per week. This allows for full knee flexion 4 to 6 weeks after surgery. We believe that the first 2 to 4 weeks after surgery constitute a very important time to restore the knee to a level of homeostasis during ACL rehabilitation.[86]

Step 5: Restore Complete Patellar Mobility

Patellar mobility not only enables the restoration of full motion, it is also needed for quadriceps function and serves to protect the patella from excessive wear and tear and prevents anterior knee pain. The loss of patellar mobility after ACL reconstruction may have various causes, including excessive scar tissue adhesions along the medial and lateral retinacula, fat pad restrictions,[58,87] and harvesting the patellar tendon for the ACL graft. The loss of patellar mobility, referred to as infrapatella contracture syndrome, results in ROM complications and difficulty activating the quadriceps.[88] Patellar mobilizations are performed by the rehabilitation specialist in the clinic and independently by patients during their home exercise program. Mobilizations are performed in the medial/lateral and superior/inferior directions, especially for those with a patellar tendon autograft, to restore the patella's ability to tilt, especially in the superior direction.

Step 6: Individualize and Adjust the Rehabilitation Program Based on the Status of the Knee

Graft type
The graft used to reconstruct the ACL should be given appropriate consideration in developing an appropriate postoperative rehabilitation program. The most commonly used graft tissue sources are the autogenous patellar bone–tendon–bone[85,89] and autogenous hamstring tendons.[90–92] In some instances physicians use allografts[93–95] or the quadriceps tendon.[96,97] Postoperative rehabilitation program need to be appropriately altered based on differences in graft tissue strength, stiffness, and the strength of fixation.

The ultimate load to failure of various tissues has been reported by several investigators.[98–101] Hamner and colleagues[98] reported that the quadrupled hamstring tendon graft is approximately 91% stronger than the native ACL and 39% stronger than the patellar tendon, whereas the patellar tendon graft is approximately 37% stronger than the native ACL. Although virtually every potential graft is stronger than the native ACL, graft fixation strength and graft size of the reconstruction must be factored into the equation when developing a rehabilitation program. The healing of bone to bone in the osseous tunnel (patellar tendon autograft), which occurs in approximately 8 weeks in most instances, is faster than the healing of tendon to bone (hamstring autograft), which takes approximately 12 weeks.[102,103] The theoretic advantage of a larger, stronger allograft that allows more aggressive rehabilitation remains unproven.[104]

The potential disadvantage of using hamstring autograft or patellar tendon allograft tissue is increased graft laxity or graft failure owing to delayed or inappropriate healing.[105] Conversely, the potential disadvantage of using a bone–patellar tendon–bone autograft is the higher rate of arthrofibrosis and anterior knee pain.[105] Both issues can be minimized or avoided by using the appropriate supervised rehabilitation program.

Our clinical approach to developing and designing a rehabilitation program based on the type of ACL graft is to initially be less aggressive with soft tissue grafts such as the quadrupled hamstring/semitendinosus graft. Therefore, the return to running, plyometrics, and sports is slightly slower with a semitendinosus graft. Additionally, we do not allow isolated hamstring strengthening for approximately 8 weeks, to allow appropriate graft site healing to occur.

Aglietti and colleagues[106] compared the outcomes of using hamstring tendon grafts versus bone–tendon–bone grafts in a consecutive series of 60 patients. The results indicated no significant difference in outcomes between the 2 types of grafts. In the patellar tendon graft group, compared with the semitendinosus group, there was a trend toward better objective stability; however, there was more knee extension motion loss and more patellofemoral complaints. These results are similar to the findings of Marder and colleagues.[107]

Our rehabilitation program for allograft reconstruction is slower than the regular program for autogenous grafts. When using allograft tissue, the limiting factor to consider is fixation of the soft tissue as it is healing within the bone tunnels. This can take longer than 4 to 6 months[108–110] and therefore may limit the patient's progression to higher level functional activities. Several authors have described the rehabilitation program after allogenous patellar tendon bone–tendon–bone grafts.[27,94,109–111] Although the initial progression is similar, the rehabilitation program for allograft tissue should be slower to progress into aggressive activities such as running, jumping, and cutting.

Medial collateral ligament injury
Hirshman and colleagues[112] reported a 13% incidence of combined ACL and medial collateral ligament (MCL) injuries in acute knee ligament injuries. Isolated MCL injuries

are often treated nonoperatively; however, when combined with ACL disruption, grade III MCL injuries may require surgical intervention owing to the loss of the ACL as a secondary restraint to valgus stress. Although individuals with grades I and II MCL sprains may not require surgical intervention for the injured MCL, they may require special attention during the rehabilitation process owing to increased pain and potential for excessive scarring of the medial capsular tissues.

The treatment approach for an ACL reconstruction with an associated nonoperative MCL injury is similar to that used for isolated ACL reconstruction, with some noteworthy special considerations. Owing to increased pain, the extent of tissue damage, and extraarticular vascularity, combined ACL and MCL injuries often present with excessive scar tissue formation[113]; thus, a slightly more accelerated progression for ROM should follow, with particular emphasis on achieving full passive knee extension because the restoration of motion can be a challenge for the clinician because of the increased pain associated with this injury.

MCL tears from the proximal origin or within the midsubstance of the ligament tend to heal with increased stiffness without residual laxity. In contrast, MCL injuries at the distal insertion site tend to have a lesser healing response, often leading to residual valgus laxity.[114] Therefore, the location of ligament damage may also affect the rehabilitation program. Injuries involving the distal aspect of the MCL may be progressed more cautiously to allow for tissue healing; in some instances, these individuals may be immobilized in a brace to allow MCL healing before ACL reconstruction. In contrast, injury to the midsubstance or proximal ligament may require a slightly accelerated ROM program to prevent excessive scar tissue formation.

Lateral collateral ligament injury

The incidence of concomitant lateral collateral ligament (LCL) injuries is far less than that of concomitant MCL injuries. Hirshman and colleagues[112] reported a 1% incidence of combined ACL and LCL injuries in acute knee injuries. ACL injuries with concomitant LCL pathology or posterolateral capsular damage usually do not exhibit the same scarring characteristics as combined ACL and MCL injuries. The progression for concomitant ACL and LCL injuries is usually slower than for combined ACL and MCL injuries to allow for adequate healing. The restoring of ROM is not altered, although WB progresses slightly slower, with full WB occurring approximately 4 weeks after surgery. Similar to the MCL, where excessive valgus stress is avoided, exercises that produce excessive varus stress should be monitored carefully for symptoms and progressed judiciously. Furthermore, if the patient exhibits a varus thrust during ambulation, then a functional medial unloader brace may be useful to control the varus moment, and isolated isotonic hamstring strengthening may be delayed for 6 to 8 weeks.

The varus and valgus stresses observed during these combined collateral injuries often results in bone bruises and articular cartilage lesions. Rehabilitation progression, particularly with impact loading, should be delayed to allow adequate bone healing in these instances.

Articular cartilage lesions

Articular cartilage lesions of the knee or bone bruises occur in approximately 70% to 92% of traumatic ACL injuries,[115–118] with another study reporting a 100% incidence of bone bruises in the ACL injured knee.[119] Generally, bone bruises occur on the lateral femoral condyle and lateral tibial plateau.[115,117,118,120,121] Bone lesions on a WB surface typically extend into the subchondral bone; in these situations, deleterious compressive forces early in the rehabilitation process must be avoided. The rehabilitation specialist should also consider delaying impact activities, such as jogging and plyometrics, until enough time has passed to allow for sufficient bone healing. Follow-up MRI is not performed routinely owing to cost constraints, but may be beneficial to determine the extent of bone healing and assist in patient progression toward higher level WB activities, requiring the rehabilitation specialist to rely on symptoms when progressing the patient. Two of the most important rehabilitation considerations in patients after ACL reconstruction with an underlying articular cartilage injury are WB restrictions and progressive ROM. Unloading and immobilization have been shown to be deleterious to healing articular cartilage, resulting in proteoglycan loss and gradual weakening off the articular cartilage.[37,122,123] Therefore, controlled WB and ROM are essential to facilitate healing and prevent articular cartilage degeneration. This gradual progression has been shown to stimulate matrix production and improve the tissue's overall mechanical properties.[124–126] Controlled compression and decompression forces observed during WB may nourish articular cartilage and provide the necessary signals within the repair tissue to produce a matrix that will match the environmental forces that are being appllied.[37,122,123] A progression of partial WB with crutches is used to gradually increase the amount of load applied to the WB surfaces of the joint. A progressive loading program that uses a pool or unloading treadmill can also be extremely beneficial in the rehabilitation progression after ACL reconstruction in a patient with a bone bruise.

PROM activities, such as continuous passive motion machines or manual PROM performed by a rehabilitation specialist, are also performed immediately after surgery with a limited ROM to nourish the healing of articular cartilage and prevent the formation of adhesions.[28,127] Motion exercises may assist in creating a smooth, low-friction surface by sliding against the joint's articular surface, and seem to be an essential component of cartilage repair.[28,128] It is these authors' opinion that PROM is a safe and effective exercise to perform immediately after surgery and has minimal disadvantageous shear or compressive forces when performed with the patient relaxed to ensure that muscular contraction does not create deleterious compressive or shearing forces. Furthermore, the use of continuous passive motion has been shown to enhance cartilage healing and long-term outcomes after articular cartilage procedures.[129,130]

The importance of communication between the surgical team and the rehabilitation team to ensure the highest quality of care for each individual cannot be overemphasized. This is particularly true when a concomitant articular cartilage procedure, such as a microfracture, is performed. Knowledge of the healing and maturation processes after these procedures will ensure that the repair tissue is gradually loaded and that excessive forces are not introduced too early in the healing process. Long-term studies are needed to better understand whether these articular cartilage lesions can lead to degenerative OA and functional disability, although, as stated, studies have reported that 40% to 90% of ACL patients will exhibit radiographic knee OA 7 to 12 years after surgery.[14,131,132]

Meniscal pathology

Meniscal injuries occur in approximately 64% to 77% of ACL injuries.[104,133] Shelbourne and colleagues[21] stated that meniscal tears in the ACL-injured knee typically occur traumatically and are not degenerative in nature compared with meniscal tears in ACL-intact knees. If meniscal pathology is present, a partial meniscectomy or meniscus repair may be necessary to alleviate symptoms. An arthroscopic partial meniscectomy does not significantly alter the rehabilitation protocol after ACL reconstruction. However, additional time may be required before initiating a running or jumping program, depending on the amount of meniscal injury. If surgical repair of the meniscus is required, alteration to the rehabilitation program is warranted. There is controversy regarding the duration of immobilization, WB progression, and the timing for return to pivoting sports, but all of these elements need to be considered in formulating a rehabilitation plan.[134,135] Cannon and Vittori[136] and other investigators[137–139] have reported an increase in meniscal healing when a concomitant ACL reconstruction was performed.

For patients undergoing concomitant ACL reconstruction and meniscus repair, ROM and WB progressions are slightly slower, depending on the extent of meniscus repair or location of meniscal injury. Although there is very limited research, we allow immediate WB on meniscus repairs with the knee brace locked in full extension. WB with the knee locked in full extension produces a hoop stress on the meniscus, which may aid in the overall healing effect. Repair of complex meniscal tears is progressed much slower than repair of isolated peripheral tears. Isotonic hamstring strengthening is limited for 8 to 10 weeks after surgery to allow adequate healing of the repaired meniscus, owing to the close anatomic relationship between the joint capsule, meniscus, and hamstrings. The patient is not allowed to squat past 60° for 8 to 12 weeks and needs to avoid squats with twisting motions for at least 16 weeks.

Specific ROM guidelines differ based on the extent and location of meniscal damage, although immediate motion with emphasis on full passive knee extension is universal. Patients with repair of a tear isolated at the periphery of the meniscus should exhibit approximately 90° to 100° of knee flexion by week 2, 105° to 115° by week 3, and 120° to 135° by week 4. Patients with repair of complex meniscal tears follow a slightly slower approach, with 90° to 100° of knee flexion by week 2, 105° to 110° by week 3, and 115° to 120° by week 4. Patients with complex meniscal repairs may also need to use crutches and partial WB for an additional 1 to 2 weeks after surgery for symptom management.

Barber and Click[134] evaluated the efficacy of an accelerated ACL rehabilitation program for patients with concomitant meniscus repairs. At follow-up (24–72 months after surgery), 92% of repairs exhibited successful meniscal healing, whereas only 67% of meniscus repairs performed in ACL-deficient knees and 67% of meniscus repairs performed in stable knees exhibited successful healing. The authors suggested that the hemarthrosis and simulated inflammatory process associated with the ACL reconstruction may enhance meniscal healing and improve the long-term results of meniscus repair.

Female athlete

Athletic females have unique rehabilitation requirements that warrant special consideration.[13,140–145] Malone and colleagues[146] reported that female college basketball players were 8 times more likely to injure their ACL than their male counterparts. Lindenfeld and colleagues[147] reported that female soccer players were 6 times more likely to sustain an ACL injury than male soccer players. There are similar data for other sports, such as volleyball and gymnastics.[148,149] It is also noteworthy that in female athletes, the vast majority of ACL injuries occur without contact.[31]

Females have unique physical characteristics that may predispose them to injury, including increased genu valgum alignment, a poor hamstring–quadriceps strength ratio, poor hip strength, running and landing on a more extended knee, a quadriceps-dominant knee posture, and hip/core complex weakness. It has also been postulated that hormonal changes associated with the female menstrual cycle may also play a role in ACL injury susceptibility.[13,140] Because a common mechanism of noncontact ACL injury is a valgus stress with rotation at the knee, it is important for the female athlete to learn to control this type of valgus moment during activity.[140,144,150] In addition to education on optimal knee alignment (keeping the knee over the second toe), exercises designed to control these valgus moments at the knee include front step-downs (**Fig. 3**), lateral step-downs with resistance (**Fig. 4**), and squats with resistance around the distal femur (**Fig. 5**). Rehabilitation should train the patient to stabilize the knee through coactivation of the quadriceps and hamstrings using various exercises, including tilt board balance exercises while performing a throw and catch. Because females tend to land with increased knee extension and decreased hip flexion after jumping, dynamic stabilization drills should be performed, with the knee flexed approximately 30° to promote better alignment and activation of the quadriceps and hamstrings.[150,151] A key rehabilitation aspect for the female athlete is to train the hip extensors, external rotators, abductors, and core stabilizers, while emphasizing a flexed knee posture during running, cutting, and jumping. We instruct the female athlete to control the knees via the hip/pelvis[152–154] and foot position.[153] Furthermore, we emphasize strength training of the hip abductors, extensors, and external rotators. We take special consideration to eccentrically train these muscle groups to help control excessive adduction and internal rotation of the femur during WB activities. Moreover, core stabilization exercises are used to aid in controlling lateral trunk displacement during functional athletic movements.[151,152,155–157] We

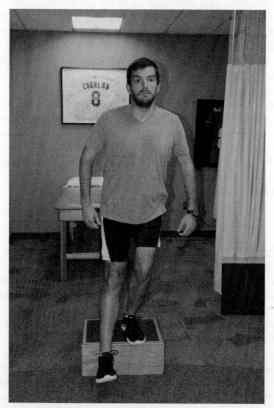

Fig. 3. Front step-down movement. During the eccentric or lowering phase, the patient is instructed to maintain proper alignment of the lower extremity to prevent the knee from moving into a valgus moment.

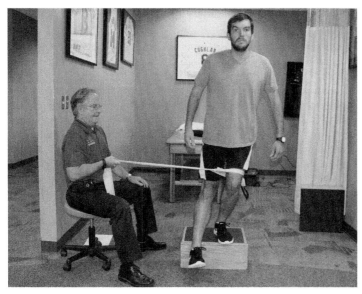

Fig. 4. Lateral step-down with resistance bands. A resistance band is applied around the inner knee to provide resistance and to control the valgus moment at the knee by recruiting hip abductors and rotators.

believe that after ACL surgery it is important that female athletes undergo a specific rehabilitation program that addresses the predisposing factors that potentially led to the injury, focusing on retraining faulty mechanics and improving muscular imbalances.

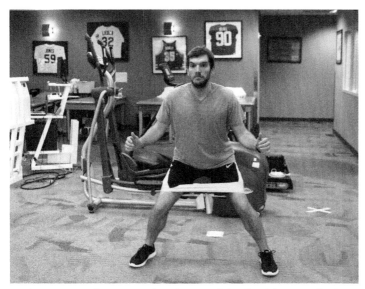

Fig. 5. Lateral stepping with resistance bands around the distal femur to further recruit hip musculature.

Step 7: Reestablish Quadriceps Activation

Inhibition of the quadriceps muscle is common after ACL reconstruction, especially in the presence of pain and effusion during the acute phases of rehabilitation. Electrical muscle stimulation and biofeedback[158] are often incorporated into therapeutic exercises to facilitate the active contraction of the quadriceps musculature. Kim and colleagues,[159] based on their recent review of the literature, concluded that using neuromuscular electrical stimulation combined with exercise was more efficient than exercise alone to improve quadriceps strength after ACL surgery.

Clinically, we use electrical stimulation immediately after surgery while performing isometric and isotonic exercises such as quadriceps sets, straight leg raises, hip adduction and abduction, and knee extensions from 90° to 40° of knee flexion.[160] Patients are instructed to actively contract the quadriceps musculature with the assistance of the superimposed neuromuscular electrical stimulation. Once independent muscle activation is achieved, biofeedback may be used to facilitate further neuromuscular activation of the quadriceps. The authors prefer electrical muscle stimulation to biofeedback for the vast majority of patients. The patient must concentrate on independently activating the quadriceps during rehabilitation.

Step 8: Restoration of Dynamic Functional Stability of the Knee Complex

We routinely begin basic proprioceptive training during the second postoperative week, pending adequate normalization of pain, swelling, and quadriceps control.[161–165] Proprioceptive training initially begins with basic exercises such as joint repositioning and weight shifting. Weight shifts may be performed in the medial/lateral direction and in diagonal patterns. Minisquats are also initiated soon after surgery. A neuromuscular training device (Monitored Rehab Systems MR Cube; CDM Sport, Fort Worth, TX; **Fig. 6**) may be used with weight shifts and minisquats to challenge the proprioception and neuromuscular system of the patient. We encourage our patients to wear an elastic support wrap underneath their brace, because several authors[81,166]

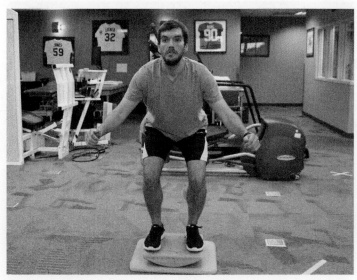

Fig. 6. Squats performed on a tilt board to improve neuromuscular control, using a Monitored Rehab Systems MR Cube. (CDM Sport, Fort Worth, TX.)

have reported that wearing an elastic bandage after surgery has a positive impact on proprioception and joint position sense.

By approximately the end of week 2, minisquats are progressed to be performed on an unstable surface, such as foam or a tilt board, if the patient exhibits good postural control and form during a double-leg squat on a solid surface. The patient is instructed to squat to approximately 25° to 30° and to hold the position for 2 to 3 seconds while stabilizing the tilt board. Wilk and colleagues[160] showed that the greatest amount of hamstring and quadriceps cocontraction occurred at approximately 30° of knee flexion during the squat. Squats may be performed with the tilt board positioned to move in the medial/lateral or anterior/posterior direction. Based on previous studies showing that muscular contraction can decrease knee varus/valgus laxity[167] and that quadriceps-to-hamstring muscle strength imbalances lead to an increased risk of ligamentous injury[11]; we believe that improving neuromuscular coactivation enhances knee stability. As proprioception improves, drills to encourage preparatory agonist/antagonist coactivation during functional activities are incorporated. These dynamic stabilization drills begin during the first 3 weeks after surgery with a single-leg stance on flat ground and unstable surfaces, cone stepping, and lateral lunge drills.

Single-leg balance exercises, performed on a piece of foam with the knee slightly flexed, are progressed by incorporating random movement of either the upper extremity or the uninvolved lower extremity to alter the position of the center of mass. Eventually, both upper and lower extremity movements may be combined in these exercises (**Fig. 7**). These single-leg balance drills with extremity movement are used to promote dynamic stabilization, improve single leg stability and recruit the activation of various muscle groups.[168] Medicine balls of progressively heavier weight can also be incorporated to provide a further challenge to the neuromuscular control system.

The patient may perform forward, backward, and lateral cone or cup step-over drills to facilitate gait training, enhance dynamic stability, and train the hip to help control forces at the knee joint. The patient is instructed to raise the knee to the level of the hip and step over a series of cones, landing with a slightly flexed knee. These cone drills may also be performed at various speeds to train the lower extremity to dynamically stabilize with different amounts of momentum. Strengthening of the hip and knee to eccentrically control the lower extremity is imperative to a return to function. These authors believe that one can improve knee stability via proximal and distal stability.

Lateral lunges are also performed to improve dynamic stability. The patient is instructed to lunge to the side, land on a slightly flexed knee, and hold that position for 1 to 2 seconds before returning to the start position. We use a functional progression for lateral lunges in which straight plane lateral lunges are performed first, then progress to multiple plane/diagonal lunges, lateral lunges with rotation, and lateral lunges onto foam (**Fig. 8**). As the patient progresses, a ball toss can be added to any of these exercises to challenge the preparatory stabilization of the lower extremity with minimal conscious awareness.

Perturbation training may also be incorporated approximately 2 to 3 weeks after surgery. Fitzgerald and colleagues[169] examined the efficacy of perturbation training in a rehabilitation program for ACL-deficient knees and reported more satisfactory outcomes and a lower frequency of subsequent giving-way episodes. Wilk and colleagues,[31] studying female patients after ACL surgery, observed improved results when a program emphasized perturbation training. Therefore, we incorporate perturbation training while the patient performs double- or single-leg balance exercises on a tilt board or an unstable surface. While flexing the knee to approximately 30°, the patient stabilizes the tilt board and begins throwing and catching a 3- to 5-lb (1.4- to

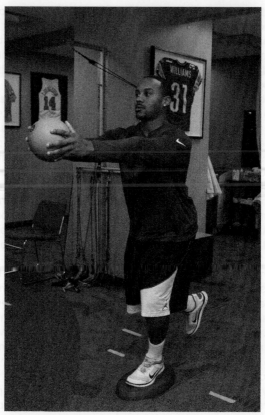

Fig. 7. Single-leg stance on foam while performing upper extremity movements using a 3.2-kg medicine ball. The clinician can perform a perturbation by striking the ball to cause a postural disturbance.

2.3-kg) medicine ball. The patient is instructed to stabilize the tilt board in reaction to the sudden outside force produced by the weighted ball. The rehabilitation specialist may also provide perturbations by striking the tilt board (**Fig. 9**) with the foot, requiring the patient to stabilize the tilt board with dynamic muscular contractions. Perturbations may also be performed during this drill by tapping the patient on the hips and trunk to provide a postural disturbance to the body. We typically use 3 levels of the tilt board to progress the patient into progressively more challenging levels of instability.

An additional goal of neuromuscular training is the restoration of the patient's confidence in the injured knee. It has been our experience that, after a serious knee injury, patients may become afraid of reinjury and returning to high-level function.[170] We believe that restoring neuromuscular control and, in particular, perturbation skill, significantly improves the patient's confidence in their injured knee.

Both WB and non-WB exercises (NWBE) have been shown to be effective for rehabilitation and return to sport after ACL surgery.[21] However, compared with NWBE, individuals who perform predominantly WB exercises tend to have less knee pain, more stable knees, generally more satisfaction with the end result, and a quicker return to sport.[21]

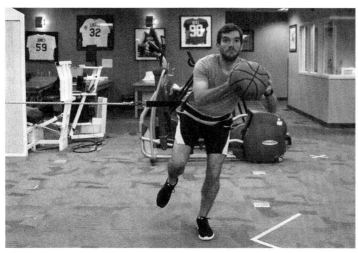

Fig. 8. Lateral lunges performed using a sport cord for resistance while landing on a foam pad and catching a ball. The patient is instructed to land and maintain a knee flexion angle of 30° during the drill.

There are differences in ACL loading between NWBE and WBE. Through a series of studies that estimated ACL loading during WBE and NWBE using the same relative exercise intensity, Wilk and colleagues[160] and Escamilla and colleagues[171–175] demonstrated higher ACL loads during NWBE (seated knee extensions). With NWBE, ACL tensile loads occurred between knee angles of 0° and 30° and peaked at approximately 150 N, compared with a peak of 50 N when performing a variety of WB exercises (barbell squats, single-leg squats, wall squats, forward and side lunges, and leg presses). These data are in agreement with in vivo ACL strain data reported by Beynnon and Fleming[176] and Heijne and colleagues,[177] who also reported a greater peak ACL tensile strain with NWBE than with WB exercises, occurring at knee flexion angles between 10° and 30°. For example, performing a leg press with 40% body weight resistance, climbing stairs, and lunging forward all produced less ACL strain than performing seated knee extension with no external resistance. Interestingly, performing seated knee extension with no external resistance (quadriceps activation only) produced the same amount of ACL strain as that measured while performing a single-leg sit-to-stand maneuver, with the latter also recruiting important hip and thigh musculature activity (eg, quadriceps, hamstrings, and gluteals), helping to stabilize the knee and protect the ACL graft.

Although it has been reported that squatting with resistance produces a similar amount of ACL strain compared with performing seated knee extension with resistance,[176] it should be noted that variations in squatting and lunging techniques can affect ACL strain.[173,174,178] For example, squatting and lunging with a more forward trunk tilt recruit the hamstrings, which helps to unload the ACL by decreasing anterior tibial translation to a greater extent than squatting and lunging with a more erect trunk.[174,178,179] Also, the gluteal musculature has higher activation in this position, which may aid in medial/lateral control at the knee. Knee flexion angles can also affect ACL loading. For NWBE and WB exercises, ACL loading primarily occurs between 0° and 50° of knee flexion; performing these exercises between 50° and 100° of knee flexion minimizes ACL loading. Finally, anterior knee translation beyond the

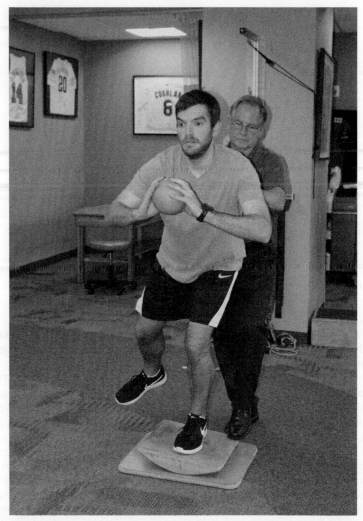

Fig. 9. Single-leg stance (knee flexed at 30°) performed on a tilt board while throwing and catching a 3.2-kg plyoball. Manual perturbations are performed by tapping the tilt board with the clinician's foot to create a postural disturbance.

toes, especially more than 8 cm, may also increase ACL loading during squatting and lunging exercises.[173,175]

WBEs performed on the involved extremity are also used to train the neuromuscular control system. Specific neuromuscular control drills designed to dynamically control valgus and varus moments at the knee include front step-downs, lateral step-downs, and single-leg balance drills. Chmielewski and colleagues[180] evaluated several WB activities in individuals with ACL-deficient and ACL-reconstructed knees and noted a strong correlation between functional outcome scores and the ability to perform the front step-down exercise.

Plyometric jumping drills may also be performed to facilitate dynamic stabilization and neuromuscular control of the knee joint, and to train for the dissipation of forces through the muscle's stretch-shortening properties.[181,182] Hewett and colleagues[150] examined the effects of a 6-week plyometric training program on the landing mechanics and strength of female athletes. They reported a 22% decrease in peak ground reaction forces and a 50% decrease in the abduction/adduction moments at the knee during landing. Moreover, significant increases in hamstring isokinetic strength, the hamstring–quadriceps ratio, and vertical jump height were reported. Using the same plyometric program, Hewett and colleagues[151] reported a statistically significant decrease in the amount of knee injuries in female athletes. It must be emphasized that with plyometric drills it is important to instruct the patient on proper jumping and landing techniques as well as the control and dissipation of forces.

Plyometric activities are typically initiated 12 weeks after a patellar tendon autograft reconstruction and delayed until 16 weeks after a semitendinosus autograft. The leg press machine is initially used to control the amount of weight and ground reaction forces as the athlete learns to correctly perform jumping drills. The patient is instructed to land softly on the toes, with the knees slightly flexed, to maximize force dissipation and avoid knee hyperextension. Plyometric drills are then progressed to flat ground and include ankle hops, jumping in place, and lateral, diagonal, and rotational jumping, bounding, and skip lunging. Flat ground plyometrics are progressed to incorporate single and multiple boxes **(Fig. 10)**. We usually begin plyometric activities with double-leg jumps, progressing to single-leg jumps. We are cautious with plyometric training because of its potential negative effects on articular surfaces, bone bruises, and the meniscus. We do not advocate the use of plyometrics for the recreational athlete.

Finally, proprioceptive and neuromuscular control has been shown to diminish once muscular fatigue occurs.[183–185] Therefore, we frequently recommend performing neuromuscular control drills toward the end of a treatment session, after cardiovascular training, to challenge neuromuscular control of the knee joint when the dynamic stabilizers are fatigued.

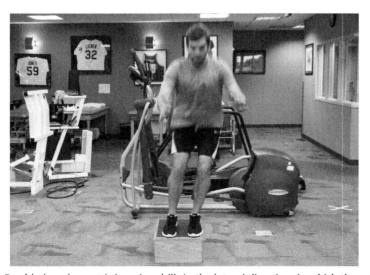

Fig. 10. Double-leg plyometric jumping drills in the lateral direction, in which the patient is instructed to land on the box and flat ground with the knee in a flexed position. These activities are initiated to allow the quadriceps musculature to create and dissipate forces at a higher level before returning to sport.

Step 9: Knee Control Must Be Provided from Both Above and Below

Stabilization of the knee joint occurs from above and below the knee, requiring a focus on restoring control of the hip complex during the rehabilitation program. Emphasis should be placed on activation and control of the hip abductors and external rotators, as well as, in strengthening the hip extensors and hamstring musculature.

Static and dynamic control and balance activities need to be incorporated aggressively with a goal of training the hip and lower leg to control dynamic valgus positions through retraining the lower quarter musculature and joint position sense to minimize or eliminate the impact of hip internal rotation and adduction moments as well as reducing the impact of foot pronation to assist in reducing valgus collapse of the knee.

Step 10: Protect the Knee Both Now and Later

The gradual increase in the amount of stress applied stress during the rehabilitation program aids in protecting the knee now and preserving it for long-term functional success with minimal to no symptoms. The majority (70%-92%) of individuals who sustain an ACL injury also have sustained a bone bruise to the lateral femoral condyle and lateral tibial plateau,[115,116] which can result in an increase in postoperative swelling, pain, and muscle inhibition.[119]

We believe that such a bone bruise could also lead to articular cartilage defects in the long term,[186] and we therefore attempt to control WB forces after surgery until the bone bruise has subsided.

This simple concept is applied to the progression of ROM, strengthening exercises, proprioceptive training, neuromuscular control drills, functional drills, and sport-specific training. For example, exercises such as weight shifts and lunges are progressed from the straight-plane anterior/posterior or medial/lateral direction to multiplane and rotational movements. Double-leg exercises, such as leg presses, knee extensions, balance activities, and plyometric jumps, are progressed to single leg exercises. This progression will also gradually increase applied loads on the ACL graft, which are believed to result in tissue hypertrophy and better tissue alignment. Persistent or increasing pain, inflammation, or swelling at any time during the rehabilitation program is an indication of an overaggressive approach. The athlete's return to sport is achieved through a series of transitional drills. The athlete is allowed to run in the pool before flat-ground running as a way to initiate a jogging program. We have found that the pool and an unloading treadmill (**Fig. 11**) are excellent options before dry-land activities. Furthermore, backward and lateral running is performed before forward running to decrease stress on the knee. Plyometric activities are performed before running and cutting drills, followed by sport-specific agility drills. The decision to return to running is based on a complex sequence of evaluations by the rehabilitation specialist and the athlete's ability to tolerate the functional progression without an increase in pain and swelling, while demonstrating good knee and hip control. Each decision regarding progression is also determined by the known concomitant injuries addressed during surgery and by adequate healing of the involved tissues.

This progression of applied and functional stresses is used to provide a healthy stimulus for healing tissues without causing damage. Our goal is to return the knee joint to its preinjury status and to the level of homeostasis described by Dye and Chew.[86]

Step 11: Objective Return to Running

"When can I start running?" This is one of the most frequently asked questions of almost any patient after ACL surgery. The simple answer for the patient is they can

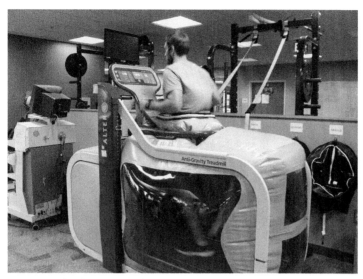

Fig. 11. Progressive loading treadmill used to initiate a walking or running program to minimize impact loading on the knee joint. (AlterG Anti-Gravity Treadmill; AlterG, Fremont, CA.)

start running when they are ready to run. Although this answer may sound flippant, it is in fact very true. Nothing is as demoralizing to a patient and produces a more problematic set back in the rehabilitation as developing reactive symptoms when trying to begin running before a patient is functionally capable. Additionally, giving a patient a specific timeframe to begin running, or any other higher level functional activity, is a critical error because the postoperative time itself is not the primary element that will determine readiness to return to running.

We advocate the use of objective criteria and the successful performance of specific tests to determine when a patient is ready to being running. Using specific criteria to progress a patient through the rehabilitation process assists in guiding the process and in progressing a patient when they are physically capable, rather than based solely on an arbitrary timeframe. The criteria we use to progress patients through their rehabilitation program has been presented in **Box 2**. The specific test and measures we administer and the scores necessary to begin running as presented in **Box 5**.

Using specific tests and predetermined criteria takes the subjective element out of patient progression and provides the patient with known measurable goals that must be achieved before progressing. This objective format serves both to motivate patients and to eliminate as much of the guess work as possible out of answering the question of, "When can I start running again?"

When the term return to play is stated, we believe there are 3 levels of return to play. The level is the return to performance training, this includes plyometrics, jump training, running and cutting, and sport-specific training. The next level is the return to practice, this includes other athletes involved with a sport specific training program. The last level is the return to sport performance, and this includes game completion.

Step 12: Objective Progression Beyond Running and Back to Sport

The last step in the sequential progression of ACL rehabilitation involves the restoration of function through sport-specific training for athletes returning to competition.

Box 5
Anterior cruciate ligament reconstruction performance progression assessment

Name: _____ Date: _____

Right/left/bilateral/procedure: _____

Group A tests: clearance to begin running

1. IKDC subjective knee evaluation form: Score_____ Pass_____ Fail_____

2. CKRS symptom rating form: Score_____ Pass_____ Fail_____

3. 30 step-and-holds (forward jump-lunge and landing): Pass_____ Fail_____

4. 10 single-leg squats to 45°: Pass_____ Fail_____

5. 1-RM on leg press: involved/uninvolved = _____/_____ = _____

6. 15-minute fast treadmill walking: Pass_____ Fail_____

7. KT-1000 or KT-2000 test (or clinical Lachman test): side to side difference _____

8. Isokinetic testing (or hand held dynamometer if available): Pass_____ Fail_____

Criteria to begin treadmill jogging
- IKDC subjective knee evaluation score of 90
- CKRS symptom rating Score of 10
- 30 step-and-holds without loss of balance or excessive motion outside sagittal plane
- 10 consecutive single-leg squats without loss of balance or excessive motion outside sagittal plane
- ≥70% 1-RM leg press involved/noninvolved
- Treadmill walking: normal gait pattern for entire 15 minutes
- KT < 2 mm involved–noninvolved
- Isokinetic fulfills criteria for quadriceps peak torque/BW ratio, H/Q ratio, bilateral peak torque comparison[a]

Group A test summary: Pass Fail

Rationale for failure:

Group B tests: clearance to begin agility drills

1. IKDC subjective knee evaluation form: Score_____ Pass_____ Fail_____

2. CKRS symptom rating form: Score_____ Pass_____ Fail_____

3. 10 single-leg squats to 45° with weight: involved/uninvolved = _____/_____ = _____

4. 1-RM on leg press: involved/uninvolved = _____/_____ = _____

5. Run 1 mile on treadmill: Pass_____ Fail_____

6. KT-1000 or KT-2000 test (or clinical Lachman test): side to side difference _____

7. Isokinetic testing (or hand held dynamometer): Pass_____ Fail_____

8. Single-leg hop tests (single-leg hop for distance, timed 6 m hop, triple cross-over hop):
   Involved/uninvolved = _____/_____ = _____
   Involved/uninvolved = _____/_____ = _____
   Involved/uninvolved = _____/_____ = _____
   Pass_____ Fail_____

Criteria to begin low-level agility drills
- IKDC subjective knee evaluation score of 90
- CKRS symptom rating score of 10
- 10 consecutive single-leg squats without loss of balance or excessive motion outside sagittal plane while holding ≥ 75% weight (dumbbells, weight vest, etc)
- Greater than 80% 1-RM leg press involved/uninvolved
- Normal running pattern on the treadmill
- KT < 2 mm involved–noninvolved (values same as prior tests)

- Isokinetic fulfills criteria for quadriceps peak torque/BW ratio, H/Q ratio, bilateral peak torque comparison[a]
- Greater than 85% Hop tests involved/noninvolved

Group B test summary: Pass Fail

Rationale for failure:

Group C tests: clearance to begin jumping

1. IKDC subjective knee evaluation form: Score _____ Pass_____ Fail_____

2. CKRS symptom rating form: Score _____ Pass_____ Fail_____

3. 10 single-leg squats to 60° with weight: involved/uninvolved = _____/_____ = _____

4. 10-RM on leg press: involved/uninvolved = _____/_____ = _____

5. Lateral shuffle, forward/backward shuttle run, and carioca: Pass_____ Fail_____

6. KT-1000 or KT-2000 test (or clinical Lachman test): side to side difference _____

7. Isokinetic testing (or hand held dynamometer if available): Pass_____ Fail_____

9. Single-leg hop tests (single-leg hop for distance, 6 m timed hop, triple cross-over hop):
    Involved/uninvolved = _____/_____ = _____
    Involved/uninvolved = _____/_____ = _____
    Involved/uninvolved = _____/_____ = _____
    Pass_____ Fail_____

Criteria to begin jumping
- IKDC subjective knee evaluation score of 90
- CKRS symptom rating score of 8
- 10 consecutive single-leg squats without loss of balance or excessive motion outside sagittal plane while holding ≥85% weight (dumbbells, weight vest, etc)
- ≥85% 10-RM leg press involved/noninvolved
- No compensation patterns with deceleration during agility drills
- KT < 2 mm involved-noninvolved (values same as prior tests)
- Isokinetic fulfills criteria for quadriceps peak torque/BW ratio, H/Q ratio, bilateral peak torque comparison, endurance values, work fatigue values[a]
- Greater than 85% hop tests involved/noninvolved

Group C test summary: Pass Fail

Rationale for Failure:

Group D tests: clearance to begin hopping and cutting

1. IKDC subjective knee evaluation form: Score _____ Pass_____ Fail_____

2. CKRS symptom rating form: Score _____ Pass_____ Fail_____

3. 10 single-leg squats to 60° with weight: involved/uninvolved = _____/_____ = _____

4. 10-RM on leg press: involved/uninvolved = _____/_____ = _____

5. Forward, lateral, and rotational jumps: Pass_____ Fail_____

6. KT-1000 or KT-2000 test (or clinical Lachman test): side to side difference _____

7. Isokinetic testing (or hand held dynamometer if available): Pass_____ Fail_____

10. Single-leg hop tests (single-leg hop for distance, 6 m timed hop, triple cross-over hop):
    Involved/uninvolved = _____/_____ = _____
    Involved/uninvolved = _____/_____ = _____
    Involved/uninvolved = _____/_____ = _____
    Pass_____ Fail_____

Criteria to begin hopping and cutting
- IKDC subjective knee evaluation score of 90
- CKRS symptom rating Score of 8

- 10 consecutive single-leg squats without loss of balance or excessive motion outside sagittal plane while holding ≥90% weight (dumbbells, weight vest, etc)
- ≥90% 1-RM on Leg Press
- No genu valgum when loading into or landing from jumps and equal weight distribution when initiating and landing the jumps
- KT test less than 2 mm involved–noninvolved (values same as prior tests)
- Isokinetic fulfills criteria for quadriceps peak torque/BW ratio, H/Q ratio, bilateral peak torque comparison, endurance values, work fatigue values[a]
- Greater than 90% hop tests involved/noninvolved

Group D test summary: Pass Fail

Rationale for failure:

Clearance criteria for return to sport
- IKDC subjective knee evaluation score of 90
- CKRS symptom rating Score of 8
- Achieves ≥90% on all strength assessments
- Displays a normal running pattern that does not increase pain
- Has practiced and displays no hesitation or compensation strategies during agility drills (particularly when decelerating) when performed at 100% effort
- Has practiced and displays normal loading (no genu valgum) and soft, athletic landings from all jumps and hops
- Has practiced and displays no hesitation or compensation strategies during cutting drills (particularly when decelerating) when performed at 100% effort
- KT test values remain unchanged
- Fulfills isokinetic testing criteria
- Demonstrates greater than 90% on hop tests

[a] Isokinetic test criteria: Quadriceps peak torque/BW ratio 180°/s: males greater than 65%, females greater than 55%, H/Q ratio 180°/s: males 66% to 72%, females 72% to 78%, Bilateral comparison: quadriceps greater than 85%, hamstrings greater than 90%, Endurance ratio 300°/s: quadriceps less than 15%, hamstrings less than 10%, No pain during test.
Abbreviations: BW, body weight; CKRS, Cincinnati Knee Rating System; H/Q, hamstring/quadriceps; IKDC, International Knee Documentation Committee; KT, knee arthrometer; RM, repetition maximum.

Many of the previously discussed drills, such as cone drills, lunges with sport cords, plyometric drills, and the running and agility progression, can be modified for the specific functional movement patterns associated with the patient's unique sport. Some sport-specific running and agility drills include side shuffling, cariocas, sudden starts and stops, zigzags, 45° cutting, and 90° cutting. The specific movement patterns learned throughout the rehabilitation program are integrated to provide challenges in a controlled setting.

Advancing functional activity needs to be more than just a return to running. Clearance tests, such as an isokinetic strength test,[46,187,188] the International Knee Documentation Committee Subjective Knee Evaluation Form,[189,190] and hop tests,[191–193] have all been advocated. In this process, the athlete must also demonstrate sufficient confidence in the affected extremity to successfully return to sport without any fears or limitations.[170,194]

Therefore, the complex nature of progressing the patient back to unrestricted athletic participation after ACL surgery should be, in and of itself, a complex progression of the key functional elements necessary for athletic performance. These elements should then be tested, measured and advanced in a sequential, criteria-driven manner. Returning an athlete to participation should be a graduated continuum that progresses from the least demanding to most demanding activities, not a single test or set of tests that releases an athlete to return to participation at 1 single point in time.

We incorporate a battery of tests applied in a sequential 5-phased performance assessment. This assessment is designed to determine activity readiness before the introduction of demanding functional athletic elements, reduce the risk of reinjury or contralateral injury, and promote psychological confidence. This program rank orders the relative demand of functional activities required for athletic participation and guides advancement back to unlimited activity via defined criteria to determine readiness for 5 key athletic elements: running, agility drills, jumping, hopping/cutting, and unrestricted sport. The tests performed and criteria to progress to each of these athletic elements is presented in **Box 5**.

This type of performance progression assessment testing provides the clinician with a useful set of tools to determine when an athlete is able to safely progress into higher level sports drills and return to unrestricted athletic activities. In addition, it may provide incentive for patients who require additional strength and neuromuscular retraining to begin simple running. The testing battery we use purposely incorporates a subjective analysis, conducted by the clinician, regarding the athlete's running, hopping, jumping/landing, and cutting maneuvers. A lack of patient confidence or any compensation strategies used during these tasks indicates an athlete who requires continued training and counseling before returning to unrestricted athletics.

SUMMARY

The rehabilitation process begins immediately after ACL injury, with an emphasis on reducing swelling and inflammation, restoring full passive knee extension, gradually restoring flexion, regaining quadriceps control, and allowing immediate WB. The goal of preoperative rehabilitation is to mentally and physically prepare the patient for surgery. Once the ACL surgery is performed, it is important to alter the rehabilitation program based on the type of graft used, any concomitant procedures performed, and the presence of an articular cartilage lesion. This aids in the prevention of several postoperative complications, such as loss of motion, patella femoral pain, graft failure, and muscular weakness. Current rehabilitation programs focus not only on strengthening exercises, but also on proprioceptive and neuromuscular control drills to provide a neurologic stimulus so that the athlete can regain the dynamic stability that is needed in athletic competition. We believe that it is also important to address any pre-existing factors, especially for the female athlete that may predispose the individual to future injury, such as hip and hamstring weakness. Our goal in the rehabilitation program after ACL surgery is to restore full, unrestricted function and to assist the patient to return to 100% of the preinjury level while achieving excellent long-term outcomes.

REFERENCES

1. Carey JL, Huffman GR, Parekh SG, et al. Outcomes of anterior cruciate ligament injuries to running backs and wide receivers in the National Football League. Am J Sports Med 2006;34:1911–7.
2. Hofmeister EP, Gillingham BL, Bathgate MB, et al. Results of anterior cruciate ligament reconstruction in the adolescent female. J Pediatr Orthop 2001;21:302–6.
3. Johnson RJ, Eriksson E, Haggmark T, et al. Five- to ten-year follow-up evaluation after reconstruction of the anterior cruciate ligament. Clin Orthop Relat Res 1984;183:122–40.
4. Matava MJ, Siegel MG. Arthroscopic reconstruction of the ACL with semitendinosus-gracilis autograft in skeletally immature adolescent patients. Am J Knee Surg 1997;10:60–9.

5. Micheli LJ, Metzl JD, Di Canzio J, et al. Anterior cruciate ligament reconstructive surgery in adolescent soccer and basketball players. Clin J Sport Med 1999;9: 138–41.
6. Shelbourne KD, Gray T. Minimum 10-year results after anterior cruciate ligament re- construction: how the loss of normal knee motion compounds other factors related to the development of osteoarthritis after surgery. Am J Sports Med 2009;37:471–80.
7. Wells L, Dyke JA, Albaugh J, et al. Adolescent anterior cruciate ligament reconstruction: a retrospective analysis of quadriceps strength recovery and return to full activity after surgery. J Pediatr Orthop 2009;29:486–9.
8. Wilk KE. Anterior cruciate ligament injury prevention and rehabilitation: let's get it right. J Orthop Sports Phys Ther 2015;45(10):729–30.
9. Wilk KE, Andrews JR, Clancy WG. Quadriceps muscular strength after removal of the central third patellar tendon for contralateral anterior cruciate ligament reconstruction surgery: a case study. J Orthop Sports Phys Ther 1993;18:692–7.
10. Ardern CL, Webster KE, Taylor NF, et al. Return to the preinjury level of competitive sport after anterior cruciate ligament reconstruction surgery: two-thirds of patients have not returned by 12 months after surgery. Am J Sports Med 2011;39:538–43.
11. Ardern CL, Webster KE, Taylor NF, et al. Return to sport following anterior cruciate ligament reconstruction surgery: a systematic review and meta-analysis of the state of play. Br J Sports Med 2011;45:596–606.
12. Spindler KP. The Multicenter ACL Revision Study (MARS): a prospective longitudinal cohort to define outcomes and independent predictors of outcomes for revision anterior cruciate ligament reconstruction. J Knee Surg 2007;20:303–7.
13. Ireland ML. The female ACL: why is it more prone to injury? Orthop Clin North Am 2002;33:637–51.
14. Pinczewski LA, Lyman J, Salmon LJ, et al. 10-year comparison of anterior cruciate ligament reconstructions with hamstring tendon and patellar tendon autograft: a controlled, prospective trial. Am J Sports Med 2007;35:564–74.
15. Fleming BC. Biomechanics of the anterior cruciate ligament. J Orthop Sports Phys Ther 2003;3(8):A13–5.
16. Busfielf BT, Kharraz FD, Starke C, et al. Performance outcomes of anterior cruciate ligament reconstructions in the National Basketball Association. Arthroscopy 2009;25(8):825–30.
17. Brophy RH, Gill CS, Lyman S, et al. Effect of anterior cruciate ligament reconstruction and meniscectomy on length of career in National Football League athletes: a case control study. Am J Sports Med 2009;37:2102–7.
18. Shah VM, Andrews JR, Fleisig GS, et al. Return to play after anterior cruciate ligament reconstruction in National Football League athletes. Am J Sports Med 2010;38:2233–9.
19. Woby SR, Roach NK, Urmston M, et al. Psychometric properties of the TSK-11: a shortened version of the Tampa scale for Kinesiophobia. Pain 2005;117(1–2): 137–44.
20. Mangine RE, Noyes FR. Rehabilitation of the allograft reconstruction. J Orthop Sports Phys Ther 1992;15:294–302.
21. Shelbourne KD, Nitz P. Accelerated rehabilitation after anterior cruciate ligament reconstruction. Am J Sports Med 1990;18:292–9.
22. Shelbourne KD, Wilckens JH, Mollabashy A, et al. Arthrofibrosis in acute anterior cruciate ligament reconstruction. The effect of timing of reconstruction and rehabilitation. Am J Sports Med 1991;19:332–6.

23. Wilk KE, Andrews JR. Current concepts in the treatment of anterior cruciate ligament disruption. J Orthop Sports Phys Ther 1992;15:279–93.
24. Wilk KE, Reinold MM, Hooks TR. Recent advances in the rehabilitation of isolated and combined anterior cruciate ligament injuries. Orthop Clin North Am 2003;34:107–37.
25. Coutts R, Rothe C, Kaita J. The role of continuous passive motion in the rehabilitation of the total knee patient. Clin Orthop 1981;159:126–32.
26. Fu FH, Woo SL-Y, Irrgang JJ. Current concepts for rehabilitation following anterior cruciate ligament reconstruction. J Orthop Sports Phys Ther 1992;15:270–8.
27. Noyes FR, Mangine RE, Barber S. Early knee motion after open and arthroscopic anterior cruciate ligament reconstruction. Am J Sports Med 1987;15: 149–60.
28. Salter RB, Simmonds DF, Malcolm BW, et al. The biological effect of continuous passive motion on the healing of full-thickness defects in articular cartilage. An experimental investigation in the rabbit. J Bone Joint Surg Am 1980;62:1232–51.
29. Wilk KE, Andrews JR, Clancy WG. Anterior cruciate ligament reconstruction rehabilitation—the results of aggressive rehabilitation: a 12-week follow-up in 212 cases. Isokin Exerc Sci 1992;2:82–91.
30. Sachs RA, Reznik A, Daniel DM, et al. Com- plication of knee ligament surgery. In: Daniel DM, Akeson WH, O'Connor JJ, editors. Knee ligaments: structure, function, injury and repair. New York: Raven Press; 1990. p. 505–20.
31. Wilk KE, Arrigo C, Andrews JR, et al. Rehabilitation after anterior cruciate ligament reconstruction in the female athlete. J Athl Train 1999;34:177–93.
32. Lephart SM, Kocher MS, Fu FH, et al. Proprioception following anterior cruciate ligament reconstruction. J Sport Rehabil 1992;1:188–96.
33. Lephart SM, Pincivero DM, Giraldo JL, et al. The role of proprioception in the management and rehabilitation of athletic injuries. Am J Sports Med 1997;25: 130–7.
34. De Carlo MS, McDivitt R. Rehabilitation of patients following autogenic bone-patellar tendon- bone ACL reconstruction: a 20-year perspective. N Am J Sports Phys Ther 2006;1:108–23.
35. Kim SJ, Kumar P, Oh KS. Anterior cruciate ligament reconstruction: autogenous quadriceps tendon-bone compared with bone-patellar tendon-bone grafts at 2-year follow-up. Arthroscopy 2009;25:137–44.
36. Mariani PP, Santori N, Adriani E, et al. Accelerated rehabilitation after arthroscopic meniscal repair: a clinical and magnetic resonance imaging evaluation. Arthroscopy 1996;12:680–6.
37. Vanwanseele B, Lucchinetti E, Stussi E. The effects of immobilization on the characteristics of articular cartilage: current concepts and future directions. Osteoarthritis Cartilage 2002;10:408–19.
38. Wilk KE. Rehabilitation of isolated and combined posterior cruciate ligament injuries. Clin Sports Med 1994;13:649–77.
39. Wright RW, Preston E, Fleming BC, et al. A systematic review of anterior cruciate ligament re-construction rehabilitation: part II: open versus closed kinetic chain exercises, neuromuscular electrical stimulation, accelerated rehabilitation, and miscellaneous topics. J Knee Surg 2008;21:225–34.
40. Howe JG, Johnson RJ, Kaplan MJ, et al. Anterior cruciate ligament reconstruction using quadriceps patellar tendon graft. Part I. Long-term followup. Am J Sports Med 1991;19:447–57.

41. Meighan AA, Keating JF, Will E. Outcome after reconstruction of the anterior cruciate ligament in athletic patients. A comparison of early versus delayed surgery. J Bone Joint Surg Br 2003;85:521–4.

42. Rubinstein RA, Shelbourne KD. Preventing complicating and minimizing morbidity after autogenous bone-patellar tendon-bone anterior cruciate ligament reconstruction. Oper Tech Sports Med 1993;1:72–8.

43. Shelbourne KD, Patel DV, Martini DJ. Classification and management of arthrofibrosis of the knee after anterior cruciate ligament reconstruction. Am J Sports Med 1996;24:857–62.

44. Birmingham TB, Kramer JF, Kirkley A, et al. Knee bracing after ACL reconstruction: effects on postural control and proprioception. Med Sci Sports Exerc 2001; 33:1253–8.

45. Risberg MA, Holm I, Steen H, et al. The effect of knee bracing after anterior cruciate ligament reconstruction. A prospective, randomized study with two years' follow-up. Am J Sports Med 1999;27:76–83.

46. Wilk KE, Romaniello WT, Soscia SM, et al. The relationship between subjective knee scores, isokinetic testing, and functional testing in the ACL-reconstructed knee. J Orthop Sports Phys Ther 1994;20:60–73.

47. Hunter RE, Mastrangelo J, Freeman JR, et al. The impact of surgical timing on postoperative motion and stability following anterior cruciate ligament reconstruction. Arthroscopy 1996;12(6):667–74.

48. Guerra JJ, Joyce ME, Wilk KE, et al. Increased prevalence and severity of intra-articular damage when ACL reconstruction is delayed. AAOS: Sports Medicine Speciality Day (62nd Annual Meeting). Atlanta (GA), Feburary 16, 1996 [Presentation].

49. Eitzen I, Moksnes H, Snyder-Mackler L, et al. A progressive 5-week exercise therapy program leads to significant improvement in knee function early after anterior cruciate ligament injury. J Orthop Sports Phys Ther 2010;11:705–21.

50. Austin JC, Phornphutkul C, Wojtys EM. Loss of knee extension after anterior cruciate ligament reconstruction: effects of knee position and graft tensioning. J Bone Joint Surg Am 2007;89:1565–74.

51. Harner CD, Irrgang JJ, Paul J, et al. Loss of motion after anterior cruciate ligament reconstruction. Am J Sports Med 1992;20:499–506.

52. Irrgang JJ, Harner CD. Loss of motion following knee ligament reconstruction. Sports Med 1995;19:150–9.

53. Rubin LE, Yeh PC, Medvecky MJ. Extension loss secondary to femoral-sided inverted cyclops lesion after anterior cruciate ligament reconstruction. J Knee Surg 2009;22:360–3.

54. Benum P. Operative mobilization of stiff knees after surgical treatment of knee injuries and posttraumatic conditions. Acta Orthop Scand 1982;53:625–31.

55. Blazevich AJ, Cannavan D, Horne S, et al. Changes in muscle force-length properties affect the early rise of force in vivo. Muscle Nerve 2009;39:512–20.

56. Knight KL, Martin JA, Londeree BR. EMG comparison of quadriceps femoris activity during knee extension and straight leg raises. Am J Phys Med 1979;58: 57–67.

57. Perry J, Antonelli D, Ford W. Analysis of knee- joint forces during flexed-knee stance. J Bone Joint Surg Am 1975;57:961–7.

58. Ahmad CS, Kwak SD, Ateshian GA, et al. Effects of patellar tendon adhesion to the anterior tibia on knee mechanics. Am J Sports Med 1998;26:715–24.

59. McClure PW, Blackburn LG, Dusold C. The use of splints in the treatment of joint stiffness: biologic rationale and an algorithm for making clinical decisions. Phys Ther 1994;74:1101–7.

60. Young A, Stokes M, Shakespeare DT, et al. The effect of intra-articular bupivicaine on quadriceps inhibition after meniscectomy. Med Sci Sports Exerc 1983;15:154.

61. DeAndrade JR, Grant C, Dixon AS. Joint distension and reflex muscle inhibition in the knee. J Bone Joint Surg Am 1965;47:313–22.

62. Spencer JD, Hayes KC, Alexander IJ. Knee joint effusion and quadriceps reflex inhibition in man. Arch Phys Med Rehabil 1984;65:171–7.

63. Fahrer H, Rentsch HU, Gerber NJ, et al. Knee effusion and reflex inhibition of the quadriceps. A bar to effective re-training. J Bone Joint Surg Br 1988;70:635–8.

64. Hart JM, Pietrosimone B, Hertel J, et al. Quadriceps activation following knee injuries: a systematic review. J Athl Train 2010;45:87–97.

65. Hopkins JT, Ingersoll CD, Krause BA, et al. Effect of knee joint effusion on quadriceps and soleus motoneuron pool excitability. Med Sci Sports Exerc 2001;33:123–6.

66. Jensen K, Graf BK. The effects of knee effusion on quadriceps strength and knee intraarticular pressure. Arthroscopy 1993;9:52–6.

67. Torry MR, Decker MJ, Viola RW, et al. Intra-articular knee joint effusion induces quadriceps avoidance gait patterns. Clin Biomech (Bristol, Avon) 2000;15:147–59.

68. DeSantana JM, Walsh DM, Vance C, et al. Effectiveness of transcutaneous electrical nerve stimulation for treatment of hyperalgesia and pain. Curr Rheumatol Rep 2008;10:492–9.

69. Prentice WE. Therapeutic modalities in sports medicine. 3rd edition. St Louis (MO): Mosby; 1994.

70. McCarthy MR, Yates CK, Anderson MA, et al. The effects of immediate continuous passive motion on pain during the inflammatory phase of soft tissue healing following anterior cruciate ligament reconstruction. J Orthop Sports Phys Ther 1993;17:96–101.

71. O'Driscoll SW, Giori NJ. Continuous passive motion (CPM): theory and principles of clinical application. J Rehabil Res Dev 2000;37:179–88.

72. Chow RT, Johnson MI, Lopes-Martins RA, et al. Efficacy of low-level laser therapy in the management of neck pain: a systematic review and meta-analysis of randomised placebo or active-treatment controlled trials. Lancet 2009;374:1897–908.

73. Haldeman S, Carroll L, Cassidy JD, et al. The bone and joint decade 2000-2010 task force on neck pain and its associated disorders: executive summary. Spine (Phila Pa 1976) 2008;33:S5–7.

74. Naeser MA. Photobiomodulation of pain in carpal tunnel syndrome: review of seven laser therapy studies. Photomed Laser Surg 2006;24:101–10.

75. Beck PR, Nho SJ, Balin J, et al. Postoperative pain management after anterior cruciate ligament reconstruction. J Knee Surg 2004;17:18–23.

76. Cina-Tschumi B. Evidence-based impact of cryotherapy on postoperative pain, swelling, drainage and tolerance after orthopedic surgery. Pflege 2007;20:258–67 [in German].

77. Ohkoshi Y, Ohkoshi M, Nagasaki S, et al. The effect of cryotherapy on intraarticular temperature and postoperative care after anterior cruciate ligament reconstruction. Am J Sports Med 1999;27:357–62.

78. Raynor MC, Pietrobon R, Guller U, et al. Cryotherapy after ACL reconstruction: a meta- analysis. J Knee Surg 2005;18:123–9.

79. Warren TA, McCarty EC, Richardson AL, et al. Intra-articular knee temperature changes: ice versus cryotherapy device. Am J Sports Med 2004;32:441–5.

80. Holcomb W, Rubley MD, Girouard TJ. Effect of the simultaneous application of NMES and HVPC on knee extension torque. J Sport Rehabil 2007;16:307–18.

81. Kuster MS, Grob K, Kuster M, et al. The benefits of wearing a compression sleeve after ACL reconstruction. Med Sci Sports Exerc 1999;31:368–71.

82. Cosgarea AJ, Sebastianelli WJ, DeHaven KE. Prevention of arthrofibrosis after anterior cruciate ligament reconstruction using the central third patellar tendon autograft. Am J Sports Med 1995;23:87–92.

83. Millett PJ, Wickiewicz TL, Warren RF. Motion loss after ligament injuries to the knee. Part I: causes. Am J Sports Med 2001;29:664–75.

84. Millett PJ, Wickiewicz TL, Warren RF. Motion loss after ligament injuries to the knee. Part II: prevention and treatment. Am J Sports Med 2001;29:822–8.

85. Shelbourne KD, Gray T. Anterior cruciate ligament reconstruction with autogenous patellar tendon graft followed by accelerated rehabilitation. A two- to nine-year followup. Am J Sports Med 1997;25:786–95.

86. Dye SF, Chew MH. Restoration of osseous homeostasis after anterior cruciate ligament reconstruction. Am J Sports Med 1993;21:748–50.

87. Atkinson TS, Atkinson PJ, Mendenhall HV, et al. Patellar tendon and infrapatellar fat pad healing after harvest of an ACL graft. J Surg Res 1998;79:25–30.

88. Paulos LE, Rosenberg TD, Drawbert J, et al. Infrapatellar contracture syndrome. An unrecognized cause of knee stiffness with patella entrapment and patella infera. Am J Sports Med 1987;15:331–41.

89. Clancy WG Jr, Nelson DA, Reider B, et al. Anterior cruciate ligament reconstruction using one-third of the patellar ligament, augmented by extra-articular tendon transfers. J Bone Joint Surg Am 1982;64:352–9.

90. Aglietti P, Buzzi R, Menchetti PM, et al. Arthroscopically assisted semitendinosus and gracilis tendon graft in reconstruction for acute anterior cruciate ligament injuries in athletes. Am J Sports Med 1996;24:726–31.

91. MacDonald PB, Hedden D, Pacin O, et al. Effects of an accelerated rehabilitation program after anterior cruciate ligament reconstruction with combined semitendinosus-gracilis auto-graft and a ligament augmentation device. Am J Sports Med 1995;23:588–92.

92. Yasuda K, Tsujino J, Ohkoshi Y, et al. Graft site morbidity with autogenous semitendinosus and gracilis tendons. Am J Sports Med 1995;23:706–14.

93. Andrews M, Noyes FR, Barber-Westin SD. Anterior cruciate ligament allograft reconstruction in the skeletally immature athlete. Am J Sports Med 1994;22:48–54.

94. Fu FH, Jackson DW, Jamison J. Allograft reconstruction of the anterior cruciate ligament. In: Jackson DW, Arnoczky SP, editors. The anterior cruciate ligament: current and future concepts. New York: Raven Press; 1993. p. 325–38.

95. Shino K, Inoue M, Horibe S, et al. Maturation of allograft tendons transplanted into the knee. An arthroscopic and histological study. J Bone Joint Surg Br 1988;70:556–60.

96. Fulkerson JP, Langeland R. An alternative cruciate reconstruction graft: the central quadriceps tendon. Arthroscopy 1995;11:252–4.

97. Harris NL, Smith DA, Lamoreaux L, et al. Central quadriceps tendon for anterior cruciate ligament reconstruction. Part I: morphometric and biomechanical evaluation. Am J Sports Med 1997;25:23–8.

98. Hamner DL, Brown CH Jr, Steiner ME, et al. Hamstring tendon grafts for reconstruction of the anterior cruciate ligament: biomechanical evaluation of the use of multiple strands and tensioning techniques. J Bone Joint Surg Am 1999;81: 549–57.

99. Race A, Amis AA. The mechanical properties of the two bundles of the human posterior cruciate ligament. J Biomech 1994;27:13–24.

100. Staubli HU, Schatzmann L, Brunner P, et al. Quadriceps tendon and patellar ligament: cryosectional anatomy and structural properties in young adults. Knee Surg Sports Traumatol Arthrosc 1996;4:100–10.

101. Woo SL, Hollis JM, Adams DJ, et al. Tensile properties of the human femuranterior cruciate ligament-tibia complex. The effects of specimen age and orientation. Am J Sports Med 1991;19:217–25.

102. Rodeo SA, Kawamura S, Kim HJ, et al. Tendon healing in a bone tunnel differs at the tunnel entrance versus the tunnel exit: an effect of graft-tunnel motion? Am J Sports Med 2006;34:1790–800.

103. Suzuki T, Shino K, Nakagawa S, et al. Early integration of a bone plug in the femoral tunnel in rectangular tunnel ACL reconstruction with a bone-patellar tendon-bone graft: a prospective computed tomography analysis. Knee Surg Sports Traumatol Arthrosc 2011;19(Suppl 1):29–35.

104. Meister K, Huegel M, Indelicato PA. Current concepts in the recognition and treatment of knee injuries. La Crosse (WI): APTA SPTS; 2000.

105. Li S, Su W, Zhao J, et al. A meta-analysis of hamstring autografts versus bonepatellar tendon-bone autografts for reconstruction of the anterior cruciate ligament. Knee 2011;18:287–93.

106. Aglietti P, Buzzi R, Zaccherotti G, et al. Patellar tendon versus doubled semitendinosus and gracilis tendons for anterior cruciate ligament reconstruction. Am J Sports Med 1994;22:211–7 [discussion 217–8].

107. Marder RA, Raskind JR, Carroll M. Prospective evaluation of arthroscopically assisted anterior cruciate ligament reconstruction. Patellar tendon versus semitendinosus and gracilis tendons. Am J Sports Med 1991;19:478–84.

108. Horstman JK, Ahmadu-Suka F, Norrdin RW. Anterior cruciate ligament fascia lata allograft reconstruction: progressive histologic changes toward maturity. Arthroscopy 1993;9:509–18.

109. Jackson DW, Corsetti J, Simon TM. Biologic incorporation of allograft anterior cruciate ligament replacements. Clin Orthop Relat Res 1996;324:126–33.

110. Jackson DW, Grood ES, Goldstein JD, et al. A comparison of patellar tendon autograft and allograft used for anterior cruciate ligament reconstruction in the goat model. Am J Sports Med 1993;21:176–85.

111. Huegel M, Indelicato PA. Trends in rehabilitation following anterior cruciate ligament reconstruction. Clin Sports Med 1988;7:801–11.

112. Hirshman HP, Daniel DM, Miyasaka K. The fate of unoperated knee ligament injuries. In: Daniel DM, Akeson WH, O'Connor JJ, editors. Knee ligaments: structure, function, injury and repair. New York: Raven Press; 1990. p. 481–503.

113. Robertson GA, Coleman SG, Keating JF. Knee stiffness following anterior cruciate ligament reconstruction: the incidence and associated factors of knee stiffness following anterior cruciate ligament reconstruction. Knee 2009;16:245–7.

114. Shelbourne KD, Patel DV. Management of combined injuries of the anterior cruciate and medial collateral ligaments. Instr Course Lect 1996;45:275–80.

115. Graf BK, Cook DA, De Smet AA, et al. "Bone bruises" on magnetic resonance imaging evaluation of anterior cruciate ligament injuries. Am J Sports Med 1993;21:220–3.

116. Johnson DL, Urban WP Jr, Caborn DN, et al. Articular cartilage changes seen with magnetic resonance imaging-detected bone bruises associated with acute anterior cruciate ligament rupture. Am J Sports Med 1998;26:409–14.

117. Rosen MA, Jackson DW, Berger PE. Occult osseous lesions documented by magnetic resonance imaging associated with anterior cruciate ligament ruptures. Arthroscopy 1991;7:45–51.

118. Spindler KP, Schils JP, Bergfeld JA, et al. Prospective study of osseous, articular, and meniscal lesions in recent anterior cruciate ligament tears by magnetic resonance imaging and arthroscopy. Am J Sports Med 1993;21:551–7.

119. Murphy BJ, Smith RL, Uribe JW, et al. Bone signal abnormalities in the posterolateral tibia and lateral femoral condyle in complete tears of the anterior cruciate ligament: a specific sign? Radiology 1992;182:221–4.

120. Fowler PJ. Bone injuries associated with anterior cruciate ligament disruption. Arthroscopy 1994;10:453–60.

121. Speer KP, Spritzer CE, Bassett FH 3rd, et al. Osseous injury associated with acute tears of the anterior cruciate ligament. Am J Sports Med 1992;20:382–9.

122. Behrens F, Kraft EL, Oegema TR Jr. Biochemical changes in articular cartilage after joint immobilization by casting or external fixation. J Orthop Res 1989;7: 335–43.

123. Haapala J, Arokoski J, Pirttimaki J, et al. Incomplete restoration of immobilization induced softening of young beagle knee articular cartilage after 50-week remobilization. Int J Sports Med 2000;21:76–81.

124. Buckwalter JA. Articular cartilage: injuries and potential for healing. J Orthop Sports Phys Ther 1998;28:192–202.

125. Buckwalter JA, Mankin HJ. Articular cartilage: tissue design and chondrocyte-matrix interactions. Instr Course Lect 1998;47:477–86.

126. Waldman SD, Spiteri CG, Grynpas MD, et al. Effect of biomechanical conditioning on cartilaginous tissue formation in vitro. J Bone Joint Surg Am 2003;85-A-(Suppl 2):101–5.

127. Mussa R, Hans MG, Enlow D, et al. Condylar cartilage response to continuous passive motion in adult guinea pigs: a pilot study. Am J Orthod Dentofacial Orthop 1999;115:360–7.

128. Shimizu T, Videman T, Shimazaki K, et al. Experimental study on the repair of full thickness articular cartilage defects: effects of varying periods of continuous passive motion, cage activity, and immobilization. J Orthop Res 1987;5:187–97.

129. Rodrigo JJ, Steadman JR, Silliman JF, et al. Improvement of full-thickness chondral defect healing in the human knee after debridement and microfracture using continuous passive motion. Am J Knee Surg 1994;7:109–16.

130. Salter RB. The biologic concept of continuous passive motion of synovial joints. The first 18 years of basic research and its clinical application. Clin Orthop Relat Res 1989;242:12–25.

131. Liden M, Sernert N, Rostgard-Christensen L, et al. Osteoarthritic changes after anterior cruciate ligament reconstruction using bone-patellar tendon-bone or hamstring tendon autografts: a retrospective, 7-year radiographic and clinical follow-up study. Arthroscopy 2008;24:899–908.

132. Nebelung W, Wuschech H. Thirty-five years of follow-up of anterior cruciate ligament-deficient knees in high-level athletes. Arthroscopy 2005;21:696–702.

133. Cerabona F, Sherman MF, Bonamo JR, et al. Patterns of meniscal injury with acute anterior cruciate ligament tears. Am J Sports Med 1988;16:603–9.

134. Barber FA, Click SD. Meniscus repair rehabilitation with concurrent anterior cruciate reconstruction. Arthroscopy 1997;13:433–7.

135. Shelbourne KD, Patel DV, Adsit WS, et al. Rehabilitation after meniscal repair. Clin Sports Med 1996;15:595–612.
136. Cannon WD Jr, Vittori JM. The incidence of healing in arthroscopic meniscal repairs in anterior cruciate ligament-reconstructed knees versus stable knees. Am J Sports Med 1992;20:176–81.
137. Krych AJ, Pitts RT, Dajani KA, et al. Surgical repair of meniscal tears with concomitant anterior cruciate ligament reconstruction in patients 18 years and younger. Am J Sports Med 2010;38:976–82.
138. Noyes FR, Barber-Westin SD. Arthroscopic repair of meniscus tears extending into the avascular zone with or without anterior cruciate ligament reconstruction in patients 40 years of age and older. Arthroscopy 2000;16:822–9.
139. Paulos L, Noyes FR, Grood E, et al. Knee rehabilitation after anterior cruciate ligament reconstruction and repair. Am J Sports Med 1981;9:140–9.
140. Hewett TE. Predisposition to ACL injuries in female athletes versus male athletes. Orthopedics 2008;31:26–8.
141. Hewett TE, Ford KR, Myer GD. Anterior cruciate ligament injuries in female athletes: part 2, a meta-analysis of neuromuscular interventions aimed at injury prevention. Am J Sports Med 2006;34:490–8.
142. Hewett TE, Myer GD, Ford KR. Anterior cruciate ligament injuries in female athletes: part 1, mechanisms and risk factors. Am J Sports Med 2006;34:299–311.
143. Hewett TE, Zazulak BT, Myer GD, et al. A review of electromyographic activation levels, timing differences, and increased anterior cruciate ligament injury incidence in female athletes. Br J Sports Med 2005;39:347–50.
144. Renstrom P, Ljungqvist A, Arendt E, et al. Non-contact ACL injuries in female athletes: an international Olympic committee current concepts statement. Br J Sports Med 2008;42:394–412.
145. Shultz SJ. ACL injury in the female athlete: a multifactorial problem that remains poorly understood. J Athl Train 2008;455:43.
146. Malone TR, Hardaker WT, Garrett WE, et al. Relationship of gender to anterior cruciate ligament injuries in intercollegiate basketball players. J South Orthop Assoc 1993;2:36–9.
147. Lindenfeld TN, Schmitt DJ, Hendy MP, et al. Incidence of injury in indoor soccer. Am J Sports Med 1994;22:364–71.
148. Chandy TA, Grana WA. Secondary school athletic injury in boys and girls: a three-year comparison. Phys Sportsmed 1985;13:106–11.
149. Ferretti A, Papandrea P, Conteduca F, et al. Knee ligament injuries in volleyball players. Am J Sports Med 1992;20:203–7.
150. Hewett TE, Stroupe AL, Nance TA, et al. Plyometric training in female athletes. Decreased impact forces and increased hamstring torques. Am J Sports Med 1996;24:765–73.
151. Hewett TE, Lindenfeld TN, Riccobene JV, et al. The effect of neuromuscular training on the incidence of knee injury in female athletes. A prospective study. Am J Sports Med 1999;27:699–706.
152. Hewett TE, Myer GD, Ford KR, et al. Biomechanical measures of neuromuscular control and valgus loading of the knee predict anterior cruciate ligament injury risk in female athletes: a prospective study. Am J Sports Med 2005;33:492–501.
153. Joseph M, Tiberio D, Baird JL, et al. Knee valgus during drop jumps in national collegiate athletic association division I female athletes: the effect of a medial post. Am J Sports Med 2008;36:285–9.
154. Powers CM. The influence of abnormal hip mechanics on knee injury: a biomechanical perspective. J Orthop Sports Phys Ther 2010;40:42–51.

155. Myer GD, Chu DA, Brent JL, et al. Trunk and hip control neuromuscular training for the prevention of knee joint injury. Clin Sports Med 2008;27:425–448 ix.

156. Zazulak BT, Hewett TE, Reeves NP, et al. Deficits in neuromuscular control of the trunk predict knee injury risk: a prospective biomechanical-epidemiologic study. Am J Sports Med 2007;35:1123–30.

157. Zazulak BT, Hewett TE, Reeves NP, et al. The effects of core proprioception on knee injury: a prospective biomechanical-epidemiological study. Am J Sports Med 2007;35:368–73.

158. Draper V, Ballard L. Electrical stimulation versus electromyographic biofeedback in the recovery of quadriceps femoris muscle function following anterior cruciate ligament surgery. Phys Ther 1991;71:455–61 [discussion 461–4].

159. Kim KM, Croy T, Hertel J, et al. Effects of neuromuscular electrical stimulation after anterior cruciate ligament reconstruction on quadriceps strength, function, and patient-oriented outcomes: a systematic review. J Orthop Sports Phys Ther 2010;40:383–91.

160. Wilk KE, Escamilla RF, Fleisig GS, et al. A comparison of tibiofemoral joint forces and electromyographic activity during open and closed kinetic chain exercises. Am J Sports Med 1996;24:518–27.

161. Barrack RL, Skinner HB, Buckley SL. Proprioception in the anterior cruciate deficient knee. Am J Sports Med 1989;17:1–6.

162. Barrett DS. Proprioception and function after anterior cruciate reconstruction. J Bone Joint Surg Br 1991;73:833–7.

163. Beard DJ, Dodd CA, Trundle HR, et al. Proprioception enhancement for anterior cruciate ligament deficiency. A prospective randomised trial of two physiotherapy regimes. J Bone Joint Surg Br 1994;76:654–9.

164. Beard DJ, Kyberd PJ, Dodd CA, et al. Proprioception in the knee. J Bone Joint Surg Br 1994;76:992–3.

165. Beard DJ, Kyberd PJ, Fergusson CM, et al. Proprioception after rupture of the anterior cruciate ligament. An objective indication of the need for surgery? J Bone Joint Surg Br 1993;75:311–5.

166. Beynnon BD, Good L, Risberg MA. The effect of bracing on proprioception of knees with anterior cruciate ligament injury. J Orthop Sports Phys Ther 2002; 32:11–5.

167. Markolf KL, Graff-Radford A, Amstutz HC. In vivo knee stability. A quantitative assessment using an instrumented clinical testing apparatus. J Bone Joint Surg Am 1978;60:664–74.

168. Paterno MV, Myer GD, Ford KR, et al. Neuromuscular training improves single-limb stability in young female athletes. J Orthop Sports Phys Ther 2004;34: 305–16.

169. Fitzgerald GK, Axe MJ, Snyder-Mackler L. The efficacy of perturbation training in nonoperative anterior cruciate ligament rehabilitation pro- grams for physical active individuals. Phys Ther 2000;80:128–40.

170. Chmielewski TL, Jones D, DayLentz TA, et al. The association of pain and fear of movement/reinjury with function during anterior cruciate ligament reconstruction rehabilitation. J Orthop Sports Phys Ther 2008;38:746–53.

171. Escamilla RF, Fleisig GS, Zheng N, et al. Biomechanics of the knee during closed kinetic chain and open kinetic chain exercises. Med Sci Sports Exerc 1998;30:556–69.

172. Escamilla RF, Fleisig GS, Zheng N, et al. Effects of technique variations on knee biomechanics during the squat and leg press. Med Sci Sports Exerc 2001;33: 1552–66.

173. Escamilla RF, Zheng N, Imamura R, et al. Cruciate ligament force during the wall squat and the one-leg squat. Med Sci Sports Exerc 2009;41:408–17.
174. Escamilla RF, Zheng N, Macleod TD, et al. Cruciate ligament forces between short-step and long-step forward lunge. Med Sci Sports Exerc 2010;42: 1932–42.
175. Escamilla RF, Zheng N, MacLeod TD, et al. Cruciate ligament tensile forces during the forward and side lunge. Clin Biomech (Bristol, Avon) 2010;25:213–21.
176. Beynnon BD, Fleming BC. Anterior cruciate ligament strain in-vivo: a review of previous work. J Biomech 1998;31:519–25.
177. Heijne A, Fleming BC, Renstrom PA, et al. Strain on the anterior cruciate ligament during closed kinetic chain exercises. Med Sci Sports Exerc 2004;36: 935–41.
178. Farrokhi S, Pollard CD, Souza RB, et al. Trunk position influences the kinematics, kinetics, and muscle activity of the lead lower extremity during the forward lunge exercise. J Orthop Sports Phys Ther 2008;38:403–9.
179. Ohkoshi Y, Yasuda K, Kaneda K, et al. Biomechanical analysis of rehabilitation in the standing position. Am J Sports Med 1991;19:605–11.
180. Chmielewski TL, Wilk KE, Snyder-Mackler L. Changes in weight-bearing following injury or surgical reconstruction of the ACL: relationship to quadriceps strength and function. Gait Posture 2002;16:87–95.
181. Wilk KE, Reinold MM. Plyometric and closed kinetic chain exercise. In: Bandy WD, editor. Therapeutic exercises: techniques for intervention. Philadelphia: Lippincott, Williams, & Wilkins; 2001. p. 179–211.
182. Wilk KE, Voight ML, Keirns MA, et al. Stretch-shortening drills for the upper extremities: theory and clinical application. J Orthop Sports Phys Ther 1993;17: 225–39.
183. Lattanzio PJ, Petrella RJ. Knee proprioception: a review of mechanisms, measurements, and implications of muscular fatigue. Orthopedics 1998;21:463–70 [discussion 470–1]; passim.
184. Lattanzio PJ, Petrella RJ, Sproule JR, et al. Effects of fatigue on knee proprioception. Clin J Sport Med 1997;7:22–7.
185. Skinner HB, Wyatt MP, Hodgdon JA, et al. Effect of fatigue on joint position sense of the knee. J Orthop Res 1986;4:112–8.
186. Oda H, Igarashi M, Sase H, et al. Bone bruise in magnetic resonance imaging strongly correlates with the production of joint effusion and with knee osteoarthritis. J Orthop Sci 2008;13:7–15.
187. Gobbi A, Francisco R. Factors affecting return to sports after anterior cruciate ligament reconstruction with patellar tendon and hamstring graft: a prospective clinical investigation. Knee Surg Sports Traumatol Arthrosc 2006;14:1021–8.
188. Mattacola CG, Perrin DH, Gansneder BM, et al. Strength, functional outcome, and postural stability after anterior cruciate ligament reconstruction. J Athl Train 2002;37:262–8.
189. Higgins LD, Taylor MK, Park D, et al. Reliability and validity of the International Knee Documentation Committee (IKDC) Subjective Knee Form. Joint Bone Spine 2007;74:594–9.
190. Mehta VM, Paxton LW, Fornalski SX, et al. Reliability of the International Knee Documentation Committee radiographic grading system. Am J Sports Med 2007;35:933–5.
191. Gustavsson A, Neeter C, Thomee P, et al. A test battery for evaluating hop performance in patients with an ACL injury and patients who have undergone ACL reconstruction. Knee Surg Sports Traumatol Arthrosc 2006;14:778–88.

192. Noyes FR, Barber SD, Mangine RE. Abnormal lower limb symmetry determined by function hop tests after anterior cruciate ligament rupture. Am J Sports Med 1991;19:513–8.
193. Reid A, Birmingham TB, Stratford PW, et al. Hop testing provides a reliable and valid outcome measure during rehabilitation after anterior cruciate ligament reconstruction. Phys Ther 2007;87:337–49.
194. Webster KE, Feller JA, Lambros C. Development and preliminary validation of a scale to measure the psychological impact of returning to sport following anterior cruciate ligament reconstruction surgery. Phys Ther Sport 2008;9:9–15.

Index

Note: Page numbers of article titles are in **boldface** type.

A

Moving?

Make sure your subscription moves with you!

To notify us of your new address, find your **Clinics Account Number** (located on your mailing label above your name), and contact customer service at:

Email: journalscustomerservice-usa@elsevier.com

800-654-2452 (subscribers in the U.S. & Canada)
314-447-8871 (subscribers outside of the U.S. & Canada)

Fax number: 314-447-8029

Elsevier Health Sciences Division
Subscription Customer Service
3251 Riverport Lane
Maryland Heights, MO 63043

*To ensure uninterrupted delivery of your subscription, please notify us at least 4 weeks in advance of move.

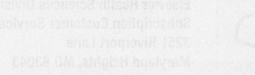

Printed and bound by CPI Group (UK) Ltd, Croydon, CR0 4YY

08/05/2025

01864696-0002